Nursing the Neonate

NURSING THE NEONATE

Second edition

Edited by

Maggie Meeks Dip Ed MB ChB MD FRCPCH

Maggie Hallsworth RSCN, RGN, ENB 405, 904, 998

Founding Editor: Helen Yeo

⊛WILEY-BLACKWELL

A John Wiley & Sons, Ltd., Publication

Library of Congress Cataloging-in-Publication Data

Nursing the neonate.— 2nd ed. / edited by Maggie Meeks, Maggie Hallsworth.
    p. ; cm.
  Includes bibliographical references and index.
  ISBN 978-1-4051-4974-7 (pbk. : alk. paper)
  1. Neonatal intensive care.   2. Newborn infants—Care. 3. Newborn infants—Diseases—Nursing. I. Meeks, Maggie.
II. Hallsworth, Maggie.
  [DNLM: 1. Neonatal Nursing. 2. Infant, Newborn, Diseases—nursing. WY 157.3 N9745 2010]
RJ253.5.N87 2010
618.92'01—dc22

                                                                                    2009012289

A catalogue record for this book is available from the British Library.

Set in 10/12.5 pt Sabon by Macmillan Publishing Solutions, Chennai, India

Printed and bound in Malaysia by KHL Printing Co Sdn Bhd

1 2010

CONTENTS

PREFACE

We were delighted to be asked to produce a new edition of Helen Yeo's classic text and called upon many of our ex and current colleagues (as well as some people that we have yet to meet) to help us do this. Neonatology continues to expand as a stimulating and emotionally challenging area of medicine and nursing. The commitment of all staff working on a neonatal unit is palpable and we both feel privileged that we have been involved in this speciality.

Our intention is that this text is considered essential reading for neonatal nurses and midwives caring for sick newborn infants. It is also intended to be a valuable resource for junior medical staff, tutors of neonatal and paediatric courses and other health care professionals working within this specialised area of practice. This edition aims to encourage the linking of theory to practice and facilitate the development of knowledge and skills that will continue to challenge and advance management strategies in the care of these infants.

A combined medical and nursing team approach has been used in order to produce an evidenced based text that will be of use for all those caring for sick newborn infants. We hope that this approach will facilitate each health care professional undertaking their own role to have an insight into the individual roles of the other professionals, and of course the parents. By working together in this way a team approach to the care of the infant will be encouraged and our mutual aims of achieving the best outcome for each individual infant on the neonatal unit will be realised.

This edition has been divided into chapters covering body systems, and of course some overlap between chapters is inevitable due to the complexities of the infants' conditions. Each chapter contains implications for practice which may be used as a quick information resource to reinforce the chapter content. It would be impossible to cover every condition that may be encountered on the neonatal unit and we have made no attempt to do this but we hope we have covered those most frequently seen.

We would like to personally thank the authors who contributed, all of whom are very busy clinical staff, and thank many other clinical colleagues who contributed with stimulating discussions and proof reading for medical content. We are also indebted to Chris Jarvis for her editing comments on the nutrition chapter and Patrick McNamara for his very helpful suggestions about the haemodynamically significant duct.

And finally, although we had both written chapters before this is our first foray into editing and if our husbands have anything to do with it, it may be our last!

Maggie Meeks
Maggie Hallsworth

INTRODUCTION

When asked, I readily agreed to write a few words of introduction to this edition. Having worked in neonatal nursing for over 20 years I have had the privilege of working alongside both editors during the past five years. I can only admire the depth (and breadth) of their personal knowledge of neonatology and their ability to impart that knowledge to nursing, midwifery and medical colleagues in both the clinical and classroom setting. They have always believed in the value of multidisciplinary education and it is an approach they have used with much success. This philosophy is reflected in the combined medical and nursing approach to the text.

The editors have many years of experience teaching and working alongside medical, nursing and midwifery colleagues and know, first hand, the challenges we face on a daily basis. They understand the imperative of delivering a book which does not provide theory in isolation, but links directly to practice. The learning outcomes identified at the beginning of each chapter and the 'implications for practice' points highlighted throughout the text ensure that this emphasis persists throughout the whole of the book.

Although both editors have now moved on to work elsewhere within neonates I look forward to being able to use this text to continue their legacy of a multidisciplinary approach to education that links theory to practice and translates into clinical care of a high standard. I can only reiterate the belief that evidence based, team approach to neonatal care is fundamental to achieving the best outcomes for babies and their families and continuing to improve standards in neonatal care.

Judith Foxon
Modern Matron
Neonatal Unit
University Hospitals of
Leicester NHS Trust

CONTRIBUTORS

ADAPT (All Dependent And PreTerm)

ADAPT is a support charity for the parents and families of premature and poorly babies needing specialist neonatal care. This support is offered to families while their baby is on the unit and continued once they go home for as long as is necessary. ADAPT was established in 1995 by Rob and Fiona Morris whose son Harry was on the neonatal unit in Leicester for nine months. The organisation now employs four part time workers and runs special 'In-B-Tweenie' groups for new mums around Leicestershire.

Belinda Ackerman RM, RN, HV, MA, PGCEA, ADM

Belinda Ackerman is a consultant midwife with a remit for promotion of normal birth. She is the lead for the 'alongside' Home from Home Birth Centre at Guy's & St Thomas' NHS Foundation Trust (GSTFT). She has a keen interest in the neonate and introduced midwifery-led examination of the newborn within the Women's Services directorate five years ago. She is a council member of the Royal College of Midwives (RCM) and represented the RCM on the recent DH Child Health Promotion Programme working group that launched its guidance in 2008. She is a member of the RCM Examination of the Newborn working group currently developing a DVD to illustrate the UK National Screening Committee 2008 *Newborn and Infant Physical Examination; Standards and Competencies* (NIPE) standards.

Eleri Adams MRCP, MRCPCH

Eleri Adams is a neonatal consultant at the John Radcliffe Hospital, Oxford and Honorary Senior Clinical Lecturer at Oxford University. She is also Lead Clinician for the South Central North Neonatal Network and Thames Valley Neonatal Transport Service. As well as supporting medical and nursing student teaching programmes, Eleri is a course director and instructor for NLS, and organises local multidisciplinary study days for the network. As part of her training she worked at the Hammersmith Hospital where she gained valuable knowledge and experience of neonatal neurological conditions, their assessment and management.

Mandy Barry RN, RM, MA, BA Hons, Dip N(Lond)

Mandy Barry is Genetic Counsellor Manager at the Clinical Genetics Unit at Birmingham Women's Hospital and has over 30 years' experience as a nurse, midwife and genetic counsellor. Her current role includes both clinical and managerial responsibilities. She is an active member of the Association of Genetic Nurses and Counsellors (AGNC) and was a committee member from 2002 to 2008 and AGNC Chair from 2005 to 2008. She has been a Registered Genetic Counsellor since 2002 and is a regular Assessor for the Registration Board. She is particularly interested in promoting genetic awareness and knowledge in health care in general.

Alison Bedford Russell BSc(Hons), FRCPCH

Alison Bedford Russell joined Birmingham Heartlands in August 2005 and is lead clinician for the SW Midlands Neonatal Network. Previously she was a part-time Consultant and Senior Lecturer at St George's, London, a training centre for paediatric infectious diseases, for nine years. She sits on the NLS (Newborn Life Support) sub-committee at the Resuscitation Council, having been involved in the evolution of the NLS course. Her ongoing research interest is in infection and immunology of the newborn, and she is the BAPM representative for the National GBS (Group B Streptococcus) sub-committee and is the neonatal advisor to the GBS support charity (GBSS). Her MD thesis was about the potential use of haematological growth factors as adjuvant therapy for neonatal sepsis, and she is currently principal investigator for a multi-centre study of PCR in the diagnosis of early onset GBS and E. coli infection.

Robert Bomont MBChB, MRCPCH

Robert Bomont works as a Consultant Neonatologist and Neonatal Tutor on the Trevor Mann Baby Unit in Brighton. He developed his interest in Neonatal Transport Medicine working with the Acute Neonatal Transport Service for the East of England and now is Operational Manager for the Sussex Transport Service. He is a member of Faculty for the PaNSTaR Course.

Elaine Boyle RGN, MBChB MD(Ed), MSc(Ed)

Elaine Boyle originally qualified as a nurse at Barts in 1982 and then worked as a theatre nurse before deciding to do medical training at Sheffield in 1987. Her MD was in neonatal pain and she had further academic neonatal training in Edinburgh and at McMaster University, Ontario, Canada. Her MSc was in epidemiology and she is currently working towards a PhD looking at feeding in preterm infants. She is currently working as a Senior Lecturer in Neonatal Medicine in Leicester and her research interests include neonatal pain, feeding in preterm infants and the problems of moderate and late prematurity.

Frances Bu'Lock MD, FRCP

Frances Bu'Lock has been a Consultant Paediatric Cardiologist and Training Programme Director at Glenfield Hospital in Leicester for the last ten years. She studied medicine in Cambridge and Oxford and developed her interest in paediatric cardiology as a student on the neonatal unit in Oxford. Her MD research in Bristol was on the echocardiographic assessment of cardiac function. She then worked at Birmingham Children's Hospital and Alder Hey Hospital, Liverpool, before moving to Leicester. She has particularly relevant expertise in foetal cardiology and the impact of complex heart disease on the newborn period.

Sonji Clarke MBBS, MRCOG, Fellow of HEA

Sonji Clarke is a Consultant Obstetrician Gynaecologist with an interest in maternal medicine and the management of teenage pregnancy. She is a Fellow of the Higher Education Academy and has a passion for teaching undergraduates and postgraduates, as well as a keen interest in exposing schools to role models from the health care professions. Dr Clarke worked for six months in a neonatal unit as part of her training in obstetrics and gynaecology and finds that this experience has been invaluable for decision making in obstetrics.

Yuet Ping Corcoran PGDip Edn, Dip Health Studies, Dip Health Services Management, SCM, SRN, ENB 402, 904, 998 and R23

Yuet Ping Corcoran has over 28 years' experience as a neonatal nurse working both clinically and within the education field. Ping worked at the Neonatal Unit, Northwick Park Hospital, before joining the Neonatal Unit at Queen Charlotte's and Chelsea Hospital, Hammersmith Hospitals NHS Trust, now Imperial College Healthcare NHS Trust in London, as a Senior Sister and then as the Practice Educator. She is an active member of the NWLPN Clinical Practice and Education Group as well as the Breastfeeding Group and the CPPD Special and Intensive Nursing Care of the Newborn based at Thames Valley University, London.

Andrew Currie DCH, FRCP(Ed), FRCPCH

Andrew Currie is a Consultant Neonatologist at the University of Leicester Hospitals NHS Trust and has over 20 years' experience in paediatrics and neonatal medicine. As the lead centre for the central newborn network Leicester neonatal service has close links with the paediatric cardiology service at Glenfield and Andy has had a long-term interest in neonatal echocardiography. Until recently he was the only neonatologist with echocardiographic skills and he still has a major role in the assessment of the significance of the ductus arteriosus. He also has an interest in neonatal transport and in 2007 he was appointed as the lead clinician for the Central Newborn Network Transport Service.

Jonathan Cusack MBChB, MRCPCH, MMedSciClinEd

Jonathan Cusack is a Consultant Neonatologist at the University of Leicester Hospitals NHS Trust with an interest in medical education. He is course director for the Newborn Life Support courses. His current educational interests involve the use of simulation in neonatal teaching and the evolving role of information technology in postgraduate education.

David Field MBBS(Hons), DCH, FRCPCH, FRCP(Ed), DM

David Field is Professor of Neonatal Medicine at the University of Leicester. He is also President of the British Association of Perinatal Medicine, Chair of the Neonatal Clinical Studies Group of the Medicines for Children Research Network and clinical lead for the Neonatal Survey. His research interests include perinatal epidemiology, the organisation of perinatal care and randomised trials in the field of perinatal medicine.

Sylvia Gomes BSc(Nursing) RGN, ENB 405, 998

Sylvia Gomes is Matron for Neonatal Services at West Hertfordshire Hospitals. She has over 15 years' experience as a neonatal nurse working both clinically on the neonatal unit and in the community. Sylvia was instrumental in setting up discharge/community services for the neonatal units at the Royal Free Hospital, London and the University Hospitals of Leicester. In her current role she continues to maintain her interest in early discharges and the extension of neonatal nursing care into the community.

Maggie Hallsworth RSCN, RGN, ENB 405, 904, 998

Maggie Hallsworth has over 30 years' experience as a neonatal nurse working both clinically and within the education field. Maggie now has a clinical role working on the Neonatal unit at the Simpson Centre for Reproductive Health in Edinburgh, but continues to maintain her education/teaching skills within the clinical area and as an NLS and STABLE instructor. Prior to relocation to Scotland she was course leader for the Neonatal Intensive Care Course at the De Montfort University in Leicester and worked as the Practice Educator for the neonatal services at University Hospitals Leicester

Lucy Hawkes BPharm(Hons), Dip ClinPharm, MRPharmS

Lucy Hawkes is a specialist pharmacist working within the neonatal unit at the Leicester Royal Infirmary. She is actively involved in the postgraduate education of clinical staff working on the neonatal unit as well as improving drug related protocols. She is also involved in the education of undergraduate pharmacy students through her role as a part time senior lecturer in pharmacy practice at De Montfort University, Leicester.

Marie Hubbard BA(Hons), RGN, RNCB, ENB 904, 405, 998

Marie Hubbard has worked in the field of neonatology for more than 20 years. Currently she works for the University Hospitals of Leicester NHS Trust as a neonatal research nurse, both as a study coordinator and principal investigator. Marie has a special interest in neurology following her involvement with the Total Body Cooling (TOBY) trial and is also very involved in developing neonatal guidelines for local use.

Kevin Hugill BSc(Hons) (Zoo), PGCE(FAHE), MSc Public Sector Management, RN, ENB 405, 998

Kevin Hugill is course leader for the neonatal undergraduate programmes at the University of Central Lancashire in Preston. He teaches on a number of undergraduate and postgraduate modules. In the past he has had a variety of neonatal clinical, managerial and educational positions mainly based in neonatal units in the West and East Midlands of the UK and has an interest in family support as well as education. He is currently completing his PhD study which explored the experiences of fathers in neonatal units.

Karissa Jowaheer RN, RM, Neonatal Nursing Certificate, ENB 934

Karissa Jowaheer has been working as a neonatal nurse/educator for the past 32 years. She is currently working as a senior lecturer/neonatal nursing degree pathway leader at Thames Valley University in London. She teaches on the neonatal specific programmes at the university for child branch students, midwifery students and post-registration students who specialise in neonatal intensive care. She is also the link tutor for neonatal nursing education for the North West London Perinatal Network.

Venkatesh Kairamkonda FRCPCH, MD, DNB, DCH, MSc

Venkatesh Kairamkonda has been a Consultant Neonatologist at University Hospitals of Leicester NHS Trusts since 2005. His main interests include the development of a neonatal electronic database and perinatal governance issues. His clinical interests include clinical cardiovascular assessment and echocardiography. His particular research interests include the role of the hormone amylin in neonatal feed intolerance and ambulatory lung function tests in infants surviving with chronic lung disease.

Andy Leslie PhD, ANNP, RSCN, RGN, ENB 405

Andy Leslie is an Advanced Neonatal Nurse Practitioner with Nottingham Neonatal Service. His background is in neonatal transport and his PhD was concerned with both the process and outcome of ANNPs assuming the lead role in transfer of critically ill infants. He has recently completed several years' post-doctoral research work as the BLISS Neonatal Research Fellow at the National Perinatal Epidemiology Unit, University of Oxford.

Maggie Meeks Dip Ed MB, ChB, MD, FRCPCH

Maggie Meeks has recently moved to Christchurch Women's Hospital New Zealand, having been educational lead for neonatology at the University Hospitals of Leicester since 2002. She has always enjoyed and prioritised education within her clinical posts of neonatology and in Leicester she was lucky enough to have undergraduate, postgraduate and nursing educational commitments from which she feels she has learnt a great deal. She has particularly enjoyed her role as an NLS Course Director and Course Assessor and Lead Instructor for STABLE. She hopes to continue her educational interest with new challenges in her new post.

Shawqui Nour MD FRCS (Paed), FRCPCH

Shawqui Nour is a Consultant Paediatric Surgeon at the University Hospitals of Leicester, where he was appointed in 1995. He trained in the paediatric surgical units at Sheffield, Leeds and Newcastle. Shawqui has a special interest in neonatal surgery, laparoscopic surgery and gastroenterology. He has done research on gastric emptying using the applied potential tomography method.

Michelle Paterson BSc Dietetics

Michelle Paterson is the Paediatric Dietician for the neonatal unit at the University Hospitals of Leicester NHS Trust. She studied at Stellenbosch University and has eight years' experience in Dietetics, specialising in Paediatric Dietetics for the last four years. Michelle has gained experience in various paediatric specialities, which include: oncology, respiratory, intensive care, metabolic disorders and neonatology.

Lynda Rafael SEN, RGN, ENB 405, 998, U05

Lynda Rafael is a Sister on the Neonatal Units at University Hospitals of Leicester NHS Trust and is also a member of the Transport Team providing Neonatal Transport for the Central Newborn Network. She has 25 years' experience nursing in Neonatal Intensive Care Units in the UK and Saudi Arabia. As one of the Senior

Sisters, Lynda plays an active part in education within the clinical areas and in respect to the transport of the sick newborn infant. She is also a member of the faculty for the Paediatric and Infant Critical Care Transport Course (PICCTS).

Inga Warren Dip COT, MSc

Inga Warren is Consultant Occupational Therapist in Neonatology and Early Intervention at St Mary's Hospital, London, part of the Imperial College Healthcare NHS Trust. She has 18 years' experience specialising in preterm and newborn development and recently set up the UK's first NIDCAP Training Centre on the Winnicott Baby Care Unit. Inga is working with neonatal services in many countries teaching developmental care, advising on programme development and collaborating with research. She takes an active role in international scientific and educational networks and was a founding member of the Brazelton Centre in the UK.

Tim Watts MBBS FRCPCH MD

Tim Watts is a full-time Consultant on the Neonatal Unit at St Thomas' Hospital, London. He has an interest in Neonatal Haematology and was awarded an MD from the University of London for his thesis 'The role of impaired megakaryocytopoiesis in thrombocytopenia in the preterm baby'. He is also involved in undergraduate teaching within the King's College London (KCL) Medical School, is the Postgraduate Medical Education and Training Lead for Paediatrics at Guy's and St Thomas' NHS Foundation Trust and has a key role in teaching neonatal nursing and midwifery staff in KCL and the Trust.

Sue Williams MIPR, CIM Cert FdA

Sue Williams has a wealth of experience in Marketing, PR and Communications and recently completed a degree course in Managing Community & Voluntary Organisations. She is currently working with the baby charity ADAPT, who support parents and families of premature and poorly babies, working in the areas of administration, fundraising and long-term development of the charity.

John Wyatt MBBS, FRCP, FRCPCH

John Wyatt is Professor of Ethics and Perinatology, University College London and Honorary Consultant Neonatologist, University College London Hospitals Foundation NHS Trust. He has undertaken research into the mechanisms, consequences and prevention of perinatal brain injury and has a long-standing interest in the philosophical, social and religious background to ethical dilemmas raised by advances in medical technology.

Zoe Wilkes MSc, BSc(Hons), RN(Child), Independent Nurse Prescriber

Zoe Wilkes is currently working as a Nurse Consultant for Children's Palliative Care for the Diana Children's Community Service within Leicester City PCT. She has worked in children's hospices both as a nurse consultant and a senior nurse practitioner. Her interest and passion for this area of nursing began while working as a staff nurse on Paediatric Intensive Care and within an in-reach pain liaison service in various hospitals across the country.

Chapter 1

THE EVOLUTION OF NEONATAL CARE

David Field and Andy Leslie

Learning outcomes

After reading this chapter the reader will be expected to be able to:

- Summarise the history of the development of neonatal care
- Explain the influences which have lead to the current model of delivery of neonatal care
- Relate the published mortality rates to the analysis of reproductive health services
- Explain the term 'evidence based practice'
- Summarise the origin of the best evidence that guides current practice
- Explain the term 'research governance'

The photo in Figure 1.1 shows an intensive care space at a modern well-designed neonatal unit that allows enough space for parental access as well as for the neonatal nurse and clinical team to provide neonatal intensive care comfortably (Christchurch Women's Hospital, New Zealand).

Introduction: historical accounts of neonatal care

Throughout history there are records of medical interventions focused on babies. In pre-modern societies, as well as in much of the developing world today, pregnancy and childbirth was the main cause of death for women of childbearing age. Infants have always been born preterm and with the other problems commonly seen on neonatal units, but it is only in the last fifty years that there has been sufficient understanding of these problems for significant effective treatments to be developed.

The problem of how to resuscitate infants at birth is a good example of these developments. It has long been recognised that some newly born infants are unresponsive and apparently lifeless. Many interventions for use in this situation were advocated by people with apparently positive experiences of their use. These included such bizarre treatments as applying onion or mustard to the infant's mouth and nose, blowing smoke into the infant's rectum and the use of an inhaled brandy mist[1]. We now understand that the apparent success of some of these treatments was simply due to the fact that most infants who do not breathe immediately at birth will go on to establish

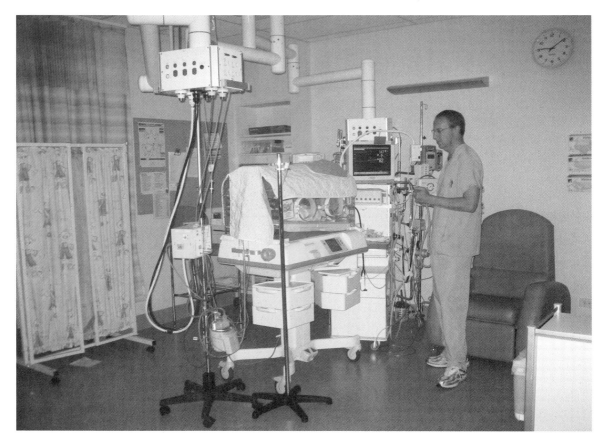

Figure 1.1 This photo shows an intensive care space at a modern well-designed neonatal unit that allows enough space for parental access as well as for the neonatal nurse and clinical team comfortably to provide neonatal intensive care (Christchurch Women's Hospital, New Zealand).

spontaneous respirations without any help at all; in other words, these historical infants were getting better *despite* what the attendants at the birth did, not *because* of it. As an understanding of the physiology of the establishment of breathing at birth was gained, so it was possible to develop effective tools and procedures to deal with infants who do not breathe immediately, and for these to be incorporated into protocolised teaching programmes that are now widely disseminated to those engaged in newborn care[2].

Similar processes, which could be characterised as a movement away from care that was based on poor understanding of physiology and towards care based on good evidence founded on well-established physiological studies, have occurred in every aspect of the care of sick newborn infants.

Implications for practice

The development of neonatal care can be summarised as occurring because of an improved understanding of the physiology of the newborn with well established physiological studies leading to evidence for the practice of effective care.

The development of modern neonatal care

Neonatology and neonatal nursing as specialty areas of work are relatively new, having largely emerged over the period since 1970. Prior to this period sick newborn infants were mostly cared for by obstetricians and midwives and there was scant specialist provision. Most hospitals did not have a dedicated unit for sick infants.

Technology

Starting slowly, clinical care has advanced ever more rapidly during the modern era. The possibility of using warmth from incubators and additional oxygen to breathe as treatments for premature infants were first explored at the end of the nineteenth century but the term 'neonatology' wasn't invented until 1960 and the first newborn ICU didn't open until 1965[3].

Innovation and new treatments have followed rapidly since this period. Some, with minor modifications, remain in use to this day. For example, the first observation that light has an effect on bilirubin levels was made in 1956 by Sister Ward, a nurse on the premature baby unit at Rochford General Hospital in Essex and remains the mainstay of treatment[4,5]. Other treatments have been adopted enthusiastically and subsequently substantially modified, most notably the use of inhaled oxygen for premature infants with respiratory distress. Early work showed that additional oxygen improved the respiratory status of infants with premature lung disease, but it needed the first ever randomised controlled trial in newborns to show that too much oxygen often led to severe visual impairment by the development of retinopathy of prematurity (ROP)[6]. Oxygen saturation monitoring for newborns was first described in 1987, and now is ubiquitous in neonatal units. It is of note, however, that the 'right' level of blood oxygen saturation for premature newborn infants has yet to be reliably established, and research continues (http://www.npeu.ox.ac.uk/boost).

Nursing

The establishment of neonatal nursing as a speciality occurred in the UK in the 1970s. The need for skilled nurses to staff newly-established neonatal units led to training courses being designed (English National Board Course 405 in Special & Intensive Care of the Newborn, and others). The nurse staffing units at this time started to come together regionally and nationally to discuss common concerns, and this led in 1977 to the formation of the Neonatal Nurses Association, and later of the Scottish Neonatal Nurses Group. While the educational framework for neonatal nursing has changed as higher education has developed, courses in universities which educate nurses in neonatal care remain a cornerstone of care provision. A number of specialist roles for nurses developed subsequently, in areas such as family support and transport.

Advanced neonatal nurse practitioners (ANNPs) have been trained in the UK since 1992[7], following earlier development of the role in the USA. ANNP training builds on the role of the neonatal nurse to produce a professional able to integrate both nursing and medical aspects of care. Differing approaches have been developed, both to the education programmes and to the subsequent deployment of ANNPs in practice. ANNPs have been evaluated in structured research projects and found to offer equivalent or better care when compared to existing caregivers in doing acute transport, resuscitation at birth and routine neonatal checks[8–10]. While their ability to provide cohesive and comprehensive care has been a strength, their identity as neither wholly medical nor nursing has hindered group development and recognition.

For nursing careers, the latest development has been the emergence of Neonatal Nurse Consultants. Envisaged as a new group giving nursing increased influence, and with diverse areas of responsibility, from transport to low dependency care, they are a group whose ability to influence quality of care is under some scrutiny and where further evaluation is needed.

Organisation

As clinical care has evolved, so has the organisation of the services in which clinical care is provided. In the UK, important steps in the establishment of neonatal care are marked by Government reports. In 1971 the Sheldon Report recommended that neonatal care be provided in some form wherever infants were being born[11]. It also recognised that not every unit would be able to provide every treatment, and so a distinction was drawn between intensive and special care units and the report recommended that expert transport facilities would be needed to move sick infants to the place best able to care for them. Subsequently, a variety of influences have helped shape the service in the UK and elsewhere. Initially, it was the enthusiasm of a small number of individuals that led to the formation of a handful of units specialising in the care of sick newborn infants. However pressure from the professions and the public encouraged successive governments in the UK to develop a service with nationwide coverage[12–17]. The rate of evolution varied around the country but, particularly during the 1980s, there was a steady move towards a three-tier service based on the health regions (populations of 2 to 4 million) that existed at the time. The intention was that each of these geographical areas would be served by three types of neonatal unit:

Level 1

- Hospitals which delivered infants expected to be well; resuscitation could be provided if necessary but no ongoing care. Infants requiring such support were transferred.

Level 2

- Hospitals with higher delivery rates capable of providing resuscitation and limited ongoing care. Infants with more complex problems were transferred.

Level 3

- Regional centres, based largely in teaching hospitals, capable of providing a full range of neonatal services.

The rationale for this approach was:

- Reasonable geographical coverage was ensured
- High throughput for the level 3 units enabled clinical skills to be maintained
- High levels of bed occupancy (in level 3 units) permitted efficient use of expensive resources

The regional centres also had additional responsibilities, including specialist training for nurses and doctors and the provision of a transport service for sick babies born elsewhere. Although this structure, which had been adopted by a number of other high-cost, low-volume specialties, appeared a sensible approach for the delivery of neonatal intensive care it was never fully established across the UK at that time. Concerns that a centralised system of care was not appropriate centred on the following:

- Infants in outlying units were disadvantaged in terms of access and availability
- Shortage of cots, leading to very long distance transfers
- Deskilling in local units
- Disruption to family life following long distance transfers

Reforms of the 1990s

By the beginning of the 1990s rising demand for neonatal intensive care generated increasing public disquiet over access to and availability of neonatal intensive care facilities. Both Government and health authorities were keen to respond to public demands for increased local services. The NHS reforms, introduced for other reasons, and an increase in the personnel with neonatal expertise available in District General Hospitals proved to be the vehicles for change. By 1992, strategic planning and funding for neonatal care (in fact for virtually all services) was reduced to Health District level (average population 500,000). By 1996 any tendency towards increasing centralisation had ceased and a quarter of neonatal intensive care was delivered in small local units (i.e. less than three intensive care cots) whilst the old regional centres (at least six intensive care cots) retained approximately one half.

The current model of care

The decentralised approach to specialist neonatal care continued until the turn of the century, when a number of factors lead to review of the service. Particularly important considerations were:

- The introduction of the European Working Time Directive, which made the medical staffing of smaller neonatal units particularly costly
- A growing shortage of specialist neonatal nurses
- Increasing complexity of care associated with improved survival of the most immature babies

A review, initiated by the Department of Health, recommended the introduction of managed clinical networks. It was envisaged that these would be based in groups of units, who between them would generally deliver 15000–30000 births, working together. Within any one network units would be designated to a particular role: level 1, level 2 or level 3, exactly in line with the three-tier model of the 1980s described above. The difference here would be that:

- Neonatal care capacity for the population would be planned
- In any one network all complex intensive care would fall to just one or two level 3 units
- Just one intensive care unit would act as the lead and take on wider responsibilities for activities such as guideline development, audit training, transport, training, etc.
- The group of hospitals would work collaboratively

It is too early to assess the success or otherwise of this particular model, but in time it will be important to look at the effectiveness of this model of care in terms of:

- Whether the increased centralisation (described in relation to the three-tier model of the 1980s) is now seen as acceptable to the public at large
- Whether outcomes are at least as good as those prior to the introduction of networks
- Whether there is increased efficiency, with higher rates of occupancy, particularly of the intensive care cots compared to when these were shared over many more units

Implications for practice

The current model of neonatal care has similarities with the three-tier system of the 1980s but involves units of different tiers working together in managed clinical networks. Its development was stimulated by changes in medical working patterns, availability of specialist nursing staff and the survival of infants with increasing complex medical needs.

The development of transport services

In any service that relies to some extent on treatment in a central unit, transport of patients becomes an essential element of the package of care. In general, families do not welcome the prospect of changing hospitals and teams at a time of anxiety and if there are other children the move may cause additional worries and impose significant cost. Referring clinicians are therefore under particular pressure to achieve the best outcome whilst exposing mother and infant to the least possible risk (see also Chapter 13).

In utero transfers

Neonatal intensive care is in the special position of often being able to choose to move the potential patient either before or after delivery. There is no doubt that it is far easier, and in general safer, to move an infant *in utero*.

While much attention has been given to the organisation of post-natal transfers (see below) there has been little increase in the sophistication of the organisation of *in utero* (or antenatal) transfers. The process usually involves a local decision that an impending infant cannot be offered care locally, for reasons of complexity of care or local workload. This decision is followed by telephone calls to obstetric, midwifery and neonatal staff at local units until both an obstetric and a neonatal bed have been found. Some networks have developed cot-finding services that appear effective in coordinating the referring and receiving units, but these are far from universal.

In utero transfer sometimes causes particular problems for the family when after moving to another hospital away from their home delivery is delayed, perhaps for several weeks.

Post-natal transfer

The same individual enthusiasm which marked the initial development of specialist neonatal units in the UK was also responsible for the provision of emergency transfer services. Units often constructed their own equipment for this purpose, with medical and nursing staff chosen ad hoc from those on duty on the neonatal unit when a transport was required. These people were often untrained in the particular constraints and issues involved in safe post-natal transfer. A number of high profile accidents highlighted the inappropriateness of this approach[18]. European standards now exist which specify very precisely the type of equipment that should be used during such transfers and the way in which it should be transported[19,20]. With regard to staff, regulation of working hours has meant that the old system of ad hoc teams could not continue and there has, since 2000, been a steady move towards the use of transport teams. Nursing and medical staff engaged in neonatal transfers now routinely receive training specifically in transport care. Many of the recently formed neonatal networks have treated getting transport provision right as a priority, and so investment in staff and supporting infrastructure for transport has been considerable in these areas.

Definitions of neonatal care

Traditionally, the work of the neonatal service has been subdivided as follows:

- Normal care – that which could reasonably be expected to be given by the parents
- Special care – for babies requiring some specialist medical or nursing input
- Intensive care (normally divided into intensive care and high dependency care) – for babies requiring continuous medical and nursing support

Within the UK, a number of definitions exist relating to this broad structure and around the world there are further variations. These systems have been developed from clinical interest to allow the work of any one unit to be monitored over time and as an aid to audit.

More recently, consideration has been given to clinical classifications as markers of cost. In the UK, Health Resource Groupings (HRGs) have been developed based on the BAPM 2001 system for describing levels of care[21]. It was envisaged that from 2008, work identified using this system would be the basis of the funding that individual neonatal units in the UK would receive.

Analysis of reproductive health services

The quality of services for mothers and babies are described by measuring particular rates. These are:

- The perinatal mortality rate: this is the number of stillbirths and the number of babies dying in the first week of life divided by the total number of births (alive and dead) for a given period. In the UK all babies born dead after 24 weeks of gestation are included in this number as stillbirths, but figures vary between countries with some using, for example, 28 weeks of gestation as the cut-off with regard to stillbirths.

- The neonatal mortality rate: this is the number of live born children dying at or before 28 days of age divided by the number of live births for a given period.
- The infant mortality rate: this is the number of live born children dying in the first year of life divided by the number of live births for a given period.

Perinatal mortality is heavily influenced by late stillbirths but all three of the above rates are heavily influenced by prematurity and congenital anomalies. In fact these are the major influences for neonatal and infant mortality[22].

These rates are typically calculated over a one-year period so that clusters of small numbers of deaths do not produce sudden major variations in the mortality rates. They are normally calculated for whole geographical population. This means that rather than looking at the results of a single hospital it is the results of the whole locality (i.e. the net effect of all the mother and baby services) that are assessed. This is done in order that some obvious biases are removed. For example, if one were to compare the perinatal mortality

results of a general hospital that booked all the women for delivery from the locality considered high risk and compared the rate to that of the local midwifery unit that delivered only low-risk women then inevitably the rate for the general hospital would be higher than that for the midwifery unit. Therefore these rates are best used to compare whether the whole service for a community with all its component parts is working better or worse than those in other parts of the country. Figure 1.2 shows trends in two of these measures over a thirty-year period.

Does this mean that individual hospitals cannot be compared? It is true that comparing hospitals fairly is complex, but systems have been developed to allow some aspects of the work of individual neonatal units to be compared. A variety of techniques have been developed which allow the babies admitted at 32 weeks gestation or less to be scored in terms of how ill they are and how likely they are to die. As a result, for each unit it is possible to calculate how many babies one would have expected to die and compare this to how many actually did die. The scoring systems are based on a variety of factors such as birthweight, gestation, oxygen requirement, temperature, etc., and the exact combination and how they are used are unique to each system. The most commonly used of these scores in the UK are CRIB (Clinical Risk Index for Babies) and CRIB II (see Table 1.1)[23,24].

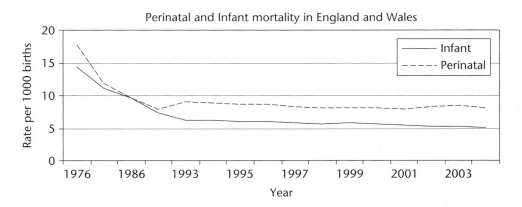

Figure 1.2 Trends in infant and perinatal mortality over 30 years (www.statistics.gov.uk).

Table 1.1 CRIB scoring system.

Physiological variable	Range of values that provided the weighting
Birthweight (g)	>1350 851–1350 701–850 ≤700
Gestation (wk)	>24 ≤24
Congenital malformation (excluding inevitably lethal malformation)	None Not acutely life-threatening Acutely life-threatening
Maximal base excess in first 12 h (mmol/L)	>−7 −7 to −9.9 −10 to −14.9 ≤−15
Minimum appropriate FIO_2 in first 12 hours (TcPO2 or PaO2 = 6.7–10.7 kPa or SaO2 = 88–95%)	≤0.40 0.41–0.60 0.61–0.90 0.91–1.00
Maximum appropriate FIO_2 in first 12 hours (TcPO2 or PaO2 = 6.7–10.7 kPa or SaO2 = 88–95%)	≤0.40 0.41–0.80 0.81–0.90 0.91–1.00

CRIB is one of a number of scores developed to help compare outcomes between units[25]. Every infant less than 32 weeks is given a numerical score based on each of the above criteria in the first 12 hours of life. Babies with higher scores are 'sicker' and therefore would be expected to have a higher risk of dying. The score allows adjustment for this fact between units. A subsequent version of this score has used a somewhat more complex approach, whilst others scores tend to be based on many more variables.

Implications for practice

The perinatal and neonatal mortality rates are used to give information that relates to the neonatal care within a particular geographical population. The use of scoring systems such as the CRIB score can be used to assess the care of a particular hospital.

Using evidence – evolution of research methods

Neonatal care can now claim to be one of the most evidence-based areas of medical practice. Most NICUs have guidelines and protocols outlining how care and treatment should be delivered, and these are usually based wholly or substantially on evidence from clinical trials. This is not to suggest that we know everything – many questions remain to be answered and many problems remain unsolved and much more research is needed, but nonetheless there is now a substantial knowledge base underpinning neonatal care.

But as we saw above in the section discussing historical practice in the resuscitation of infants at birth, it is only in the recent past that it has been possible to base clinical practice on good evidence. To understand how we got from a time when there was little evidence, and practice was governed by the beliefs of the practitioner, to the situation now, where discussion of evidence in the clinical setting is commonplace, it is necessary to consider both the regulatory and social contexts in which both care and research were undertaken and also improvements in research methods.

Research methods

The knowledge base is advanced by several distinct types of study. Basic science research is concerned to understand physiological processes. For example, in neonatal care important work was done in 1960s to work out what the problem was in premature infants that caused them to have breathing difficulties. For some time the patent ductus arteriosus was thought to be the cause, and treatment strategies were developed for this. It was the work of Mary Ellen Avery which led to an understanding that the key issue was surfactant deficiency[26].

Once physiological processes are understood it becomes possible to develop rational treatment strategies. However, simply because a new drug or treatment has been developed from basic science research does not mean that it will be effective. The most important development in clinical research has been the ability to do good randomised controlled trials.

Randomised controlled trials (RCTs)

The RCT has become the cornerstone of clinical research. Before RCTs it was common for new treatments to simply be given to a selected group of patients and some simple short-term outcome data collected. These treatments often appeared effective, especially when compared with a selected group of patients given the 'old' treatment. Many problems became evident with these methods. Groups of patients given the old and new treatments were not comparable, studies were very small, the researchers knew who had received which treatment so might have been biased in favour of the patients receiving the new one and outcome measures were often very short term. Modern RCTs aim to produce evidence that is as unbiased and as widely applicable as possible. In order to do this, researchers take a number of important steps. First, the study is designed with sufficient numbers of patients to reduce the possibility of an erroneous conclusion. When studies are very small it is possible to achieve apparently strikingly significant results which are actually incorrect because by chance there are a larger than expected number of treatment successes or failures in one of the groups. Larger studies minimise these problems. Second, wherever possible researchers seek to achieve comparability between the two groups of patients in the study, those receiving the new treatment and those not. This is best done by randomly assigning patients to receive one or other treatment. Additionally, in order to reduce bias it is best if none of the team caring for the patient (or family) or the researchers are aware of which treatment group the patient is in. This helps reduce the possibility for any possibly unconscious bias when patients are being assessed. Finally, studies are designed

with outcome measures that are important. For example, a new treatment for hypotension could be shown to raise blood pressure when compared to standard treatment. While this finding might be interesting to researchers, what clinical staff and families want to know is whether this results in more infants surviving NICU care and surviving with neurodevelopment that is equal or better than infants treated without the new drug.

Cochrane

The most significant recent development in RCTs is the improvements in the methods available for pooling the results of several studies. Each individual study in a particular area has limitations, maybe in the number of infants enrolled or their severity of illness or their ethnic background, etc. The Cochrane Library of Systematic Reviews is a web-based resource comprising meta-analyses of similar studies. A meta-analysis is where several similar studies are analysed together in an attempt to elicit whether the increase in numbers of patients available for analysis by this pooling of data reveals more reliable findings than from the individual studies alone. For example, using these methods established unequivocally the effectiveness of antenatal steroid treatment for maturing the lungs of premature infants[27].

Other research methods

While interventions such as new drugs and treatments may be readily studied using RCTs, other aspects of care require different approaches. Much neonatal nursing research has been directed toward understanding the experience of being a parent of an NICU infant. Qualitative research methods are the appropriate tool to use in this setting, and a diverse range of approaches have been developed.

Rather than try to produce definite results like in a drug trial, qualitative research aims to develop an authentic understanding of the lived experience of the subjects. A number of methods have been developed to both collect and analyse qualitative data. Some data collection methods aim to reproduce the rigour of quantitative studies, for example by using scales to quantify attitudes and feelings. Others reject attempts at quantification, claiming this area of research is unsuitable for numerical analysis, and use observation, interview and recordings of conversations to collect data.

While these types of research are often criticised for their subjectivity when compared to quantitative studies, it seems unlikely that attitudes and feelings can be reliably reduced to numerical analysis. In fact there is now a large body of nursing research attempting to understand various aspects of the parental experience. The challenge now is to attempt to draw these together and build a greater understanding based on many individual studies.

Implications for practice

The evidence for neonatal care was historically based on scientific physiological studies as well as observation. These methods had a number of weaknesses and have been replaced by the use of randomised controlled trials which aim to provide quantitative information of an unbiased nature that provides evidence to advance neonatal care.

Evolution of research regulation

The climate in which research is undertaken has changed completely over the period of the evolution of modern neonatal care.

In the early days of neonatal research, projects were usually undertaken entirely at the whim of the academic involved. A new treatment could be developed and tested on sick newborn infants with little external scrutiny of whether it was a sound idea, whether the study was well constructed and likely to yield a result, whether it might result in harm for the patient and certainly without seeking consent for participation from the infant's family.

In the wider social context of the time, this was not an unusual attitude. All kinds of medical treatments were delivered by paternalistic doctors to passive patients, both parties believing that 'doctor knows best'. The relationship between the medical professions and the public has altered substantially and hand in hand with that the research climate has evolved too. In particular, widely reported instances of problems with research both in neonates and elsewhere have led to ever greater regulation of how research is done. A substantial legislative and procedural framework ('research governance') now exists, which governs every aspect of how research is undertaken. For a research project to proceed now formal applications for approval will have to be made, both locally and possibly nationally, to ethics committees, research and development departments of hospitals, to funding bodies, research coordination networks and others. The process is intensely bureaucratic, repetitive and time-consuming. The days of the amateur researcher, the clinician who dabbles, are largely over. There have been a number of important benefits from the changes in the research climate. Better constructed, larger studies are being done, and because such multicentre studies often need local coordination there are opportunities for nurses and others to get involved in research. Nurse academics with their own research programmes are also established now, both in the UK and elsewhere.

Implications for practice

The term 'research governance' is a term that encompasses the policies and procedures that now surround the application and delivery of research, which have been brought in to raise standards and protect patients.

Conclusion

Nurses have always believed that nursing care makes a difference for babies in intensive care, and while there is some evidence for this the nature of what constitutes 'best care' remains to be elicited in many areas[28]. The challenge in the coming era for both clinical neonatal nurses and for those engaged in research is to strive to make neonatal nursing a speciality that has a sound research base and where the connections between researchers and clinical nurses mean that the care that is delivered is based on this research evidence.

References

1. O'Donnell CPF, Gibson AT, Davis PG (2006) Pinching, electrocution, ravens' beaks, and positive pressure ventilation: a brief history of neonatal resuscitation. *Archives of Disease in Childhood – Fetal and Neonatal Edition*, **91** (5), F369–F373.
2. Resuscitation Council (UK) (2005) *Newborn Life Support Provider Course Manual*. Resuscitation Council (UK), London.
3. Neonatology on the Web, Timeline of Neonatology – Information for Parents Residents, Students and Teachers (www.neonatology.org/tour/timeline.html).
4. Cremer RJ, Perryman PW, Richards DH (1958) Influence of light on the hyperbilirubinaemia of infants. *Lancet*, **271** (7030), 1094.
5. Dobbs RH, Cremer RJ (1975) Phototherapy. *Archives of Disease in Childhood*, **50** (11), 833.
6. Kinsey V (1956) Retrolental fibroplasia. Cooperative study of retrolental fibroplasia and the use of oxygen. *Arch Ophthalmol*, **56** (4), 481–543.
7. Redshaw M, Harvey M (2001) Education for a new role: a review of neonatal nurse practitioner programmes. *Nurse Education Today*, **21** (6), 468–476.
8. Leslie A, Stephenson T (2003) Neonatal transfers by advanced neonatal nurse practitioners and paediatric registrars. *Archives of Disease in Childhood Fetal & Neonatal Edition*, **88**, F509–F512.
9. Aubrey W, Yoxall C (2001) Evaluation of the role of the neonatal nurse practitioner in resuscitation of preterm infants at birth. *Archives of Disease in Childhood Fetal & Neonatal Edition*, **85** (2), F96–F99.
10. Lee T, Skelton R, Skene C (2001) Routine neonatal examination: effectiveness of trainee paediatricians compared with advanced neonatal nurse practitioners. *Archives of Disease in Childhood Fetal & Neonatal Edition*, **85** (2), F100–F104.
11. Sheldon Report (1971) *Report of the Expert Group on the Special Care of Babies. DHSS Report on Public Health and Medical Subjects*, No. 127. HMSO, London.
12. Report by the Comptroller and Auditor General (1990) *Maternity Services*. HMSO, London.
13. House of Commons Committee of Public Accounts (1990) *35th Report Maternity Services*. HMSO, London.
14. House of Commons Health Committee Session 1991–1992 (1992) *Second Report: Maternity Services*. HMSO, London.
15. Liaison Committee of the British Paediatric Association and the Royal College of Obstetricians and Gynaecologists (1977) *Recommendations for the Improvement of Infant Care During the Perinatal Period in the UK*. BPA/RCOG, London.
16. Social Services Committee (1980) *Perinatal and Neonatal Mortality. Second Report from the Social Services Committee*. HMSO, London.
17. Royal College of Physicians (1988) *Medical Care of the Newborn in England and Wales. A Report by the Royal College of Physicians*. Royal College of Physicians London.
18. CEN TC 239. Rescue systems – Transportation of incubators – Part 1: Interface conditions. 2001. prEN 13976-1.2 (http://www.cen.eu/cenorm/homepage.htm).
19. Madar RJ, Milligan DWA (1994) Neonatal transport: safety and security. *Archives of Disease in Childhood Fetal and Neonatal Edition*, **71**, F147–F148.
20. CEN TC 239. Rescue systems – Transportation of incubators – Part 2: System requirements. 2001. prEN 13976-2.2 (http://www.cen.eu/cenorm/homepage.htm).
21. British Association of Perinatal Medicine (2001) *Standards for Hospitals Providing Neonatal Intensive and High Dependency Care*, 2nd edn. BAPM, London.
22. Dorling JS, Field DJ, Manktelow B (2005) Neonatal disease severity scoring systems. *Archives of Diseases in Childhood Fetal and Neonatal Edition*, **90** (1, Jan.), F11–F16.
23. The International Neonatal Network (1993) The CRIB (Clinical Risk Index for Babies) score: a tool for assessing initial neonatal risk and comparing performance of neonatal intensive care units. *Lancet*, **342**, 193–198.
24. Parry G, Tucker J, Tarnow-Mordi W and UK Neonatal Staffing Study Collaborative Group (2003) CRIB II: an update of the clinical risk

index for babies score. *Lancet*, **361** (9371), 1789–1791.

25. The International Neonatal Network (1993) The CRIB (Clinical Risk Index for Babies) score: a tool for assessing initial neonatal risk and comparing performance of neonatal intensive care units. *Lancet*, **342**, 193–198.

26. Avery ME (2000) Surfactant deficiency in hyaline membrane disease: the story of a discovery. *American Journal of Respiratory and Critical Care*, **161** (41), 1074–1075.

27. Roberts D, Dalziel S (2006) Antenatal corticosteroids for accelerating fetal lung maturation for women at risk of preterm birth. *Cochrane Database of Systematic Reviews*, Issue 3. Art. No.: CD004454. DOI: 10.1002/14651858. CD004454.pub2.

28. Hamilton KE, Redshaw ME, Tarnow-Mordi W (2007) Nurse staffing in relation to risk-adjusted mortality in neonatal care. *Archives of Diseases in Childhood Fetal & Neonatal Edition*, **92** (2), F99–F103.

Chapter 2

OBSTETRIC ISSUES RELATING TO NEONATAL CARE

Belinda Ackerman and Sonji Clarke

Learning outcomes

After reading this chapter the reader will be expected to be able to:

- Recognise the role of the neonatal team in counselling families in the antenatal period

- Identify some of the generic factors that are important in preconception counselling and explain why these are important

- Summarise the antenatal screening tests that are currently available and the types of ultrasound scanning that may be performed

- Explain the risks to the neonate in common medical conditions, pregnancies that are complicated by hypertension, pre-eclampsia and maternal diabetes

- Have an understanding of the effects on the newborn of the less common medical conditions, pregnancies complicated by maternal epilepsy, haemoglobinopathies, SLE and anti-phospholipid syndrome, thyroid disease and obstetric cholestasis

---

Introduction

In considering the obstetric issues relating to neonatal care, it is important to begin prior to pregnancy itself, with preconception counselling. This has emerged over the years as having an increasingly important role, not only for obstetricians and midwives, but for physicians, geneticists, GPs and other members of the multidisciplinary team involved in the care of the pregnant woman.

Routine antenatal care in England and Wales has now been standardised to ensure that every woman is offered screening and referral for diagnostic tests and treatment, if necessary, prior to the birth of the baby[1]. The timing of diagnosis and treatment of a maternal medical condition is crucial in relation to its effect on the developing embryo, foetus and ultimately the neonate.

Close communication between the obstetricians, midwives and neonatologists is essential in planning the management of a high-risk labour and to ensure the running of a safe and effective labour ward and maternity unit. The service that is provided should be able to cope with the multidisciplinary management of preterm deliveries, multiple births, instrumental and operative deliveries as well as with the unexpected diagnoses.

This chapter will discuss the diagnosis and management of common maternal medical conditions and review the outcome to the neonate. Care planning by the multiprofessional team to ensure the optimum outcome will be reviewed, including antenatal care and treatment, labour care, the most effective mode of birth and subsequent neonatal care.

Preconception care and early counselling

The aim of preconception counselling is to achieve the best outcomes for any ensuing pregnancy and it includes:

- Lifestyle advice
  - Smoking, alcohol, recreational drugs
  - Dietary manipulations, e.g. avoidance of soft cheeses and uncooked meats
- Information about maternal medical conditions: e.g. Diabetes, epilepsy, renal disease, Marfan syndrome
- Management of medications in pregnancy
  - e.g. anticonvulsants, antidepressants
  - advice regarding non-prescription medications
- Screening: screening takes place for abnormalities in the foetus but also for abnormalities in the mother
- Neonate: —Nuchal scans and serum screening for Down's syndrome and other chromosomal abnormalities
- Mother: maternal HIV testing, blood pressure measurement and urinalysis are all screening tools that may ultimately affect the health and well-being of the neonate

Counselling for screening involves helping the parents understand probabilities and relating those to their individual situation – a personalised risk assessment. Once an abnormality has been diagnosed through antenatal screening, the obstetrician should discuss the options with the family, ranging from termination of pregnancy, to what may happen after delivery should the pregnancy continue. The obstetrician should also be expected to make the appropriate referrals to other clinicians able to provide more information regarding prognosis. This area can involve lia

ising between the parents and neonatologists, paediatricians, geneticists and surgeons.

Risk assessment in pregnancy

The NICE Antenatal Care guideline 2003 recommended that women should have a needs and risk assessment at booking, in order to give appropriate, individualised care[2]. This should take place at every visit and modifications should be made regarding care accordingly. This recommendation was further emphasised in the CEMACH (Confidential Enquiry into Maternal and Child Health) report 2004, *Why Mothers Die*[3], which encouraged strengthening and developing interdisciplinary communication and working. Whilst these recommendations were made in a report concerning maternal deaths, they remain pertinent for perinatal morbidity. These recommendations also echo the *Maternity Standard of the National Service Framework for Children, Young People and Maternity Services* (2003), the CEMACH *Perinatal Mortality Report* (2005) and *Maternity Matters* (DoH 2007)[4–6].

Antenatal care

Booking and risk assessment

Adequate risk assessment is supported when the GP is able to provide full and correct information to the midwife and/or obstetrician prior to booking. Within the information obtained from the full history, demographic details (see below) are as important as the past medical and family history, as indicators of risk.

Age

There is increasing evidence that extremes of reproductive age are associated with poor pregnancy outcome. Preterm delivery, intra-uterine growth restriction (IUGR), stillbirth and neonatal deaths are more common in women under 20 years old and women aged 40 years and over[7,8].

Marital status

There is evidence that partner support has an influence on pregnancy outcome, as women who are unmarried and/or unsupported may have worse pregnancy outcomes than those described as married or cohabiting. This information can prompt enquiry about social exclusion and domestic violence, allowing appropriate referral to social care for needs assessment and advice and for child protection issues. Neonatologists and paediatricians should be made aware of the issues at the earliest opportunity, as recommended in *Every Child Matters*, 2003[9].

Assisted conception

Paternity and conception method is also important to record, e.g.

- Artificial insemination by donor (AID)
- *In vitro* fertilisation (IVF) pregnancy with donated egg/sperm
- IVF and intracytoplasmic sperm injection (ICSI)

All are associated with a significantly increased risk of pre-eclampsia and a higher risk of poor pregnancy outcome[10,11].

BMI

Obesity (Body Mass Index (BMI) > 35), is associated with poor perinatal outcome. There is increased risk of medical conditions in the mother, which increase perinatal morbidity and mortality, and a concomitant increase in congenital anomaly, macrosomia and unexplained stillbirth. Early pregnancy outcome is also worse in these women[12,13].

Family history

Family history alerts the clinician to the risk in both mother and infant of hereditary conditions. The following are some factors which may alert the clinician to increased risk:

- A family history of diabetes or hypertension, particularly on the maternal side of the family.
- A family history of pre-eclampsia (PET) in a first-degree sibling or mother[14].
- A personal or family history (usually in the first-degree relatives) of a genetic or chromosomal condition, e.g. Marfan's syndrome, Huntingdon's chorea. If such a condition is found, then referral to the regional genetic centre and foetal medicine unit can be made.

Previous obstetric, medical and gynaecological history

Poor previous obstetric history obviously highlights a need for greater surveillance and reassurance, whether the history relates to preterm labour or recurrent pregnancy loss. The obstetrician and midwife should also be aware of the woman who has had previous cervical surgery (e.g. loop biopsy). Recurrent termination of pregnancy, or mid-trimester termination of pregnancy, may increase the risk of preterm delivery or mid-trimester loss.

Demographic data

Housing and social circumstances remain an important part of risk assessment of the pregnant woman. Important issues include:

- Whether housing is permanent or temporary
- Ethnicity
  - Some categories are difficult to define and therefore risk assessment is difficult (i.e. Black British)
  - Year of arrival in the country
  - Country of birth

First-generation immigrants have an increased risk of pregnancy complications and this is compounded if they are asylum seekers or socially excluded. Some of these women will not be legally entitled to benefits or help with housing which further worsens perinatal outcome.

There is no doubt that perinatal mortality is higher in some postcodes compared to others and being aware of the underlying social issues and demographic factors helps the perinatal team assess the risk and mobilise the necessary help[15].

Implications for practice

Antenatal screening is a valuable tool for prenatal assessment of both the mother and foetus.

Screening

Antenatal screening begins on the day that the pregnancy is booked. One of the first antenatal screening tests to be established was the identification of maternal blood group and the measurement of Rhesus antibodies against the D antigen (see Chapter 17). Anti D is now offered routinely to mothers that are rhesus D negative at 28 weeks gestation as well as after delivery if the baby is found to be Rhesus positive[16]. Screening for infection also takes place, following the appropriate counselling (see Box 2.1).

Ultrasound

Ultrasound has become a very important tool in the obstetrician's management of pregnancy (see Figure 2.1 and Box 2.2).

Scans measuring cervical length are used to determine the risk for preterm labour and are used for placental localisation in major placenta praevia.

Box 2.1 Examples of antenatal screening blood tests

Screening for infection

- HIV: HIV testing is now carried out routinely throughout the antenatal clinics in the United Kingdom and requires the patient to opt out.
- Hepatitis B (HBV): identification of hepatitis B (HBV) infection allows immunisation to be given to the newborn following delivery as well as passive immunoglobulin in high risk cases.
- Syphilis: untreated syphilis can lead to congenital syphilis in the neonate. In the last few years the prevalence of syphilis has increased greatly in the community, but once disclosed can be very effectively treated, usually with penicillin, such that congenital syphilis is rarely seen today.
- Group B streptococcal (GBS): GBS infection may sometimes be implicated as the cause of late miscarriages and intrauterine death. Nevertheless, routine screening for GBS is not carried out [17], but treatment given during labour on the basis of risk factors, as suggested by the RCOG Green Top guideline (see Chapter 16) [18]. The neonatal team should be informed of maternal GBS carriage when called to examine the baby.

Screening for haemoglobinopathy

Haemoglobinopathy screening is carried out using haemoglobin electrophoresis. The exact method varies depending on the area in which the family live as in some areas screening is universal and in others it occurs in' risk groups' only. When heterozygosity for haemaglobinopathy is found, then referral to a haemoglobinopathy counsellor is made and the partner tested. If the partner is found to be heterozygous or homozygous for a haemoglobinopathy, appropriate counselling should take place and diagnostic testing offered in the form of chorionic villus sampling (CVS) or amniocentesis.

Screening for chromosome anomaly and spina bifida

Screening for chromosomal anomaly and spina bifida can now be offered through various combinations of tests, in the first and second trimesters. The serum screening tests most widely available are carried out in the second trimester between 15 weeks and 22 weeks of pregnancy. Should the screening test give a positive result (e.g. giving a probability of Down's syndrome as > 1: 250), invasive testing and referral to a foetal medicine specialist should be offered. A dating scan will still be a requirement for this test to be applied with any accuracy, but there is greater flexibility in provision of the screening as there is a wider time frame.

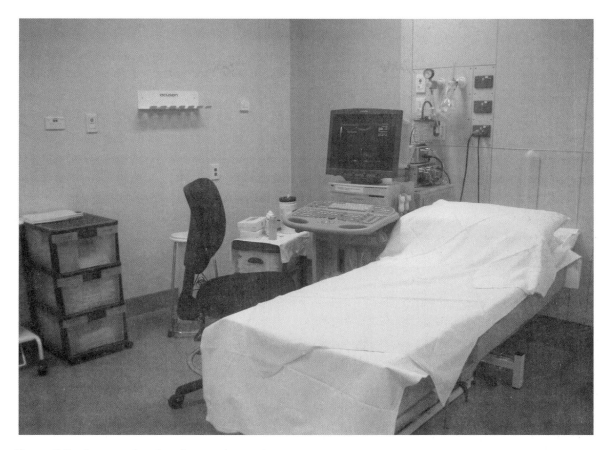

Figure 2.1 A room set up for ultrasound screening.

Foetal medicine unit

Foetal medicine units perform detailed foetal assessment to screen for congenital conditions. These include interventional procedures such as amniocentesis, chorionic villus sampling (CVS) and foetal blood sampling, as well as tertiary level ultrasonography. Maternal complications include a 1% risk of miscarriage for amniocentesis and 2% for CVS, in addition to possible sepsis which may require delivery, either through termination of pregnancy or induction if the pregnancy is viable. Early amniocentesis (< 14 weeks) is associated with postural limb deformities, club foot and hip dislocation[21]. There was no increased risk of preterm delivery[22].

Maternal medical conditions

Hypertension and pre-eclampsia (PET)

Maternal diagnosis and management
Hypertension is the most common medical complication seen in pregnancy and the following conditions increase the risk of hypertension and PET in pregnancy:

- Obesity
- Chronic hypertension
- Multiple pregnancy
- Renal disease
- Diabetes types I and II
- Anti-phospholipid syndrome (APS)

Box 2.2   Examples of antenatal ultrasound screening

- Foetal viability scans: for bleeding in the first and sometimes the second trimester.
- Dating scan: this is useful if the menstrual dates are unclear, but it is also used to ensure accuracy of serum screening and determine that the pregnancy is not multiple gestation.
- Nuchal scan: this is indicated for chromosomal anomaly screening, but may also indicate a cardiac diagnosis in a baby with normal chromosomes. It can be combined with first and second trimester serum screening to improve the reliability of chromosomal anomaly screening. It is carried out between 11 weeks and 13 weeks and 6 days of pregnancy [19]. These early scans can also allow the determination of chorionicity in multiple gestations by the finding of a lambda sign (dichorionic), or T sign (monochorionic).
- Anomaly scan: this scan looks for the major anomalies in the baby, between 18 and 22 weeks. During this scan women considered to be at risk of pre-eclampsia (PET) or foetal growth restriction (IUGR) may have uterine artery Doppler studies carried out, looking for the positive finding of notching in the wave form or a raised resistance

index (RI) [20]. If notching or a raised RI is identified at 20 weeks, low dose aspirin may be given, (if not already prescribed) and a repeat scan arranged for 24 weeks. If the uterine artery waveform is normal at that time, the patient is considered to be low risk for PET and IUGR.
- Foetal cardiology scan: this may be indicated following detection of an aberration in the anomaly scan. It may also be indicated in a woman being treated with anti-epileptic drugs (AEDs) or in a woman with pre-existing diabetes; foetal cardiology scans should be arranged for the increasing numbers of women with congenital heart disease who become pregnant.
- Growth scans: this may be a single scan at approximately 32 weeks, for a foetus found to have a two-vessel cord, or a woman with a BMI < 19. Serial growth scans are required for women with early onset PET or with pre-existing diabetes. These usually begin at 28 weeks. Multiple gestations, e.g. dyzygotic twins should be scanned each month starting from 28 weeks, but monozygotic twins will be scanned from as early as 16 weeks every two weeks, because of the risk of twin to twin transfusion.

- Rare causes include:
  - HIV on HAART
  - Uncontrolled hyperthyroidism
  - Coarctation of the aorta
  - Endocrine disease (CAH, Cushing's syndrome, Conn's syndrome, phaeochromocytoma)

Chronic hypertension predating pregnancy may be undiagnosed until the blood pressure (BP) is taken in the first trimester and found to be > 120/ 80 mmHg. This level of BP requires a thorough assessment and should prompt regular surveillance carried out at the GP surgery as part of the antenatal care pathway. With known hypertension, treatment should be reviewed and maximised appropriately for pregnancy. Women managed with diuretics, ace inhibitors or angiotensin II receptor antagonists should stop this medication as soon as pregnancy is diagnosed. Medications most commonly used for treatment of blood pressure in pregnant women are:

- methyldopa
- calcium channel antagonists (Nifedipine MR)
- ß blockers (labetalol)
- α blockers (doxazasin)

There is an increased risk of both IUGR and PET in this group of women and low dose aspirin (LDA) should be recommended and commenced after 12 weeks. Aspirin has been found to reduce the risk of PET by approximately 15% and perinatal death by a similar amount[23]. Uterine artery Doppler studies should be arranged for 20 to 24 weeks and growth scans as necessary. There should be regular surveillance for worsening blood pressure and proteinuria throughout pregnancy.

Some women develop gestational hypertension (PIH) without proteinuria late in the third trimester without any other features. This is usually accompanied by a good perinatal outcome.

In women with early proteinuria, the diagnosis of PET tends to be made if there has been a doubling of proteinuria in 24 hours. Whilst this diagnosis may not prompt delivery, it may prompt admission for observation related to an increased risk of abruption and stillbirth with PET, which is not present with essential hypertension or PIH. Additional therapeutic measures include:

- Daily CTGs
- Prophylactic dose of low molecular weight heparin (LMWH)
- Thromboembolic compression stockings
- High dose antenatal steroids if < 34–36 weeks gestation
- Plan for delivery in the thirty-eighth week of pregnancy

A plan for the birth should also be established and discussed with the woman.

Consider delivery if:

- Platelets < 100 x 10^9/l
- Creatinine > 100 µmol/l
- ALT > 80 iu/l
- Albumin < 20gm/L
- Deranged clotting (PT, APTT and fibrinogen < 3.0)
- Oliguric (< 25 mls/hour over 4 hours)
- Persistent headache
- Visual symptoms
- Epigastric pain
- Uterine tenderness ± bleeding suggesting abruption
- Reduced foetal movements
- Epigastric pain
- Eclampsia (convulsions)

Delivery is the only measure which cures the disease and if fulminating PET occurs at any gestation, delivery will be required for the mother's safety whether the foetus is viable or not.

HELLP syndrome (haemolysis elevated liver enzymes and low platelets) is a severe variant of PET with an increased risk of perinatal and maternal morbidity and mortality. Other conditions with poor perinatal outcome which should be excluded are:

- Acute fatty liver of pregnancy (AFLP)
- Haemolytic uraemic syndrome (HUS)
- Thrombotic thrombocytopenic purpura (TTP)

All of these conditions warrant delivery of the foetus for the mother's safety and may therefore result in preterm delivery by emergency LSCS.

In early onset and severe PET which is associated with stillbirth or abruption, a thrombophilia screen should take place and thrombophilia markers should be sent[24]:

- Antiphospholipid syndrome
- Antithrombin deficiency
- Protein S deficiency
- Protein C deficiency
- Factor V Leiden
- Homocysteinuria

Implications for practice

Maternal medical assessment is needed to try to predict and prevent potential foetal compromise.

Care planning for labour and birth

For women with uncomplicated PIH and essential hypertension, the aim is to allow spontaneous labour. Women should take their normal medication while in labour. If antihypertensives have not been required during pregnancy but hypertension occurs during labour (mean arterial pressure of 125 mmHg or a systolic blood pressure >160 mmHg), then management is commonly with labetalol.

For women with PET, if symptomatically well controlled with well managed blood pressure, the aim would be to deliver them electively at term, by induction of labour (IOL). Both CEMACH and the RCOG recommend that protocols for the management of PET should guide admission and subsequent clinical management through the antenatal period, labour and delivery[25,26]. In severe PET, HELLP syndrome or eclampsia, magnesium sulphate therapy should be given for 24–48 hours after delivery.

The pain relief method of choice for women with PET during labour is an epidural, as it helps with blood pressure control and pain relief post-delivery[27].

Women < 32 weeks gestation are likely to require delivery by LSCS, although IOL has been attempted successfully at 32 weeks and less. Regional anaesthesia is the preferred method although general anaesthesia may be required in the following situations:

- Immediate delivery for foetal compromise
- Low platelets ($< 75 \times 10^9$/l)
- DIC

The mother's condition must be stabilised prior to delivery of the foetus, and this can sometimes lead to perinatal death[28].

Neonatal outcome of a woman with PET

IUGR

Women with PIH have a higher risk of having a baby with asymmetrical growth restriction (IUGR) due to an effect on the functioning of the placenta. These infants have relatively normal head circumference and length but minimal subcutaneous fat.

In the absence of complications, including perinatal asphyxia and respiratory distress, neonates may be managed on the post-natal ward with the mother. Skin-to-skin care helps in maintaining temperature and facilitates breast-feeding. Feeding the newborn within the first hour of life can prevent hypoglycaemia[29]. Term small for dates (SFD) infants do not usually pose serious difficulties because they have no problems in breast-feeding. However, these infants are at risk of comorbidities and should be monitored regularly for hypoglycaemia and polycythaemia in the first 24–48 hours.

Prematurity

Prematurity is a risk factor following early induction of labour or planned caesarean section for pre-eclampsia. Care plans for admission to the neonatal unit should be made early and discussed with the parents.

Meconium aspiration

During the birthing process the foetus needs to be monitored for foetal distress. A foetus with late decelerations is showing signs of foetal hypoxia and as a result may relax the anal sphincter and pass meconium *in utero*. Aspiration of meconium can occur *in utero*, or during the labour. It is important to note that while many infants have the onset of symptoms at birth, some infants have an asymptomatic period of several hours before respiratory distress becomes apparent. Thus, all babies should continue to have respiratory rate observed[30]. Observations should include:

- Chest movements
- Nasal flaring
- Skin colour (including perfusion)
- Feeding
- Muscle tone
- Temperature
- Heart rate
- Respirations; hourly for two hours, then two-hourly until 12 hours

If there is evidence of expiratory grunting, sternal or subcostal recession, tachypnoea or lethargy, the baby should be transferred to a transitional care ward or neonatal unit. A sick newborn with meconium aspiration will have alveolar atelectasis and require intensive care treatment.

Respiratory distress syndrome (RDS)

If maternal PIH has resulted in induction of labour prior to 37 weeks gestation, the baby will be born with structural immaturity of the lungs, including surfactant deficiency, resulting in pulmonary dysfunction. Without surfactant, the surface tension of the alveolar sacs is high, leading to an increased tendency of the alveoli to collapse. Expiratory grunting is the new-born's attempt to maintain the pressures and gas volume within the lung. See Box 2.3 below.

Medication related
Maternal labetalol may lead to hypoglycaemia in the neonate.

Vitamin K
If there has been maternal HELLP syndrome, thrombocytopenia or neutropenia, IM Vitamin K should be recommended for the baby[31].

Diabetes

Maternal diagnosis and management
Diabetes is a maternal medical condition that clearly demonstrates almost all of the obstetric issues relating to neonatal care. Preconception counselling can make a significant improvement to perinatal outcome by emphasising the following points:

- The need for tight blood sugar control peri-conception and throughout pregnancy, to reduce the risk of foetal anomaly and later complications: clear blood sugar targets should be discussed[32]; women should aim for capillary glucose between 4 and 5 mmol/l pre-meal and less than 7–7.5 mmol/l post-meal
- High dose folic acid (5 mg) should be rec-ommended for at least three months prior to conception, and throughout the first trimester, because of an increased risk of neural tube defect in the foetus
- If maternal nephropathy and or retinopa-thy are present, this increases the risk of pre-term delivery and implies a worse perinatal outcome
- Changes in lifestyle, related to exercise, smok-ing, alcohol use and weight loss should be encouraged where necessary
- Optimise the management of comorbidities, e.g. hypertension, renal disease: medication should be reviewed and adjusted to reduce the risk of teratogenicity, i.e. stop an ace inhibitor and change to methyldopa or calcium channel antagonist
- Perinatal risk should be discussed and likely outcomes explored
- Discuss the use of low dose aspirin (LDA) fol-lowing conception, to reduce the risk of PET and IUGR

Once the pregnancy is booked, care should be provided through a multidisciplinary team. Discussions regarding the plan for maternal and neonatal care should take place in early pregnancy and include meeting members of the neonatal team and a visit to the neonatal unit. The following are important aspects of man-agement in women with diabetes. See Box 2.4 below.

Publication of the ACHOIS trial in 2005[34], clearly demonstrated a reduction in perinatal morbidity and mortality following intervention with treatment in women with gestational dia-betes and has widened the debate about which method to use to screen for gestational diabetes.

Antenatal steroids for women at risk of preterm delivery can cause particular prob-lems in women with diabetes, as they are high dose and will derange glycaemic control. The greatest danger remains for women with poorly controlled pre-existing diabetes, relating to the risk of diabetic ketoacidosis, which may result in severe morbidity for the mother and significantly increase the risk of intra-uterine (IUD) death.

Box 2.3   Expiratory grunting

The newborn employs a coping mechanism which involves partially closing the glottis during exhalation to maintain alveolar distending pres-sure. This can only be tolerated for a short space of time as retained carbon dioxide leads to res-piratory distress. Surfactant reverses this process. The phospholipids and surfactant related proteins contained in surfactant, spread along the air liq-uid interface to decrease alveolar surface tension.

Box 2.4   Management of diabetes in pregnancy

- Women with type II diabetes currently stop oral hypoglycaemic drugs and transfer to insulin.
- Baseline renal function should be taken at booking and during each trimester as pregnancy can accelerate the decline of function in women with nephropathy.
- Serum screening cannot be used in women with diabetes.
- Scans should be arranged, including the nuchal scan, foetal cardiology, anomaly, and serial growth scans. Uterine artery Dopplers should be carried out at the 20 week scan.
- Serial growth scans are arranged from 28 weeks until delivery, at monthly intervals. Polyhydramnios, macrosomia or IUGR may be demonstrated in these scans, sometimes in spite of excellent glycaemic control and should therefore prompt closer surveillance which may then inform timing of delivery [33].

Box 2.5   Features associated with poor pregnancy outcome

- Maternal social deprivation.
- Lack of contraceptive use for 12 months preceding pregnancy.
- No folic acid in preceding 12 months.
- Sub-optimal self-management of diabetes.
- Sub-optimal preconception care.
- Sub-optimal glycaemic control at any stage before or during pregnancy.
- Sub-optimal antenatal or diabetic care whilst pregnant.
- Sub-optimal foetal surveillance of big babies.

However, whilst diabetic ketoacidosis is to be avoided, the maternal deaths related to diabetes, in 2000–2002, were all attributed to hypoglycaemia, not hyperglycaemia.

Care planning for labour and birth

Preconception care and multidisciplinary team working is universally recommended as the most effective way of delivering effective care for the pregnant woman with diabetes, both pre-existing and gestational[35]. Particular features associated with poor pregnancy outcome are set out in Box 2.5.

A care plan should be prepared by the obstetrician and the diabetic team for labour and delivery and placed in the notes at 36 weeks of pregnancy. Women with diet controlled gestational diabetes and normal foetal growth can await spontaneous labour, although some units will recommend delivery at 40 weeks.

Women managed on insulin tend to be delivered during the thirty-eighth week, with 50–70% of these pregnancies delivered by caesarean section, whether labour is induced or spontaneous[36,37]. The presence of macrosomia, polyhydramnios or growth restriction reinforces the plan to deliver at 38 weeks, as the risk of unexplained stillbirth is five times that of the general population. Shoulder dystocia and associated birth trauma are also a potential concern. It has been argued that in the presence of excellent glycaemic control and a normally grown baby, there is a good reason to allow for spontaneous labour, or deliver electively at 40 weeks. Nevertheless, the recent CEMACH report has shown that 36% of pregnancies in women with diabetes end preterm[38].

Women with insulin controlled diabetes requiring elective caesarean section, should ideally be delivered first in the morning, as they will have been starved overnight and require an insulin sliding scale and dextrose infusion. If the mother's blood sugar is poorly controlled at the time of delivery, neonatal hypoglycaemia is likely to be a significant problem. It is essential that electronic foetal monitoring be used continuously during labour for women with diabetes.

Neonatal outcome of a diabetic mother
Hypoglycaemia
The neonate of a well-controlled diabetic mother during pregnancy and labour is likely to have a positive outcome but must be observed for signs of hypoglycaemia. There should be a written

policy for the management of the baby and the policy should assume that babies will remain with their mothers in the absence of complications and therefore routine admission of babies to the neonatal unit is not indicated[39]. All babies of women with diabetes should be offered skin-to-skin contact immediately after birth and breast-feeding within one hour of birth should be encouraged[40]. Early blood glucose testing should be avoided in the 'well' baby and a plan of care agreed with the mother should be documented in the records. The infant of a less well-controlled diabetic mother is commonly large for gestational age (macrosomic) and may not feed well. Pre-feed glucose testing is indicated in these babies.

Thermoregulation

Thermoregulation plays a vital part of care planning at birth. The macrosomic neonate has a large body surface area, which leads to greater heat loss and interference with surfactant function, increasing the risk of respiratory distress.

Pulmonary disease

The baby of a poorly controlled diabetic woman has a higher incidence of pulmonary disease. Delivery by caesarean related to macrosomia also increases the risk for transient tachypnoea of the newborn, while polycythaemia predisposes the infant to persistent pulmonary hypertension. Even allowing for a slightly higher than expected incidence of preterm birth, surfactant deficient lung disease is more common at all gestational ages where there is abnormal maternal glucose tolerance. This may be related to delay, or even abnormalities, in the maturation of the pulmonary surfactant system.

Congenital malformations

Foetal congenital malformations increase with poor maternal glucose control during the first trimester of pregnancy and are ten times greater than in the normal population[41]. See Box 2.6 below.

Box 2.6 Congenital malformations related to poor glucose control

- Congenital cardiovascular anomalies include cardiomyopathy with intraventricular hypertrophy. Symptoms usually resolve within two to four weeks. These infants are also at an increased risk of congenital heart defects, including ventricular septal defect (VSD) and transposition of the great arteries (TGA).
- Musculoskeletal deformities such as the rare syndrome of caudal regression syndrome may occur. This is characterised by the absence of the sacrum, and defects of variable portions of lumbar spine[24].
- Congenital central nervous system malformations include anencephaly, spina bifida and caudal dysplasia. If one birth defect is discovered, it is obligatory to assess all other organ systems to rule out other associated anomalies.

Birth trauma

The macrosomic baby may sustain trauma from shoulder dystocia at birth, which can result in:

- Fractured clavicle
- Brachial plexus injury (Erb's palsy (C4 and C5) or Klumpke's palsy (C8 –T1))
- Birth asphyxia

Brachial plexus injury is more common than a fracture and is caused by traction to the neck. The incidence is 0.5 to 2 per 1000 live births[43]. Care plans for the neonate who has sustained an injury should include prompt assessment and referral to a neonatal registrar with further referral to the orthopaedic surgeon or neurologist as required.

Implications for practice

Infants of diabetic mothers need to be fed early and closely monitored within a thermoneutral environment in order to minimise potential complications.

In contrast to the macrosomic babies, infants of mothers with significant vascular problems may be small for gestational age, and may have suffered chronic hypoxia and be polycythaemic, as discussed previously. Hypoglycaemia from hyperinsulinaemia may also be a problem. Prompt neonatal referral should be made and a plan of care documented.

Neurological

Epilepsy

Maternal diagnosis and management

Epilepsy is the most common chronic neurological disorder encountered in pregnancy, affecting 1:200 women of childbearing age. A diagnosis of epilepsy will usually predate pregnancy but if a fit occurs during pregnancy, further investigation is required.

The most important issue for women with epilepsy is not the condition itself, but the medication required to control it. However, there is a possibility of harm to the foetus if status epilepticus occurs, related to maternal hypoxia and possible trauma[44]. Preconception counselling is very important for women with epilepsy and may have a significant impact on perinatal outcome. Both preconception counselling and multidisciplinary care have been recommended by CEMACH and NICE as best practice[45,46]. A preconception visit should encompass the following points:

- Use of high dose folic acid before conception and throughout pregnancy to reduce the risk of neural tube defects and the risk of folate deficiency anaemia[47].
- A discussion regarding treatment with anti-epileptic drugs should also take place as these are the greatest concern relating to perinatal outcome. It may be possible, if the woman has been fit free for more than two years, to stop anti-epileptic medication (AED) following a clear discussion of all the implications surrounding that decision. If medication is

necessary then there are certain measures that can be taken to reduce risk to the foetus and child:
  ○ Monotherapy rather than poly-pharmacy reduces the risk of major congenital anomalies and AED syndrome.
  ○ Sodium valproate should be avoided, not only because it is the drug with the greatest risk of anomaly, but there is also significant risk of neurodevelopmental problems. Reduction of risk can also be gained by giving long-acting preparations of the medication and trying not exceed the doses of lamotrigine (LTG) or valproate (VPA), which are known to be associated with a higher risk of anomaly (1000 mg for VPA and 200 mg for LTG).

Once pregnancy is confirmed the following should be offered:

- Serum screening
- Nuchal screening
- Women taking AEDs should be offered further scans for foetal cardiology and anomaly
- It may be prudent to check drug levels of AED during pregnancy as confirmation of compliance, but also to confirm therapeutic levels because of nausea and vomiting in the first trimester
- If the pregnant woman has not had seizures for some time, and has chosen to continue her medication throughout pregnancy, one should aim to manage her on the lowest dose possible, changing if seizure frequency increases
- Women who are taking the enzyme inducing drugs, carbamazepine, phenytoin (phenobarbitone), Oxcarbazepine and topiramate should be given Vitamin K 10 mg daily from 34–36 weeks of pregnancy, to reduce the risk of haemorrhagic disease of the newborn.

If a new fit occurs after 20 weeks pregnancy then eclampsia should be excluded because of its association with poor perinatal outcome and the risk to the mother. If eclampsia is diagnosed, the woman will require management with magnesium sulphate and delivery once stable.

Care planning for labour and birth

When counselling women with epilepsy regarding labour and delivery, it should be emphasised that she should be accompanied at all times. Labour may increase seizure risk due to several factors:

- Tiredness
- Dehydration
- Stress
- Pain
- Fear

It should be stressed that medications should be taken normally during labour. Should a seizure occur, they are usually self-limiting but if medication is required for a prolonged fit then IV lorazepam 4 mg may be given or diazepam 10–20 mg rectally with oxygen by mask. The neonatal doctor should be informed that they have been given if administered before delivery because of possible effects on the newborn infant. Women with epilepsy should expect to deliver vaginally. There is no increased risk of caesarean section or preterm delivery

Neonatal outcome

A care plan should be drawn up prior to the birth and discussed with the woman, to include giving the baby IM Vitamin K to prevent haemorrhagic disease of the newborn which may occur in the first 24 hours of life.

Congenital malformations

The initial and full neonatal examination within the first 72 hours should involve careful examination for unusual facial features, cleft lip or cleft palate, abnormalities of the fingers and spinal defects. Neural tube defects occur in 1–2% neonates who have been exposed to valproate or carbamazepine, with a slightly increased frequency with phenytoin and phenobarbital[48].

Withdrawal

In the newborn period one of the other important implications is that of withdrawal from the AEDs. In term newborns the half-life of phenytoin is 21 hours (adult 11–29 hours), the half-life of phenobarbital is 82–199 hours (adult 24–140 hours) and half-life of carbamazepine is 8–28 hours (adult 21–36 hours)[49]. Occasionally the newborn neonate will be irritable or have a 'fit' following withdrawal of the drugs and observations over the first 24 hours for withdrawal symptoms; if the woman has had to remain on higher therapeutic doses of AEDs during pregnancy it should be included in the care plan. In preterm infants there will be reduced metabolism and excretion of these drugs and an increased risk of toxicity.

Implications for practice

Preconception counselling is strongly advised and screening of the foetus for anomalies is vital if the expectant mother is taking medication for epilepsy.

Connective tissue disease

Systemic lupus erythematosus

Maternal diagnosis and management

Systemic lupus erythematosus (SLE) is a multisystem disease which affects more women than men and is particularly seen during the reproductive years. It may affect skin, joints, brain, heart, kidneys, the haematological system and serosal surfaces like the pleura and pericardium. It can be characterised by a number of signs and symptoms but the following are the most relevant to foetal and neonatal well-being:

- 30% of women with lupus will have antibodies to extractable nuclear antigens (ENAs) including anti-Ro and anti-La, both associated with a risk of congenital heart block in the foetus

- Other important antibodies associated with poor perinatal outcome in pregnancy are the antiphospholipid antibodies (APAs), anticardiolipin antibody and lupus anticoagulant, which will be discussed at greater length later in the chapter
- Lupus nephritis is a particularly malignant form of the condition and women would be advised to wait until they have been in remission for six months before conceiving and ideally would want to wait until their creatinine level is within the optimum range and associated blood pressure is adequately treated

This is a condition where preconception counselling and multidisciplinary care during pregnancy is extremely beneficial. During preconception counselling, the following information should be discussed:

- Increased risk of an excerbation of the SLE, particularly post-partum[50]
- Safety of commonly used medications in lupus for pregnancy and breast-feeding[51], i.e. azathioprine, hydroxychloroquine, prednisolone
- Joint pain may be managed with paracetamol as NSAIDS carry a risk to the foetus of oligohydramnios and closure of the ductus arteriosus, particularly after 32 weeks of pregnancy
- Women with lupus nephritis should be made aware of their risk of PET, worsening blood pressure and therefore of the risk of preterm delivery. They should be advised to start low dose aspirin (LDA) 75 mg from 12 weeks until delivery. This risk increases significantly if the baseline creatinine at the time of booking is >120 µmol/l.
- Antibody status should be known, as the presence of anti-Ro and La, ACL and LA requires specific management.
- Medication for hypertension should be appropriate for pregnancy, therefore ACE inhibitors should be avoided. It is not necessary to avoid using methyldopa or hydralazine.
- For women with known APAs, the anomaly scan should be extended to include uterine artery Dopplers. If notching is present at 20 weeks, it should be repeated at 24 weeks and LDA commenced, if not already given. The presence of APAs also warrants a growth scan at 32 weeks and some advocate serial growth scans from 28 weeks.
- For those women with ENAs, referral to foetal cardiology should be made because of the risk of congenital heart block. CHB usually occurs after 20 weeks gestation. Appropriate surveillance will then be arranged between foetal cardiology and the foetal medicine unit.

Finally, women with SLE who have been in remission for more than six months without APS antibodies or ENAs should be reassured that their perinatal risk is equivalent to that of the general population. Those with renal involvement, hypertension or APAs have an increased risk of PET, IUGR, stillbirth and preterm delivery.

Care planning for labour and birth

Women with SLE who are in remission should be managed by a multidisciplinary team and, if all continues to be well, allowed to go into spontaneous labour. For those with hypertension or growth restriction, elective delivery may be necessary by induction of labour, or caesarean section if very preterm. For some women with antiphospholipid syndrome, they may have the misfortune of experiencing very early onset PET, such that the pregnancy may need to be curtailed before the foetus is viable either in terms of estimated foetal weight (< 700 g) or less than 24 weeks.

In a situation where congenital heart block has been found, the major issue during labour and delivery is the inability to monitor foetal well-being, using the cardiotocograph (CTG). This may mean that delivery would be electively by caesarean section, but successful labour and delivery of these babies has taken place, with subsequent pacing as necessary.

Neonatal outcome
Cutaneous lupus and neonatal heart block

In women who test positive for either anti-Ro, or anti-La antibodies the risk of cutaneous lupus in the neonate is around 5%, with congenital heart block (CHB) affecting about 2%. The neonatal risk is increased if there is a previously affected sibling. The affected neonate with cutaneous neonatal lupus will start to become symptomatic within the first two weeks of life. Skin lesions around the face and neck appear after exposure to the sun and disappear after six months of age. Phototherapy should therefore be avoided[52]. For neonates diagnosed with CHB who have been delivered early by caesarean section, there is a 19% perinatal mortality rate. Out of the survivors, 50–60% are treated by fitting a pacemaker and make good progress.

Implications for practice

Ensure that infants who develop heart block are evaluated for antibodies associated with this and that mothers are evaluated for SLE.

Antiphospholipid syndrome

Maternal diagnosis and management
Antiphospholipid syndrome (APS) is classed as one of the thrombophilias, i.e. a condition where the affected person has an increased risk of venous and arterial thromboses. The diagnosis of antiphospholipid syndrome requires the presence of clinical features as well as antiphospholipid antibodies. The clinical features include:

- \> 3 consecutive miscarriages at < 10 weeks gestation
- Maternal venous thrombosis
- Maternal arterial thrombosis
- A foetal death (> 11 weeks gestation) with documented foetal heart seen prior to foetal demise
- Preterm delivery associated with PET
- Severe IUGR

Women should be investigated for APS when there are any of the above features. Once the syndrome has been diagnosed, then low dose aspirin (LDA) is prescribed and should ideally be taken prior to conception until delivery[53].

APS can be further divided into two main categories:

- Those with recurrent early miscarriages (secondary to delay in placentation)
- All others

It is rare for women who have had APS diagnosed following recurrent miscarriage to develop problems with thromboembolic disease. They also have a lower risk of preterm delivery related to IUGR and PET. In contrast women with APS and a previous poor obstetric history have a 30–40% risk of preterm delivery and significant risk of IUGR, abruption and PET.

Some women may require low molecular weight heparin (LMWH) prophylaxis during pregnancy as well as LDA. This includes women who have been treated with warfarin prior to conception (women with cerebral manifestations of the disease). They will require therapeutic doses of heparin during the pregnancy and, in particularly high risk cases, may require warfarin in the second and third trimesters, with its attendant risk to the foetus of intracerebral bleeding and abruption.

In women with APS that are at high risk of foetal growth restriction, scans may be carried out at 20–24 weeks to look for uterine artery notches or high resistance index and serial growth scans will also be performed. Serial scans for foetal well-being should also be carried out for those women who need to continue on warfarin.

Care planning for labour and birth
For women with APS relating to recurrent miscarriage, with no other complications, the plan for labour and delivery is to await spontaneous labour. There would be no need to stop the once daily LDA dose, as there are no risks to the foetus and there should be no contraindication to regional anaesthesia.

If LMWH is being used for treatment and there are no other complications, then the woman would be advised to refrain from taking her heparin once there is evidence that labour may be starting. If elective delivery is planned, then heparin should be withheld, allowing a 12-hour window for regional anaesthesia for labour or elective delivery by caesarean section. This reduces anaesthetic risk to the mother and the risk of delivery of an anaesthetised baby.

Neonatal outcome
IUGR
Following delivery, attention should be paid to thermoregulation and the establishment of early regular feeding in view of the intra-uterine growth restriction (IUGR). Pre-feed blood glucose testing will be required if the baby's weight is below the third centile.

Medication related complications
The neonate of a woman with APS, taking warfarin, will be at higher risk of intracranial bleeding due to maternal anticoagulant therapy. Therefore IM Vitamin K 1 mg would be recommended in line with the NICE post-natal guidelines[54]. In addition, neonates may be affected by thrombocytopenia from maternal platelet specific antibodies (foetal allo-immune thrombocytopenia – FAITP). This may present with intracranial haemorrhage and seizures, petechiae or bruising. Infusion of HPA compatible platelets would be given as first line treatment over 2–5 days and recovery is spontaneous, between 1–6 weeks[55].

Alloimmune neutropenia
Alloimmune neutropenia is rare and occurs when the mother produces IgG neutrophil alloantibodies. However, the commonest cause of neutropenia is prematurity and IUGR. Affected neonates often have additional thrombocytopenia and polycythaemia but it resolves spontaneously in 2–3 days after birth[56].

Thyroid disease

Maternal diagnosis and management
Thyroid disease is the most common endocrine disease seen in pregnancy after diabetes. Hypothyroidism (prevalence 1%) and hyperthyroidism (prevalence 0.2%) are usually diagnosed before pregnancy. Hypothyroidism is treated with thyroid replacement therapy and, as long as replacement is adequate, perinatal outcome should be excellent. In rare cases hypothyroidism may be caused by TSH receptor blocking antibodies and these may cross the placenta, leading to neonatal goitre and hypothyroidism. Where pregnancy occurs in women with untreated hypothyroidism, then there may be adverse perinatal outcome which includes:

- Maternal anaemia and consequent effects on the foetus and neonate
- IUGR
- Early and late miscarriage
- Stillbirth
- PET

Hyperthyroidism potentially has more malignant effects on pregnancy for several reasons. If the woman begins the pregnancy euthyroid, the perinatal outcome is likely to be excellent. Most cases have a diagnosis predating pregnancy and should therefore be adequately treated, but if thyrotoxicosis presents in pregnancy, it is usually in the late first or second trimester[57]. There may be some difficulty in diagnosis, as many of the symptoms of hyperthyroidism and pregnancy overlap, but if the following signs or symptoms occur, thyroid function tests should be carried out and treatment instituted:

- Tremor
- Weight loss
- Persistent tachycardia
- Lid lag
- Exophthalmos

Untreated thyrotoxicosis has similar perinatal outcomes to untreated hypothyroidism, with the additional risk of preterm labour and an increased risk of stillbirth (up to 50%). In Graves' disease or thyroid disease with high antibody titres there is risk of the antibodies (thyroid stimulating antibodies), crossing the placenta and leading to poor perinatal outcome. Fortunately, for most women, hyperthyroidism improves during pregnancy and antibodies tend to fall.

Active hyperthyroidism is treated with propylthiouracil or carbimazole, which both cross the placenta. The aim should therefore be to manage mothers on the lowest effective dose throughout pregnancy. Agranulocytosis is a potential complication, in the mother taking carbimazole, with a consequent risk of infection which may in turn cause preterm labour, or foetal demise. ß blockers may be used following the initial diagnosis of hyperthyroidism for symptomatic treatment, and for short periods of treatment do not seem to be related to adverse neonatal or foetal outcome. Surgery is not recommended treatment for hyperthyroidism in pregnancy[58]. Radioiodine therapy cannot be used in pregnancy due to the risks relating to radioactivity.

Care planning for labour and birth

Special planning for labour and delivery is unnecessary in the euthyroid mother. Vaginal delivery should be expected apart from the normal obstetric indications. Concern occurs in labour and delivery only in the case of the woman with uncontrolled thyrotoxicosis as foetal tachycardia may be present and lead to the diagnosis of a suspicious trace requiring delivery by caesarean. In this situation the multidisciplinary team will need to be involved, including a senior anaesthetist, physician, obstetrician and neonatologist.

Neonatal outcome

The neonate can present prematurely and with IUGR.

Neonatal thyrotoxicosis

Neonatal thyrotoxicosis is usually secondary to thyroid stimulating antibodies but is relatively rare. Clinical features include:

- Enlarged thyroid gland (goitre)
- Staring eyes with lid-retraction
- Tachycardia
- Excessive appetite with weight loss

- Thrombocytopenia
- Petechiae
- Sweating
- Acrocyanosis
- Hepatosplenomegaly[59]

The baby will also be restless and jittery. Treatment with anti-thyroid drugs would need to be commenced immediately as mortality rates are high.

Hypothyroidism

Screening for congenital hypothyroidism is carried out through neonatal blood spot screening at 7–8 days. Transient hypothyroidism which is not clinically significant is seen in 0.12% of LBW or 0.4% VLBW neonates.

Obstetric cholestasis

Maternal diagnosis and management

Obstetric cholestasis (OC) is a pregnancy specific condition which can result in a poor perinatal outcome and requires increased foetal surveillance once it has been diagnosed. Women usually present in the third trimester of pregnancy complaining of pruritus and specifically pruritus on the palms of the hands and soles of the feet. With this history, the following investigations are carried out:

- Renal function
- Liver function
- Bile acids

If the liver function tests are abnormal then further investigations are carried out to exclude common liver conditions. If the itching is unbearable; liver function is significantly deranged, or bile acids are raised > 14 µmol/l, ursodeoxycholic acid (UCDA) may be given[60]. This usually helps modify the pruritus and is also associated with an improvement in the bile acid and liver enzyme levels. Twice weekly blood tests are carried out to monitor the trend of the disease. If liver function deteriorates significantly then earlier delivery may be indicated. Vitamin K should be given from 34 weeks onwards due to the increased risk of haemorrhagic disease of the newborn, related to relative vitamin K deficiency (due to malabsorption).

Care planning for labour and birth

Women with OC have an increased risk of stillbirth at term, meconium present during labour and also increased risk of foetal distress; therefore delivery during the thirty-seventh week should be discussed. This would usually be by induction of labour, unless vaginal delivery is contraindicated[61]. The foetal heart rate should be continuously monitored. Preterm labour and preterm rupture of membranes can occur in this group of women and should be managed with GBS prophylaxis when in labour[62]. If caesarean is planned during the thirty-seventh week, antenatal steroids may be given to aid foetal lung maturity, in the hope of reducing the risk of admission to the neonatal unit with respiratory distress syndrome[63].

Neonatal outcome

The neonate should be offered IM Vitamin K as prevention for haemorrhagic disease of the newborn and appropriate observation should meconium have been present in the liquor, at delivery.

Haemoglobinopathies

Maternal diagnosis and management

The haemoglobinopathies refer to disorders of haemoglobin synthesis or the presence of haemoglobin variants which are inherited through an autosomal recessive pattern. If both parents are found to have evidence of a haemoglobinopathy trait then there is a 25% risk of the foetus inheriting the full haemoglobinopathy. In this situation, prenatal diagnosis will be discussed and offered through the foetal medicine unit. If the foetus is found to be affected following invasive testing, then counselling regarding pregnancy and neonatal outcome should take place and may include the option of terminating the pregnancy.

α thalassaemia

If the foetus is found to have α thalassaemia, this is not compatible with extra-uterine life and foetal hydrops (heart failure secondary to anaemia) is likely to develop. There is also a significant risk of severe PET in the mother, thus increasing the risk of preterm delivery. The presence of hydrops may also heighten the risk of birth trauma in this situation[64].

β thalassaemia major

Women with β thalassaemia major are likely to have difficulty conceiving but there are many with β thalassaemia trait who conceive with good perinatal outcome. The main problem in this situation will be management of maternal anaemia and appropriate iron stores. This is important for the iron status of the foetus and infant in the first year of life[65].

Sickle cell disease

Sickle cell disease is the other major haemoglobinopathy seen during pregnancy. During pregnancy maternal sickle cell disease can manifest itself in different ways with foetal and maternal consequences. These are shown in Table 2.1.

It is important that the analgesia given for bone crises is sufficient for the mother's needs, but recurrent crises may result in problems with opiate dependence. If several crises occur during pregnancy, then exchange transfusion may be given. Treatment with folic acid (5 mg) and iron helps modify the anaemia. Women with sickle cell disease should also be receiving penicillin V

Table 2.1 Effects of sickle cell disease in pregnancy.

Maternal	Foetal
Bone pain	Miscarriage
Haemolysis → anaemia	IUGR
Acute chest syndrome	Stillbirth
Urinary tract infection	Preterm delivery
Avascular necrosis of joints	Opiate withdrawal
Issues with analgesia	Neonatal death
Exchange transfusion	
PET	
Thrombosis	
Maternal death	

to protect against infection with pneumococcus. Because of the risk of PET and IUGR, low dose aspirin should be considered and prophylactic LMWH given during any admission to hospital.

Care planning for labour and birth

Labour and delivery is a high-risk time for maternal crises to occur, and for that reason warmth, adequate hydration and oxygen should be ensured and care given following a plan produced by the multidisciplinary team. Continuous electronic foetal monitoring should be used, but it is likely that vaginal delivery will be achieved by most women. For those who have experienced a significant number of crises during pregnancy or required exchange transfusion, it is likely that the pregnancy will not be allowed to go beyond 38 weeks and elective delivery by IOL will be planned. Use of regional analgesia should be encouraged, as an epidural during labour means that general anaesthesia, with its attendant risks, can be avoided if caesarean section is required.

Neonatal outcome

Care plans for prematurity and admission to neonatal unit should be considered and discussed with the multiprofessional team during the pregnancy.

Neonatal haemoglobinopathy

Sickle cell disease and β thalassaemia do not cause problems in the neonate during the first four to eight weeks of age due to the high proportion of HbF (which consists of two alpha and two gamma chains). However, α thalassaemia will become apparent straight away due to the alpha chain production controlled by two pairs of genes[66].

Neonatal prophylactic treatment of Penicillin V 62.5 mg twice daily and folic acid 500 mcg per kg per day should be commenced once sickle cell anaemia has been identified through the neonatal screening programme[67].

Medication complications

A plan for observation of symptoms and signs of drug withdrawal should be commenced on the neonate if maternal opiates have been prescribed for sickle cell crises.

Implications for practice

An infant born to a mother who regularly takes medication known to cross the placenta should be observed for signs of withdrawal.

IM Vitamin K should be recommended to counteract aspirin and heparin treatment during pregnancy[68].

Management of the birth and neonatal outcome

Induction of labour

IOL includes stimulation of labour following pre-labour rupture of membranes. If labour is to be stimulated, then by definition the membranes are no longer intact. The RCOG have defined prolonged ruptured membranes as > 18 hours and recommend that GBS prophylaxis should be given during labour at term under these conditions[69].

Stimulation of labour can be required at any gestation and may be carried out using an oxytocin infusion, or by preceding the infusion with prostaglandin in order to prime the cervix. The risks of induction include hyperstimulation of the uterus, which can be stopped using a ß sympathomimetic, or by stopping/reducing the oxytocin infusion. Foetal distress and birth asphyxia are likely to be the result of prolonged hyperstimulation.

Induction of labour is used from 41 weeks and 3 days to deliver women and avoid the excess risk of stillbirth. The following should be assessed prior to IOL:

- Estimated date of delivery and correct gestation (preferably using the dates given by an ultrasound scan prior to 20 weeks)
- Presentation (abdominal palpation)
- Foetal well-being (CTG)

Cervical assessment will then determine the method for IOL.

Prematurity

The gestation at the time of birth is a strong determinant of perinatal morbidity and mortality and much research is focused on finding predictors and causes of preterm delivery. If delivery seems likely to occur between 24 and 34 weeks, there is clear evidence supporting the giving of antenatal corticosteroids for maturation of the foetal lungs. In a planned preterm delivery (e.g. for IUGR), steroids should be given as a matter of course and the timing of delivery planned appropriately. In a spontaneous preterm labour, this presents a problem. It has therefore become a relatively common practice to give tocolytic agents for 48 hours to allow steroids time to become effective. Nifedipine and atosiban are now recommended for use and have little adverse effect on the foetus when used in this way. There remains some debate about giving antenatal steroids between 34 and 36 weeks of pregnancy, but it may confer some benefit for those babies who are to be delivered by caesarean section, reducing the risk of admission to the neonatal unit with breathing difficulties[70]. The evidence for antenatal steroids suggests, that no more than one course should be given, as animal studies have shown deleterious effects on brain growth and maturation with multiple administration[71].

Antibiotics to cover GBS should be given during all preterm labour[72]. If preterm rupture of membranes occurs without labour and the mother is known to have a positive culture for GBS in this pregnancy, then 48 hours of benzyl penicillin should be given alongside erythromycin as this was shown by the ORACLE trial to prolong pregnancy. Following ORACLE it may also be advisable to avoid the use of co-amoxyclav during pregnancy, because of the excess risk of necrotising (NEC) in the preterm foetus[73].

The issue of viability is a complicated one for both obstetricians and neonatologists. By definition, the gestation at which a foetus is deemed viable is 24 weeks, but the public knows that babies have survived after being born at 22 and 23 weeks and find it difficult to comprehend why intensive resuscitation is not given to a foetus when delivered at these gestations. Many obstetricians will not carry out caesarean section for obstetric indications in gestations below 26 weeks or with an estimated foetal weight of < 700 g, because:

- Classical caesarean section is likely to be required
- This increases risk for future pregnancies
- High risk of severe perinatal and long-term morbidity and mortality

Type of delivery

Vaginal birth is associated with the lowest overall risk to mother and neonate, but planned vaginal birth of a breech presenting baby is now unusual following the publication of the term breech trial[74]. The risk of head entrapment may possibly be greater in preterm breech births but there is no strong evidence currently suggesting that delivery by caesarean for the preterm breech improves outcome. There is also an increased risk of cord prolapse and thus asphyxia with breech presentation. The current recommendation of ECV (external cephalic version) at term for breech presentations[75], is aimed at increasing vaginal birth and reducing short and long-term, maternal and foetal risks.

The most recent debate has arisen over the delivery of twins vaginally, relating to poor perinatal outcome for the second twin[76]. In practical terms, for both vaginal twin and breech deliveries, it is essential that the attendants (midwives and obstetricians) are well trained and confident in the conduct of these deliveries and are conversant with the evidence and guidelines related to the management of these deliveries. When managing a twin birth, the obstetrician must be confident enough to carry out breech extraction, external cephalic version and internal podalic version.

For babies that are classed as macrosomic, there are concerns about shoulder dystocia, and its related birth trauma and asphyxia; however, most shoulder dystocia occurs with babies of normal weight and cannot be anticipated.

Forceps

Instrumental delivery rates are approximately 11% in England, with forceps deliveries accounting for 4% of those. The vacuum instrument, however, tends to be the instrument of choice as recommended by the Royal College of Obstetricians and Gynaecologists (RCOG)[77].

Where assisted vaginal delivery is required for the preterm foetus, the forceps is the recommended instrument until 34 to 35 weeks of gestation, because of the risk of cerebral trauma associated with the vacuum cup. Forceps may also be used to deliver the after coming head, during an assisted, vaginal breech delivery or to deliver a face presentation.

Rotational forceps (Kiellands) has now largely been replaced by rotational vacuum delivery, but may still be the instrument of choice in particular situations, e.g. deep transverse arrest in a preterm infant. Manual rotation may also be employed to deliver a foetus with a malposition (transverse or occiput-posterior position) and is associated with minimal injury to the foetus, when used in conjunction with lift out forceps or non-rotational ventouse.

Ventouse

The incidence of ventouse delivery has increased in the last 20 years. It accounts for approximately 7% of all deliveries. However, there is no doubt that vacuum assisted delivery brings a higher risk of neonatal morbidity than delivery with forceps. The risk of neonatal trauma, particularly haemorrhage increases with:

- Total time cup attached to the foetal scalp
- Cup detachments
- Technique

- o Incorrect placement of the cup (not over the flexion point)
- o Prolonged traction with a high head
- o Cup placement over the anterior fontanelle
- o Use of multiple instruments

It is important for obstetricians to minimise risk to the foetus by selection of the appropriate instrument for delivery in each case. Ventouse delivery requires good maternal effort to enable traction on the foetal scalp to be kept to a minimum. In situations where delivery needs to be effected very quickly, forceps may be the most appropriate instrument to use, as the delivery process is not as dependent on maternal effort.

Possible neonatal sequelae

These are discussed in Table 2.2.

LSCS

Caesarean section has been rising over the last few decades and has now reached a prevalence of approximately 23.5% in the UK[78]. There are few situations where caesarean section is recommended:

- Breech presentation
- HIV with viral load > 50 copies/ml
- Multiple pregnancies > twins
- Twins with non-cephalic presentation of the presenting twin
- Major placenta praevia

Table 2.2 Possible neonatal sequelae.

Ventouse	Forceps
Neonatal headache	Forceps marks on face
Scalp lacerations	Facial lacerations
Cephalhaematoma	Facial nerve palsy
Subgaleal haemorrhage	Brachial plexus injury
Intracerebral bleeding (increased risk with preterm infants)	Skull fracture
Retinal haemorrhages	Smaller risk of haemorrhage (see under ventouse)

- Tumours of various types obstructing descent of the presenting part
- Abnormal foetal lie (transverse)

Increased caesarean section rates have been identified in women with diabetes of all types and they have been increasing due to women having undergone previous caesarean sections. Increasing evidence of adverse maternal and perinatal outcome following caesarean, is emerging. In women having their first caesarean, particularly if they have not laboured, there is a risk of breathing difficulties in the neonate which may necessitate admission to the neonatal unit and sometimes treatment with surfactant, at term. It is for this reason that most units now carry out elective caesarean section during the thirty-ninth week, rather than between 37 and 39 weeks. The risk of neonatal breathing difficulties is not as high in women who have emergency caesarean sections in labour (unless there are risk factors for birth asphyxia). Recently, the idea of giving antenatal steroids was explored through the ASTECS trial, which suggested that this reduced the incidence of TTN and RDS in term newborns, delivered by elective LSCS[79].

With the rise in caesarean sections, there is a consequent increase in pregnancies where the woman has undergone previous caesarean section. In counselling regarding the risks for the pregnancy, a 3:1000 risk of scar dehiscence is quoted and perhaps a 1:200 risk of perinatal death as a result of scar rupture[80]. This risk is increased where prostaglandin has been used to induce labour [81]. There also seems to be an excess risk of stillbirth in pregnancies following caesarean section[82, 83].

There is a minor risk of direct trauma to the foetus, through scalpel cuts and limb fractures, but these are rare and usually the benefit to the infant of LSCS outweighs the risk. The issues surrounding LSCS tend to exist where elective LSCS is carried out for maternal request and without obstetric indication[84].

The mounting evidence regarding short and long-term maternal and perinatal morbidity and mortality, should be discussed with mothers when exploring this decision, so that any decisions made regarding elective caesarean without obstetric indication, can be through informed choice. For the obstetrician, 24–26 weeks gestation remains a difficult time to decide whether it is beneficial for the foetus and mother for caesarean section to be carried out.

Neonatal care planning following instrumental vaginal birth or LSCS

Observations
The neonate is at increased risk of developing jaundice from bruising caused by trauma in instrumental birth. Additionally, the neonate may have transient tachypnoea caused by slow clearance of lung fluid with reduced adrenaline release. Vital observations should be carried out for 24 hours: hourly observation for four hours, then four hourly for the remaining 24 hours.

Medication
Adequate analgesia must be prescribed for the neonate following a traumatic birth, e.g. oral paracetamol.

Feeding
The baby should be assisted to have skin-to-skin contact as soon as possible following the birth, in order to facilitate regular breathing. This should help the rooting reflex and assist with latching on and breast feeding. The baby should be latched on to the breast while the mother is still in theatre following LSCS unless she has had a general anaesthetic.

Multiprofessional working

Communication
Communication across the multiprofessional team is the single most important factor in improving the care of the woman and therefore the baby. The CEMACH report *Why Mothers Die* recommends joint management of the woman with a medical condition in pregnancy[85]. This includes care planning for mode and time of

birth and for the presence of the neonatologist to support respiratory adaptation of the newborn.

The NHS Litigation Authority sets out standards for the maternity services through the Clinical Negligence Scheme for Trusts (CNST) which includes regular labour ward forum meetings between the obstetric, anaesthetic, neonatal and midwifery teams to risk assess, plan joint care and produce joint operational and clinical guidelines[86]. Joint audit of guidelines should then be facilitated to ensure good standards of practice are maintained. This ensures transparency within the service and includes input from lay representatives.

Local maternity service liaison committees provide an additional open forum for the multiprofessional team to work in partnership with users of the maternity services. Development of patient information leaflets and guidelines on maternity services and neonatal care can be produced through this route, ensuring everyone has a voice and meeting the requirements of the *Maternity Standard of the Children's National Service Framework*[87].

Organisation of perinatal care

In a level 3 unit, the long-term planning for infants of women with medical conditions on the antenatal ward can be facilitated by the neonatologist joining the weekly ward round. Arrangements for induction of labour, or planned caesarean section for medical complications relating to mother or baby, should be agreed to take place at the optimum time of day, with the optimum obstetric, anaesthetic and neonatal team[88]. Where this is not possible within the host unit, *in utero* transfer arrangements should be made using the neonatal networks.

It is good practice to have twice daily updates between the senior obstetrician on the labour ward and the senior neonatologist on the neonatal unit. This ensures good forward planning for cots required within a 24-hour period. The neonatologist can arrange to meet a woman in preterm labour and discuss the neonatal care plan with her midwife and obstetrician. This facilitates a smoother transition for the woman and her family.

Implications for practice

Setting up a system to facilitate effective communications between the maternity and neonatal services will ensure a robust clinical governance framework.

Standards, guidelines and relevant multiprofessional forums should be in place across both tertiary and primary care sectors to ensure a seamless service.

Joint weekly meetings involving maternity and neonatal teams should be held to discuss and review perinatal mortality and morbidity cases in order to agree good practice points and make recommendations to improve quality of care.

Conclusion

Provision of excellence in neonatal care relies on the neonatal team's prior knowledge of the maternal antenatal condition and its effects on the foetus and neonate, a detailed knowledge of the labour, type of birth (normal vaginal or instrumental), immediate assessment of the newborn, clear documentation and care planning. Communication with the multiprofessional team is essential.

References

1. National Institute of Health and Clinical Excellence (2003) *Antenatal Care: Routine Care for the healthy pregnant woman.* RCOG Press, London (www.nice.org.uk or www.rcog.org.uk).
2. National Institute of Health and Clinical Excellence (2003) *Antenatal Care: Routine Care for the healthy pregnant woman.* RCOG Press, London (www.nice.org.uk or www.rcog.org.uk).
3. Confidential Enquiry into Maternal and Child Health (2004) *Why Mother's Die, 2000–2002,* Sixth Report of Confidential Enquiries into Maternal Deaths in UK. RCOG Press, London.
4. Department of Health (2004) *Maternity Standard National Service Framework for Children, Young*

People and Maternity Services. Department of Health, London.

5. Confidential Enquiry into Maternal and Child Health (2007) *Perinatal Mortality 2005, England, Wales and Northern Ireland.* CEMACH, London.

6. Department of Health (2007) *Maternity Matters: Choice, Access and Continuity of Care in a Safe Service.* Department of Health, London.

7. Confidential Enquiry into Maternal and Child Health (2007) *Perinatal Mortality 2005, England, Wales and Northern Ireland.* CEMACH, London.

8. Wellings K (2007) Causes and consequences of teenage pregnancy. In: Baker P, Guthrie K, Hutchinson C (eds) *Teenage Pregnancy and Reproductive Health.* RCOG Press, London.

9. Department for Education and Skills 2003 *Every Child Matters.* Cm 5860: Department of Health, London (http://www.everychildmatters.gov.uk/_files).

10. McVeigh J, Kurinczuk J (2007) *Perinatal Risks Associated with IVF,* Royal College of Obstetricians and Gynaecologists. Scientific Advisory Committee Opinion Paper 8. RCOG Press, London.

11. Trogstad L (2003) The paternal role in pre-eclampsia. In: Critchley H, Maclean A, Poston L, Walker J (eds), *Pre-eclampsia.* RCOG Press, London.

12. Confidential Enquiry into Maternal and Child Health (2007) *Perinatal Mortality 2005, England, Wales and Northern Ireland.* CEMACH, London.

13. Yu CKH, Teoh TG, Robinson S (2006) Obesity in pregnancy. *BGOG,* **113** (10), 1117–1125.

14. Nelson-Piercy C (2003) Pre-eclampsia: the women at risk. In: Critchley H, Maclean A, Poston L, Walker J (eds). *Pre-eclampsia.* Martin Dunitz Ltd, London.

15. Confidential Enquiry into Maternal and Child Health (2007) *Perinatal Mortality 2005, England, Wales and Northern Ireland.* CEMACH, London.

16. National Institute for Clinical Excellence (NICE) (2002) *Guidance on the Use of Routine Antenatal Anti-D Prophylaxis for RhD-negative Women.* NICE, London.

17. National Institute of Health and Clinical Excellence (2003) *Antenatal Care: Routine Care for the healthy pregnant woman.* RCOG Press, London (www.nice.org.uk or www.rcog.org.uk).

18. Royal College of Obstetricians and Gynaecologists (2003) *Prevention of Early Onset Neonatal Group B Streptococcal Disease,* Guideline No. 36: RCOG Press, London.

19. Whitlow BJ, Economides DL (2000) Screening for foetal anomalies in the first trimester. In: Studd J (ed.) *Progress in Obstetrics and Gynaecology* 14. Churchill Livingstone, London.

20. O'Neill AM, Burd ID, Sabogal JC, *et al.* (2006) Doppler ultrasound in obstetrics: current advances. In: *Progress in Obstetrics and Gynaecology.* Churchill Livingstone, London.

21. Cederholm M, Haglund B, Axelsson O (2005) Infant morbidity following amniocentesis and chorionic villus sampling for prenatal karyotyping. *BJOG,* **112** (4), 394–402.

22. Cederholm M, Haglund B, Axelsson O (2005) Infant morbidity following amniocentesis and chorionic villus sampling for prenatal karyotyping. *BJOG,* **112** (4), 394–402.

23. Nelson-Piercy C (2003) Pre-eclampsia: the women at risk. In: Critchley H, Maclean A, Poston L, Walker J (eds). *Pre-eclampsia.* Martin Dunitz Ltd, London.

24. Kupferminc M (2003) Pre-eclampsia and inherited thrombophilias. In: Critchley H, Maclean A, Poston L, Walker J (eds). *Pre-eclampsia.* RCOG Press, London.

25. Confidential Enquiry into Maternal and Child Health (2004) *Why Mother's Die, 2000–2002,* Sixth Report of Confidential Enquiries into Maternal Deaths in UK. RCOG Press, London.

26. Nelson-Piercy C (2003) Pre-eclampsia: the women at risk. In: Critchley H, Maclean A, Poston L, Walker J (eds). *Pre-eclampsia.* Martin Dunitz Ltd, London.

27. Clarke S, Nelson- Piercy C (2005) Pre-eclampsia and HELLP syndrome. *Anaesthesia and Intensive Care,* **6** (3), 96–100.

28. Clarke S, Nelson- Piercy C (2005) Pre-eclampsia and HELLP syndrome. *Anaesthesia and Intensive Care,* **6** (3), 96–100.

29. UNICEF UK Baby Friendly Initiative (2007) Guidance on the Development of Policies and Guidelines for the Prevention and Management of Hypoglycaemia of the Newborn, UNICEF (www.babyfriendlyinitiative.org.uk).

30. NICE (2007) *Intrapartum Care.* NICE, London.

31. NICE (2007) *Intrapartum Care.* NICE, London.

32. Confidential Enquiry into Maternal and Child Health 2007 *Diabetes in Pregnancy: Are We Providing the Best Care?* England, Wales and Northern Ireland CEMACH, London.

33. Crowther CA, Hiller JE, Moss JR, *et al.* (2005) Australian Carbohydrate Intolerance Study in Pregnant Women (ACHOIS) trial group. Effect of treatment of gestational diabetes mellitus on pregnancy outcomes. *NEJM,* **352** (24), 2477– 2486.

34. Crowther CA, Hiller JE, Moss JR, *et al.* (2005) Australian Carbohydrate Intolerance Study in Pregnant Women (ACHOIS) trial group. Effect of treatment of gestational diabetes mellitus on pregnancy outcomes. *NEJM*, **352** (24), 2477–2486.

35. Confidential Enquiry into Maternal and Child Health 2007 *Diabetes in Pregnancy: Are We Providing the Best Care?* England, Wales and Northern Ireland CEMACH, London.

36. Confidential Enquiry into Maternal and Child Health 2007 *Diabetes in Pregnancy: Are We Providing the Best Care?* England, Wales and Northern Ireland CEMACH, London.

37. Black RS, Gillmer MD (2003) Diabetes in pregnancy. *The Obstetrician and Gynaecologist*, 5, 143–148.

38. Confidential Enquiry into Maternal and Child Health 2007 *Diabetes in Pregnancy: Are We Providing the Best Care?* England, Wales and Northern Ireland CEMACH, London.

39. Confidential Enquiry into Maternal and Child Health 2007 *Diabetes in Pregnancy: Are We Providing the Best Care?* England, Wales and Northern Ireland CEMACH, London.

40. Confidential Enquiry into Maternal and Child Health 2007 *Diabetes in Pregnancy: Are We Providing the Best Care?* England, Wales and Northern Ireland CEMACH, London.

41. Rennie JM (ed.) (2005) *Robertons's Text Book of Neonatology*, 4th edn. Elsevier Churchill-Livingstone, New York.

42. Tappero EP, Honeyfield ME (2003) *Physical Assessment of the Newborn*, 3rd edn. NICU INK Publishers, California USA.

43. Tappero EP, Honeyfield ME (2003) *Physical Assessment of the Newborn*, 3rd edn. NICU INK Publishers, California USA.

44. Nelson-Piercy C (2006) *Handbook of Obstetric Medicine*, 3rd edn. Informa Healthcare, London.

45. Confidential Enquiry into Maternal and Child Health (2004) *Why Mother's Die, 2000–2002*, Sixth Report of Confidential Enquiries into Maternal Deaths in UK. RCOG Press, London.

46. NICE Clinical Guideline (2004) CG20 *Epilepsy in Adults and Children: Full Guideline*, Appendix D. National Institute of Health and Clinical Excellence, London.

47. Nelson-Piercy C (2006) *Handbook of Obstetric Medicine*, 3rd edn. Informa Healthcare, London.

48. Johnston PGB, Flood K, Spinks K (2003) *The Newborn Child*, 9th edn. Churchill Livingstone, Edinburgh.

49. Blackburn ST (2003) *Maternal, Fetal & Neonatal.* Saunders, St Louis.

50. Nelson-Piercy C (2006) *Handbook of Obstetric Medicine*, 3rd edn. Informa Healthcare, London.

51. Sau A, Clarke S, Bass J, Kaiser A, Marinaki A, Nelson-Piercy C (2007) Azathioprine and breastfeeding – is it safe? *BJOG*, **114** (4), 498–501.

52. Nelson-Piercy C (2006) *Handbook of Obstetric Medicine*, 3rd edn. Informa Healthcare, London.

53. Nelson-Piercy C (2006) *Handbook of Obstetric Medicine*, 3rd edn. Informa Healthcare, London.

54. National Institute of Clinical Excellence (2006) *Routine Postnatal Care of Women and Their Babies.* NICE, London.

55. Rennie JM (ed.) (2005) *Robertons's Text Book of Neonatology*, 4th edn. Elsevier Churchill-Livingstone, New York.

56. Rennie JM (ed.) (2005) *Robertons's Text Book of Neonatology*, 4th edn. Elsevier Churchill-Livingstone, New York.

57. NICE Clinical Guideline (2004) CG20 *Epilepsy in Adults and Children: Full Guideline*, Appendix D. National Institute of Health and Clinical Excellence, London.

58. Nelson-Piercy C (2006) *Handbook of Obstetric Medicine*, 3rd edn. Informa Healthcare, London.

59. Rennie JM (ed.) (2005) *Robertons's Text Book of Neonatology*, 4th edn. Elsevier Churchill-Livingstone, New York.

60. Royal College of Obstetricians and Gynaecologists (2006) *Obstetric Cholestasis*, RCOG Greentop Guideline No. 43 January. RCOG, London.

61. Roncaglia N, Arreghini A, Locatelli A, Bellini P, Andreotti C, Ghidini A (2002) Obstetric cholestasis: outcome with active management. *European Journal of Obstetric & Gynaecology Reproductive Biology*, 10 Jan, **100** (2), 167–170.

62. Royal College of Obstetricians and Gynaecologists (2003) *Prevention of Early Onset Neonatal Group B Streptococcal Disease*, Guideline No. 36: RCOG Press, London.

63. Stutchfield P, Whittaker R, Russell I (2005) Antenatal betamethasone and incidence of neonatal respiratory distress after elective caesarean section: pragmatic randomised trial. Antenatal steroids for Term Elective Caesarean section (ASTECS) research team. *BMJ*, **331** (7518), 662–670.

64. Letsky EA (1999) Anaemia. In: James DK, Steer PJ, Weiner CP, Gonik B (eds) *High Risk Pregnancy Management Options*. WB Saunders, London.

65. Letsky EA (1999) Anaemia. In: James DK, Steer PJ, Weiner CP, Gonik B (eds) *High Risk Pregnancy Management Options*. WB Saunders, London.

66. Blackburn ST (2003) *Maternal, Fetal & Neonatal*. Saunders, St Louis.

67. Rennie JM (ed.) (2005) *Robertons's Text Book of Neonatology*, 4th edn. Elsevier Churchill-Livingstone, New York.

68. Royal College of Obstetricians and Gynaecologists (2006) *Obstetric Cholestasis*, RCOG Greentop Guideline No. 43 January. RCOG, London.

69. Royal College of Obstetricians and Gynaecologists (2003) *Prevention of Early Onset Neonatal Group B Streptococcal Disease*, Guideline No. 36: RCOG Press, London.

70. Stutchfield P, Whittaker R, Russell I (2005) Antenatal betamethasone and incidence of neonatal respiratory distress after elective caesarean section: pragmatic randomised trial. Antenatal steroids for Term Elective Caesarean section (ASTECS) research team. *BMJ*, **331** (7518), 662–670.

71. Kelly TF, Resnik R (2005) Antenatal corticosteroids: the controversy continues (Adrenal cortex). *Current Opinion in Endocrinology and Diabetes*, **12** (3), 237–241.

72. Royal College of Obstetricians and Gynaecologists (2003) *Prevention of Early Onset Neonatal Group B Streptococcal Disease*, Guideline No. 36: RCOG Press, London.

73. Kenyon SL, Taylor DJ, Tarnew-Mardi W (2001) Broad-spectrum antibiotics for preterm, pre-labour rupture of foetal membranes: the ORACLE I randomised trial. *Lancet*, 357, 978–988.

74. Hannah ME, Hannah WJ, Hodnett ED, *et al.* (2000) Planned caesarean section versus planned vaginal birth for breech presentation at term: a randomised multicentre trial. *Lancet*, 356 (9239), 1375–1383.

75. National Institute of Health and Clinical Excellence (2003) *Antenatal Care: Routine Care for the healthy pregnant woman*. RCOG Press, London (www.nice.org.uk or www.rcog.org.uk).

76. Smith G, Fleming K, White I (2007) Birth order of twins and risk of perinatal death related to delivery in England Northern Ireland and Wales 1994–2003. A retrospective cohort study. *BMJ*, **334** (7593), 576.

77. Royal College of Obstetricians and Gynaecologists (2005) Green top guideline No. 26: *Operative Vaginal Delivery*. RCOG Press, London.

78. 2005–2006 *Maternity Statistics for England* (2007) (http://www.ic.nhs.uk).

79. Letsky EA (1999) Anaemia. In: James DK, Steer PJ, Weiner CP, Gonik B (eds) *High Risk Pregnancy Management Options*. WB Saunders, London.

80. Smith GC, Pell J, Pasupathy D, Dobbie R (2004) Factors predisposing to perinatal death related to uterine rupture during attempted vaginal birth after caesarean section: retrospective cohort study. *BMJ*, **329** (7462), 375–381.

81. 2005–2006 *Maternity Statistics for England* (2007) (http://www.ic.nhs.uk).

82. Smith GC, Pell JP, Dobbie R (2003) Caesarean section and risk of unexplained stillbirth in subsequent pregnancy. *Lancet*, **36** (2), 1779–1784.

83. Gray R, Quigley MA, Hockley C, *et al.* (2007) Caesarean delivery and risk of stillbirth in subsequent pregnancy: a retrospective cohort study in an English population. *BJOG*, **114** (3), 264–270.

84. National Collaborating Centre for Women's and Children's Health (2004) *Caesarean Section*. Clinical guideline 13. National Institute for Clinical Excellence, London.

85. Confidential Enquiry into Maternal and Child Health (2004) *Why Mother's Die, 2000–2002*, Sixth Report of Confidential Enquiries into Maternal Deaths in UK. RCOG Press, London

86. NHS Litigation Authority (2007) Clinical Negligence Scheme for Trusts. *Maternity Clinical Risk Management Standards* (April). NHSLA, London.

87. Department of Health (2004) *Maternity Standard National Service Framework for Children, Young People and Maternity Services*. Department of Health, London.

88. National Collaborating Centre for Women's and Children's Health (2004) *Caesarean Section*. Clinical guideline 13. National Institute for Clinical Excellence, London.

Chapter 3

NORMAL ADAPTATION TO THE POST-NATAL ENVIRONMENT

Maggie Meeks and Maggie Hallsworth

Learning outcomes

After reading this chapter the reader will be expected to be able to:

- Reproduce or accurately label a diagram of the foetal circulation

- Explain the way in which the anatomy or function of the kidneys may affect liquor volume

- Describe the effect of an infant's first gasp together with clamping of the cord on the blood flow through the heart

- Justify a neonatal guideline that discouraged measurement of glucose in a healthy well grown term infant

- Recommend ways in which a normal term infant should be supported following delivery in order to maximise the chances of successful:

  ○ Cardiorespiratory adaptation

  ○ Nutritional adaptation

  ○ Thermoregulation

Introduction

Birth is a physiologically challenging event both for the mother and the foetus. An understanding of the physiology of foetal adaptation to the post-natal environment by midwifery and neonatal staff is essential if this adaptation is to be supported.

Some of the principles of post-natal adaptation can be understood by comparing details of the anatomy and physiology of the foetus with that of the newborn infant after birth. This chapter will therefore begin by reviewing the situation *in utero*, specifically the anatomy

and physiology of the foetal circulation, and the normal physiology of foetal adaptation. It will then discuss the assessment and support of a newborn infant that successfully adapts to extra-uterine life.

Physiology of intrauterine life

Foetal circulation

One of the fundamental principles behind understanding the way in which the blood flows around the body of the foetus is to remember that it is the maternal/placental unit which provides the foetus with their metabolic needs prior to birth. These needs include:

- Oxygenation and clearance of carbon dioxide: a function of the cardiorespiratory system after birth
- Provision of glucose, protein and lipid: a function of the gastrointestinal system and liver after birth
- Fluid balance and clearance of metabolites: a function of the kidneys after birth

A diagram of the foetal circulation is shown in Figure 3.1 and this is explained in more detail in the following paragraphs.

A comparison of the foetal circulation, or *in utero* circulation, with the fully adapted *exutero*, or adult circulation, reveals the following differences.

The foetal circulation has three 'short cuts' or 'shunts' which are described below:

- The ductus arteriosus allows blood from the pulmonary arteries to pass directly into the aorta and therefore bypass the lungs
- The ductus venosus allows much of the blood to bypass the liver
- The foramen ovale allows blood to pass from the inferior vena cava into the right atrium and directly into the left atrium rather than into the right ventricle, which has two effects:
  - It allows the most oxygenated blood from the placenta to flow to the head of the infant
  - It also serves to bypass the lungs

This is elaborated in the sub-sections below:

Oxygenation and clearance of carbon dioxide
Cardiovascular circulation

Oxygenated blood is supplied to the foetus from the maternal circulation and placenta through the umbilical *vein*. Blood leaves the foetus to return to the placenta through the umbilical *artery*. These are important points to remember in the interpretation of cord gases.

An umbilical venous gas should be more highly oxygenated than the umbilical arterial gas as it indicates the condition of the blood entering the foetus to supply the foetus with oxygen and nutrients. The umbilical arterial gas shows the condition of the blood leaving the foetus after giving up oxygen and nutrients to meet the metabolic demands of the foetus. This often causes confusion as it should be the only time that a vein has blood within it that is more highly oxygenated than that within the artery. The reason for this is that although this is the situation *in utero* the umbilical artery will be the supplier of oxygen and nutrients to the infant once delivery has occurred and there has been separation from the maternal/placental unit.

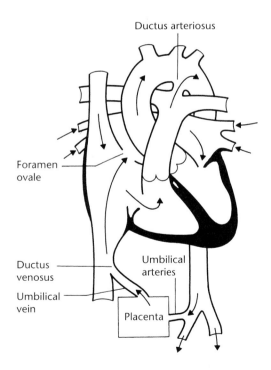

Figure 3.1 Fetal circulation showing that the oxygenated blood from the umbilical vein flows as a priority across the foramen ovale in to the left side of the heart to ensure that the systemic circulation receives oxygenated blood (adapted from Rees *et al.*(1989)).

Implications for practice

A blood gas taken from the umbilical vein should be more highly oxygenated than that taken from the umbilical artery and indicates the condition of the blood entering the foetus.

Oxygen diffuses from the maternal circulation across the placenta into the foetal vessels and the umbilical vein. This diffusion is facilitated by the differences between the adult haemoglobin of the mother and the foetal haemoglobin of the foetus: foetal haemoglobin has an increased oxygen affinity compared to adult haemoglobin which means that it forms tighter links with the oxygen molecules at lower oxygen concentrations (partial pressures)[1,2]. This allows the foetus to ensure that oxygen released from the adult haemoglobin is taken up and bound to the foetal haemoglobin. This principle is illustrated in Figure 3.2.

The oxygen saturation of foetal haemoglobin is higher than that of adult haemoglobin when exposed to an identical oxygen tension. For example at 30 mmHg (4KPa) partial pressure of oxygen adult haemoglobin is saturated to 50%, while foetal haemoglobin is saturated to almost 80%[3].

The oxygenated blood from the umbilical vein passes up the body to reach the inferior vena cava and the right atrium (see Figure 3.1) where it is diverted through the foramen ovale, one of the essential shunts, into the *left* atrium and then *left* ventricle. From here it passes up into the aorta to supply the upper end of the systemic circulation of the infant with oxygen directly from the placenta. This occurs via the right subclavian and carotid arteries which leave the arch of the aorta prior to the ductus arteriosus. This ensures that the brain receives the most highly oxygenated blood. The anatomy of the arch of the aorta is an important point to remember when considering the application of preductal and postductal saturation monitors; the right arm is the only limb that will always measure preductal oxygenation (see Chapter 11).

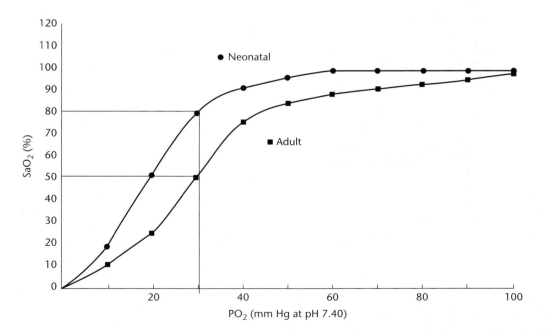

Figure 3.2 A comparison of foetal/neonatal and adult oxygen saturation curves. Reprinted from Rennie, J, *Roberton's Textbook of Neonatology*, copyright 2005 by kind permission of Elsevier.

Implications for practice

A preductal oxygen saturation probe should be sited on the right arm in order to guarantee preductal oxygen saturations.

The less oxygenated blood from the superior vena cava also passes into the right atrium and mixes with some of the oxygenated blood from the inferior vena cava before passing into the right ventricle and up into the pulmonary artery. Although some of this blood will pass into the lungs to provide lung tissue with oxygen and essential nutrients, much of it will bypass the lungs via the ductus arteriosus, which connects the pulmonary artery to the aorta. In the foetal circulation the direction of flow across the ductus arteriosus is right to left from the pulmonary artery, a high pressure circuit, into the aorta and the systemic circulation, a low pressure circuit. The direction of flow through a patent ductus arteriosus after birth depends on the pressure of the pulmonary and systemic circuits. The common situation in preterm infants is that the blood flows from the systemic circuit to the pulmonary circuit (left to right). In this situation there will be an increase in blood flow through the left side of the heart leading to heart failure. If the pulmonary blood pressure remains high and there is blood flow from the pulmonary circuit to the systemic circuit (right to left) there will be cyanosis as the lungs are being bypassed in a similar way to how they are *in utero*. This is the situation that occurs in pulmonary hypertension (persistent foetal circulation). These two situations will be discussed in more detail in Chapter 11.

Foetal lung

The foetal lung develops predominantly over the third trimester in preparation for delivery. This involves formation of the major bronchi, each of which then divides to form segmental bronchi and further serial branching ultimately produces

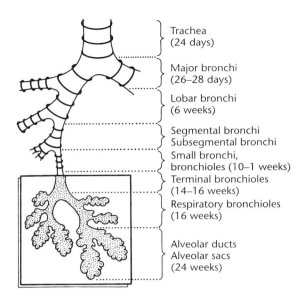

Figure 3.3 Respiratory tract with approximate gestational ages of formation (adapted from Korones and Lancaster, 1986).

the bronchioles and alveoli (see Figure 3.3). This is discussed further in Chapter 8.

The main phases involved in the development of the alveoli are[4]:

- Embryonic (0–7 weeks): the lungs form as a diverticulum from the ventral portion of the endodermal foregut at about four weeks' post-conceptual age. This leads to the formation of the bronchi.
- Glandular (7–16 weeks): there is rapid proliferation of the airways during this stage.
- Cannalicular (17–27 weeks): this refers to the development of the respiratory bronchioles and acinar as well as the vascular channels that are closely opposed to the potential air spaces. This development is critical for gas exchange.
- Saccular (28–35 weeks): this refers to the development of alveolar ducts which give rise to terminal sacs (hence the name saccular) and type I and type II pneumocytes differentiate during this period.

- Alveolar: this final developmental stage results in a significant increase in the surface area available for gas exchange and alveoli will continue to increase in number until the age of three years.

The term gaseous exchange refers to the diffusion of oxygen from the lung into the capillaries and the diffusion of carbon dioxide out of the capillaries and into the lung. This necessitates that there is a close anatomical relationship between the developing alveoli and the developing capillary network so that ventilation and perfusion are closely linked.

In utero the alveoli are filled with alveolar fluid secreted by the pulmonary epithelium. The formation of this fluid involves the secretion or active transport of chloride by type I pneumocytes[5], which is followed by the passive diffusion of other electrolytes and water. As the infant prepares for birth these pneumocytes will change from secretory to absorbent, which will contribute to the clearing of the lung fluid[6,7]. Type II pneumocytes are those that secrete surfactant. Surfactant is a phospholipid that helps to prevent alveolar collapse by lowering their surface tension (in a similar way to the action of detergents) and reducing the amount of pressure required to keep each alveolar open. It is consequently extremely important in helping the infant maintain a functional residual capacity. Surfactant is produced by the type II pneumocytes in small quantities from 20 weeks gestation but it is not until 34 weeks gestation that it is produced in amounts large enough to exert a physiological effect.

Implications for practice

Surfactant production is important to ensure normal physiological postnatal adaptation by the lungs.

Hypothermia is one of the factors that can affect surfactant production and one of the complications of hypothermia is alveolar collapse

Table 3.1 Table of factors associated with a decrease in surfactant production (increased risk of respiratory distress syndrome) or an increase in surfactant production (decreased risk of respiratory distress syndrome).

Factors associated with an increase in surfactant production and *decreased* risk of RDS [8]	Factors associated with a decrease in surfactant production and/or *increased* risk of RDS [9]
Maternal factors	**Maternal factors**
*Maternal steroids (used in preterm deliveries) [10]	*Maternal diabetes
*Narcotic/cocaine use	*Chorioamnionitis
*Pregnancy induced hypertension	**Foetal/infant factors**
*Increased thyroid hormone	*Hypoxia/acidosis
*Prolonged rupture of membranes	*Hypothermia
Foetal/infant factors	
*Intrauterine growth restriction	*Meconium
*Twin gestation	*Congenital abnormality of surfactant production (e.g. surfactant protein B deficiency

and persistent pulmonary hypertension (previously known as a persistent foetal circulation). The importance of maintaining a normal temperature in a newborn infant cannot be overestimated. Other factors that affect surfactant production are discussed in Chapter 8 and listed in Table 3.1.

Provision of glucose, protein and lipid

In the foetus a large proportion of the blood bypasses the liver through the ductus venosus before passing into the inferior vena cava. In a similar way to that which happens with the lungs the liver receives enough blood to supply its cells with essential oxygen and nutrients, but the majority of its functions can be accomplished by the placenta (and maternal liver) so blood is shunted past.

During foetal life the infant is dependent on both glucose, ketone bodies and lactate as the fuel or energy needed to perform its metabolic functions[11]. It receives a constant supply of glucose through the placenta to provide energy for its metabolic functions and growth[12]. The placenta supplies this glucose at 4–6 mg/kg/day and foetal blood glucose levels are approximately 70–80% of maternal levels[13]. Insulin is present in the foetal pancreas from 8–10 weeks with increasing levels as the foetus approaches term and appears to have a role in foetal growth as well as the regulation of glucose uptake into the cells. Insulin cannot cross the placenta. The role of glucagon in the foetus is unclear but it has been identified from as early as 15 weeks gestation, the physiological action being to raise blood glucose levels. It is important to be aware that the regulation of foetal insulin and glucagon levels are determined by the foetal blood glucose level which in turn is determined by the maternal blood glucose level.

In the foetus of a mother with diabetes the glucose delivery may not be as constant in view of her own diabetic control during pregnancy and throughout labour, as well as other factors[14]. An excessive glucose supply to the foetus will result in stimulation of the foetal pancreas to produce insulin and this hyperinsulinaemia state may persist following birth to cause significant problems with glucose control even in those with gestational diabetes[15]. Unfortunately, good control in itself may not prevent neonatal hypoglycaemia[16].

Fluid balance and clearance of metabolites

Water accounts for a significant proportion of the foetus and is commonly considered as:

- Intracellular: this is the water within the cells
- Extracellular: this is the water outside of cells including:
  - Intravascular and lymphatics
  - Interstitial: water between cells

The water within the foetus is predominantly extracellular and the proportion of the foetus that is water will decrease towards term (see Chapter 7).

There is no shunt within the foetal circulation to bypass the kidneys as the kidneys do produce urine but the blood flow to the kidneys will increase following birth (see below). Foetal urine makes a significant contribution to the liquor surrounding the foetus. The amount of liquor can often give an indication to concerns within the renal or gastrointestinal tracts in the following way; liquor surrounding the foetus is swallowed and passes through the gastrointestinal tract to aid the foetus in the development of the physiological coordination of peristalsis that will be necessary during post-natal life. The amount of liquor is therefore influenced by both the anatomy and function of the GIT as well as the anatomy and function of the genitourinary system. Oliguria will occur as a result of limits in the amount of urine produced by the kidneys or due to an obstruction to urinary flow after the kidney. Polyhydramnios will occur due to an inability in swallowing which may be anatomical (for example oesophageal atresia) or physiological (muscle disease preventing coordinated swallowing). Although the kidneys do produce urine they do not perform a major excretory function prior to delivery – this is performed by the maternal placental unit.

Implications for practice

The kidneys produce urine in the foetus *in utero* which contributes to the amniotic fluid volume.

Some of the reasons for oligohydramnios include renal problems such as:
- Absent kidneys
- Poorly functioning kidneys
- Obstructed kidneys

The physiological adaption to birth

Changes in ventilation and circulation during and following delivery

Labour is usually spontaneously initiated at around 38 weeks after conception in singleton pregnancies, 37 weeks in twin pregnancies and earlier in more multiple pregnancies[17]. It is defined as the onset of regular painful contractions associated with dilatation of the cervix and occurs because of the complex interaction between a number of factors, some of which also have a role in preparing the infant for birth. The detail of this complex interaction remains elusive but it is known that an increase in hormones such as cortisol and oestrediol together with a decrease in progesterone affect the myometrial activity of the uterine muscle and stimulate resorption of foetal lung fluid to prepare the infant for birth[18,19].

For the foetus each contraction during labour is a mildly hypoxic event and in most cases the normally grown term infant is able to cope with this. During a contraction there is a reduction in blood flow from the maternal circulation to the placenta and this is followed by a reactive hyperaemia or increase in blood flow to the placenta once the contraction has ceased. This does not usually affect the umbilical venous blood flow, although changes can be demonstrated when the infant is responding with variable or late decelerations[20]. Healthy appropriately grown term infants will tolerate the mild degree of hypoxia which occurs because of the contractions. However, it may not be so well tolerated in infants that are already compromised, such as those with intrauterine growth retardation or preterm infants and this is one of the reasons why it is useful to identify these infants before labour.

The foetal lungs are obviously filled with alveolar fluid prior to and during delivery. There is some evidence from animal studies that the volume of fluid begins to decrease prior to the onset of labour as a result of the hormonal changes[21], but a small amount of fluid remains. Although some of the fluid is cleared from the oropharynx during a normal vaginal delivery this is not clinically significant and most of the fluid is rapidly reabsorbed into the bloodstream and lymphatics[22-24].

Following delivery there are two important physiological events that precipitate the

necessary changes for physiological adaption to the *ex utero* environment:

- The infants' cries: crying involves a significant inspiration followed by expiration against a closed glottis
  o This inflates the lungs, displacing the alveolar fluid into the lymphatics and establishing a functional residual capacity of air within the lungs over the course of a few minutes
  o This also has the effect of reducing the resistance to blood flow in the pulmonary circulation and consequently reducing the pressure on the pulmonary side of the heart
- The cord is clamped (the umbilical artery and vein will spontaneously constrict if the cord is not artificially clamped): clamping the cord effectively removes the placenta from the systemic side of the infant's circulation
  o This increases the resistance of systemic circulation and the systemic blood pressure therefore increases
  o The blood stops flowing through the umbilical vein and the ductus venosus starts to close

The result of the fall in pulmonary blood pressure, increase in systemic blood pressure and increase oxygenation is that the foramen ovale and ductus arteriosus begin to close so that blood no longer bypasses the lungs but flows through the right side of the heart to the lungs and then into the left side of the heart and to the systemic circulation (see Figure 3.4).

Provision of glucose, protein and lipid

In utero the infant had been used to receiving an almost constant supply of nutrients from the placenta, but with the clamping of the cord this supply ceases. This results in a mild physiological hypoglycaemia that stimulates an endocrine response to break down glycogen and fat in order to provide glucose, lactate and ketones for the infant's cells to metabolise[25]. Some of the glycogen within the liver and the brain may have been broken down during labour but a normal

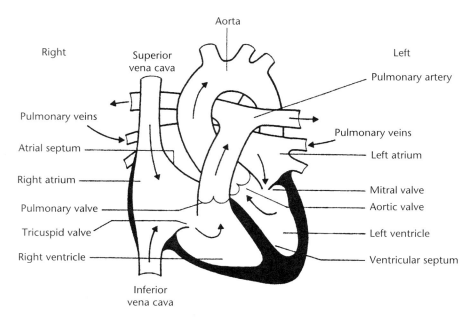

Figure 3.4 Adult circulation with physiological closure of the foramen ovale (and also of the ductus arteriosus) (adapted from Rees *et al.*).

term infant will have laid down fat supplies during the last trimester to provide fuel for the first few days. These forms of fuel are essential as the transition is made from the continuous placental supply to the intermittent milk supply of the post-natal infant. The routine measurement of glucose in healthy term infants shortly after birth is therefore no longer recommended in view of this physiological hypoglycaemic response[26].

There are several hormonal and metabolic changes which facilitate the post-natal adaptation in maintaining glucose levels. These include a rise in:

- Catecholamine levels (e.g. epinephrine/adrenalin)
  - This occurs due to the fall in environmental temperature and also due to loss of the placenta
  - Increased catacholamine levels stimulate lipolysis releasing fatty acids which may be used as an energy source
- Glucagon levels which activate hepatic glycogen phosphorylase which induces glycogenolyisis

- Cortisol levels which rise at the time of delivery and the falling glucose concentration stimulate hepatic glucose –6 phosphatase activity, producing an increase in hepatic glucose release

This release of hormones acts to maintain normoglycaemia and to produce ketones as a food supply for the first few days[27]. The production and release of insulin also matures to enable the glucose to be utilised for energy and stored for future energy. Insulin is produced by the beta cells of the islets of the pancreas and acts to transport glucose from the blood into the cells and also to convert glucose into glycogen for storage (glycogenesis) and to lay down fat (lipogenesis).

Fluid balance and clearance of metabolites

There are two main consequences of the fall in pulmonary blood pressure: increase in systemic blood pressure and closure of the foramen ovale and ductus arteriosus (outlined above) as far as the kidneys and fluid balance are concerned. These are:

- The blood flow to the kidneys increases, which has a direct effect on urine production
- The blood flow returning to the left atrium increases and this dilatation of the left atrium causes the release of a hormone called atrial natriuretic hormone, which acts to decrease the extracellular fluid and to cause the excretion of sodium with an accompanying diuresis (water loss)

The clinical result is that the newborn infant has a diuresis shortly after birth as well as a physiological loss of weight that is due to the contraction of the extracellular fluid space and diuresis. A weight loss of 5–10% is normal. In infants that have respiratory distress syndrome, where the pulmonary blood pressure remains high until surfactant is either produced or administered, this diuresis is delayed because of the delay in the dilatation of the left atrium and release of atrial natriuretic hormone. The remaining physiological challenge is for the infant to maintain his/her temperature, which is discussed in Chapter 6.

Care of the infant to aid successful adaption at birth

Cardiorespiratory

The importance of preparation prior to the delivery of any newborn infant cannot be overemphasised. The need for resuscitation cannot be reliably predicted, which is why all professionals attending the birth of an infant should be competent in the skills of basic life support (www.resus.org.uk). It is important for the obstetric and neonatal team to be aware of the mechanisms of foetal adaption in order for them to work together to try to prevent the infant experiencing known triggers that may hinder this adaption process.

The neonatal nurse should have a key role within the resuscitation team and has a responsibility to work with others to ensure that optimum conditions are met. The types of delivery at which a nurse is likely to be present will include:

- Birth of term infants in whom problems during delivery have been identified
  - Infants with congenital abnormalities
  - Infants in whom foetal distress has been identified
- Birth of preterm infants

One of the most important areas of care to be considered during the delivery of any infant is that of thermoregulation. This is covered in detail in Chapter 6 but its importance cannot be overemphasised and yet it remains a common reason for admission of term or mildly preterm infants to the neonatal unit. In maintaining the infant's temperature at 37°C there are factors involving both the infant and the surrounding environment that have an effect. These are discussed below.

Infant factors
- A newborn infant is small with a large surface area to volume ratio allowing for rapid heat loss by evaporation, radiation, convection and conduction
- A newborn infant is born covered in liquor which will significantly increase heat loss by evaporation unless the infant is rapidly dried

Environment factors
- The ambient temperature of the room in which the infant is delivered should be 25–28°C; this may be slightly uncomfortable for the parents during delivery but the temptation to reduce the temperature must be resisted
- It is common on labour ward for staff to move in and out of a delivery room and the opening of doors will increase the risk of convective heat loss

- Any towels that will be used to dry the infant should already have been prewarmed to minimise conductive heat loss

An infant that is successfully adapting to birth will not require resuscitation. The infant should be kept warm by placing in skin to skin contact with the mother or if the need for resuscitation is being assessed he/she should be dried and wrapped in a warm towel (or placed in a polythene bag if preterm and within the hospital environment) and clinically assessed by noting the following four signs:

- Colour
- Tone
- Breathing
- Heart rate

A healthy infant will be born with a heart rate of > 100 beats per minute, a good tone and a vigorous cry. The infant's colour will be blue initially but will rapidly change to pink although the peripheries may remain blue for up to 48 hours. It is not unusual for a less vigorous infant to take up to three minutes to establish regular respirations and become centrally pink. The role of those attending the delivery in these circumstances is to ensure that the infant remains warm and that the airway is patent.

Every newborn infant should be assessed following delivery. This is usually the responsibility of the midwifery team but if the neonatal team have been present then they share this responsibility and obviously all neonates that are admitted to the neonatal unit should be accurately assessed. This is especially important when there have been clinical concerns on antenatal assessment as these need to be more fully evaluated.

Nutrition

Glucose

The normal well-grown term infant should not need routine glucose monitoring during the first few hours following birth as alternative fuels such as ketones and lactate are also utilised. There is some evidence that these alternative fuels are suppressed by formula feeds which is a relative contraindication to the use of formula feeds in infants establishing breast-feeds as long as there is no medical indication to do so[28]. This ketogenic response and metabolic adaption may not be as effective in preterm or small for gestational age infants[29]. Infants of 34–37 weeks gestation are increasingly managed on the PNW as are small for gestational age infants > 1.5 kg and there should be strict guidelines for the management of these infants with attention to temperature, establishment of feeds and regular glucose monitoring. Some of these infants will require admission to the neonatal unit for more intensive monitoring.

Implications for practice

Glucose should not be measured in the first few hours after birth in the well-grown term infant as the hypoglycaemia at this stage is physiological not pathological[30].

Breast-feeding

The infants should be placed skin to skin as soon as possible after delivery in order to facilitate the establishment of breast-feeding as part of the post-natal adaption to extra-uterine life. The principle hormone promoting lactation is prolactin, secreted from the anterior pituitary gland under the control of the hypothalamus. Its release is stimulated by thyrotropin releasing hormone and inhibited by dopamine. Prolactin is produced in increasing amounts throughout the pregnancy but milk production is suppressed due to the levels of oestrogen and progesterone. Following delivery, when the levels of these hormones fall, milk production will start. The infant sucking at the breast is the principal stimulus for maintaining prolactin levels and sucking also stimulates the posterior pituitary gland to produce oxytocin which induces the 'let down' reflex and ejection of milk[31]. This may take from 30–60 seconds after the infant has commenced sucking at the breast.

Fluid balance

The infant should be cared for in a thermon-eutral environment and should be protected from situations where trans-epidermal fluid loss is likely to increase, as even term infants are quite vulnerable to dehydration. A term infant can adjust to varying intakes of water during the first few days of life as long as they receive a minimum intake that will cover urinary and insensible losses.

Implications for practice

The weight and urine output of a newborn infant should be used to assess hydration.

Conclusion

The successful adaption to extra-uterine life involves a complex system of cardiorespiratory and metabolic adaptive systems. Knowledge of this normal physiology allows a more complete understanding of the nursing care needed to facilitate successful adaption of the newborn infant to post-natal life.

References

1. Polin RA, Fox WW (eds) (1998) *Foetal and Neonatal Physiology*. WB Saunders, Philadelphia, USA.
2. Rennie JM, Roberton NRC (eds) (2000) *Textbook of Neonatology*. Harcourt Brace, London.
3. Rennie JM, Roberton NRC (eds) (2000) *Textbook of Neonatology*. Harcourt Brace, London.
4. Polin RA, Fox WW (eds) (1998) *Foetal and Neonatal Physiology*. WB Saunders, Philadelphia, USA.
5. Bland RD, Nielson DW (1992) Developmental changes in lung epithelial ion transport and liquid movement. *Annu Rev Physiol*, 54, 373–394 (accession number 1314041).
6. Polin RA, Fox WW (eds) (1998) *Foetal and Neonatal Physiology*. WB Saunders, Philadelphia, USA.
7. Walters DV, Olver RE (1978) The role of catecholamines in lung liquid absorption at birth. *Pediatr Res*, 12 (3), 239–242.
8. Gomella TL (2004) *Neonatology*, 5th edn. Lange Medical Books, New York.
9. Gomella TL (2004) *Neonatology*, 5th edn. Lange Medical Books, New York.
10. Crowley P, Chalmers I, Keirse MJ (1990) The effects of corticosteroid administration before preterm delivery: an overview of the evidence from controlled trials. *Br J Obstet Gynaecol*, 97 (1), 11–25.
11. Rennie JM, Roberton NRC (eds) (2000) *Textbook of Neonatology*. Harcourt Brace, London.
12. Hauguel, S, Desmaizieres V, Challier JC (1986) Glucose uptake, utilization, and transfer by the human placenta as functions of maternal glucose concentration. *Pediatr Res*, 20 (3), 269–273.
13. Rennie JM, Roberton NRC (eds) (2000) *Textbook of Neonatology*. Harcourt Brace, London.
14. Schwartz R, Teramo KA (2000) Effects of diabetic pregnancy on the foetus and newborn. *Semin Perinatol*, 24 (2), 120–135.
15. Gonzalez-Quintero VH, Istwan NB, Rhea DJ, et al. (2007) The impact of glycemic control on neonatal outcome in singleton pregnancies complicated by gestational diabetes. *Diabetes Care*, 30 (3), 467–470.
16. Evers IM, de Valk HW, Visser GH (2004) Risk of complications of pregnancy in women with type I diabetes: nationwide prospective study in the Netherlands. *BMJ*, 328 (7445), 915.
17. Henderson C, Macdonald S (eds) (2004) *Mayes Midwifery. A Textbook for Midwives*, 13th edn. Balliere Tindell, London.
18. Jeschke U, Mylonas T, Richter DU, et al. (2005) Regulation of progesterone production in human term trophoblasts in vitro by CRH, ACTH and cortisol (prednisolone). *Arch Gynecol Obstet*, 272 (1), 7–12.
19. Sfakianaki AK, Norwitz ER (2006) Mechanisms of progesterone action in inhibiting prematurity. *J.Matern Foetal Neonatal Med*, 19 (12), 763–772.
20. Murakami M., Kanzaki T, Utsu M, Chiba Y (1985) Changes in the umbilical venous blood flow of human foetus in labor. *Nippon Sanka Fujinka Gakkai Zasshi*, 37 (5), 776–782.
21. Polin RA, Fox WW (eds) (1998) *Foetal and Neonatal Physiology*. WB Saunders, Philadelphia, USA.
22. Bland RD, Nielson DW (1992) Developmental changes in lung epithelial ion transport and liquid

movement. *Annu Rev Physiol*, **54**, 373–394 (accession number 1314041).

23. Resuscitation Council (2006) *Newborn Life Support*, 3rd edn. Resuscitation Council, London.

24. Lind J (1962) Initiation of breathing in the newborn infant. *J Ir Med Assoc*, **50**, 88–93.

25. Hawdon JM, Ward Platt MP, Aynsley-Green A (1992) Patterns of metabolic adaptation for preterm and term infants in the first neonatal week. *Arch Dis Child*, **67** (4 Spec No.), 357–365.

26. Williams AF (2005) Neonatal hypoglycaemia: clinical and legal aspects. *Semin Foetal Neonatal Med*, **10** (4), 363–368.

27. Hawdon JM, Ward Platt MP, Aynsley-Green A (1992) Patterns of metabolic adaptation for preterm and term infants in the first neonatal week. *Arch Dis Child*, **67** (4 Spec No.), 357–365.

28. de Rooy L, Hawdon J (2002) Nutritional factors that affect the postnatal metabolic adaptation of full-term small- and large-for-gestational-age infants. *Pediatrics*, **109** (3), E42.

29. Hawdon JM, Ward Platt MP, Aynsley-Green A (1992) Patterns of metabolic adaptation for preterm and term infants in the first neonatal week. *Arch Dis Child*, **67** (4 Spec No.), 357–365.

30. Polin RA, Fox WW (eds) (1998) *Foetal and Neonatal Physiology*. WB Saunders, Philadelphia, USA.

31. Tay CC, Glasier AF, McNeilly AS (1996) Twenty-four hour patterns of prolactin secretion during lactation and the relationship to suckling and the resumption of fertility in breast-feeding women. *Hum Reprod*, **11** (5), 950–955.

Chapter 4

THE NEONATAL ENVIRONMENT AND CARE OF FAMILIES

Kevin Hugill with contributions from ADAPT

Learning outcomes

After reading this chapter the reader will be expected to be able to:

- Describe the sources of stress and anxiety for parents with a baby in a neonatal unit

- Reflect upon the impact, limitations and contribution of theories of social bonding to neonatal care and the promoting of positive parent-infant outcomes

- Critically explore the needs and perspectives of parents within a neonatal unit care setting

- Appreciate the ways in which parents' life experiences, their gender and staff behaviours affect an individual parent's needs and help seeking behaviours

- Critically discuss nursing interventions that contribute to optimising parents experiences in the neonatal unit

- Produce recommendations for developing own and own unit's practice to improve the delivery of care for parents

---

Introduction

No book that intends to consider the nursing care of infants in a neonatal unit is complete without some consideration of the needs and care of parents and families. In this book, there are specific chapters that consider in detail parents' needs during bereavement and their role in contributing to the optimisation of their baby's developmental outcomes. This chapter complements this material by focusing upon some more general aspects of the care of parents within the neonatal unit. Some interventions are considered that we know help parents and families increase their coping strategies, enhance their experiences of parenthood in a neonatal unit and support the integration of

these experiences into their self-identity. Finally, some implications for practice are suggested and a summary draws all of these points together.

Becoming a parent

Becoming a parent marks an important life-course transition for women and men[1-4]. The transition to parenthood affects an individual's sense of self-identity and esteem[5-8]. In the UK around 8–13% of all newborn babies will be admitted to a neonatal unit, with approximately 1–3% requiring the full utilisation of intensive care resources that a neonatal intensive care unit (NICU) can provide[9-12]. Consequently, in the UK this means that around

80,000 families per year will experience becoming a parent for the first or subsequent time whilst also having to cope with the challenges of their child being admitted to a neonatal unit.

Despite considerable progress in reducing mortality and morbidity, preterm birth remains an important epidemiological concern[13–16]. There is also evidence of persistent socioeconomic deprivation in families of babies born with low birthweight or at less than thirty-two weeks gestation[17–22]. As a consequence, some families in the neonatal unit may already be facing the effects of pre-existing socioeconomic disadvantage and admission to the neonatal unit may exacerbate or create additional social, economic and emotional burdens for these families.

One of the central characteristics of parenthood transition is the development of social bonds between parents and their children. The human infant social bond starts in early pregnancy, through the embodied experience of pregnancy and childbirth, changes in social status (the expectant mother and father) and pregnancy confirmation through technology[23,24]. These social bonds tend to strengthen through time following birth and throughout life. The structure of these social bonds is influenced by a number of factors, including gender, socioeconomic status and life experiences within an evolving cross-cultural belief system. Within maternity and neonatal care, two separate, yet linked social theories have received widespread acceptance and informed clinical practice. These are:

- 'Attachment theory'
- 'Bonding theory'

Social theories

Attachment theory

In 1965 John Bowlby, a psychoanalyst, published the second edition of an abridged and amended version of the 1951 World Health Organisation report, *Maternal Care and Mental Health* that he had previously authored[25,26]. According to Bowlby, differences between individuals' 'security' of attachment during childhood are important in later life, in that they provide a template for future adult relationships. Bowlby supports his theory with reference to a considerable number of empirical studies by researchers within psychoanalysis and other fields[27–29]. His work has become highly influential in shaping practices within health care, including maternity and neonatal care.

Bonding theory

The central concept of Klaus and Kennell's 'bonding theory' was that early physical contact between a mother and infant acted as a trigger for innate attachment behaviours, and that separation during the 'critical' or 'sensitive' period shortly after birth could alienate mothers from their infants[30]. Unfortunately, Klaus and Kennell's early work contains flaws, both methodically and conceptually; their original research consisted of a small sample size of only 28 mothers and they developed their theory from animal studies that may not have had direct relevance to primates. Nevertheless, Klaus and Kennell's work has become highly influential in many maternity and neonatal units[31,32]. For example, their nine steps to promoting bonding, including such steps as pregnancy confirmation, seeing, touching and caregiving have become widely established within practice.

It is important to point out that there is not a single theory of social bonding or attachment. Earlier ideas have being elaborated upon and modified (either by design or accident) to reflect changing social norms, experiences, expectations and understandings by other writers[33]. These theories can be interpreted as perpetuating the view that women are and should be, responsible for both childbearing and childrearing and that fathers' roles should exist on the margins of childcare. Whilst such views concerning gender based parenting distinctions exist, they no longer retain their once universal status. In part, this erosion of 'traditional' gender based role distinction has come about due to a number of pervasive changes in society that have taken place within the latter part of the twentieth century. These include key social changes such as increased urbanisation and mobility, geographical, social and economic. In addition, at a personal level the last fifty years have seen increasing diversity of family structures and increased participation of women in paid work outside the home, all of which have an effect upon parenting roles.

Newer ideas and models of parenting, particularly relating to fatherhood have become established in recent years[34-37]. These newer paradigms of parenthood bring into question some ideas about the formation of social bonds between infants and their parents, a situation acknowledged in part by changes to the titles of Klaus and Kennel's books and contents of later editions of Bowlby's work[38,39-41]. However, despite these criticisms and misgivings, both attachment and bonding theory have made significant contributions to improving the experiences of parents and their children in hospital institutions, including neonatal units.

Experiences of parents in neonatal units

The admission of a baby to a neonatal unit is a stressful event in parents' lives. This conclusion is supported by a considerable body of empirical research[42,43-56]. In research, more attention has been paid to the experiences and needs of mothers of healthy full-term infants within maternity care than with mothers of preterm infants. In the past, fathers' experiences also received relatively less detailed study[57]. However, increasingly exceptions exist where fathers have formed the focus of studies. Some of these studies have focused upon fathers' experiences in the early neonatal period or neonatal units[58-64].

The precise nature of the expectations and aspirations of parents of infants within neonatal units remains poorly understood. Much of the neonatal

parent research has focused upon identifying and measuring sources of stress and anxiety in parents. Earlier studies[65-74], identified a number of common features that prompted anxiety in parents. These included:

- Communication with professionals
- Ambiguity of roles
- Power and control
- Concerns over morbidity, mortality and the appearance of the infant

Later studies[75-95], using different methods and approaches have replicated and added to our understanding. Because of this research activity, the experience of stress by parents in the neonatal unit is widely recognised to consist of a number of components related to:

- The neonatal environment
- The individual emotional experiences
- Parents' perceptions
- Parents' previous experiences and experiences in the neonatal unit
- Parents' personal characteristics
- The reasons for the infant's admission
- The infant's premature appearance

The effects of the environment

Parents' perceptions of the neonatal environment have an important bearing upon their experiences in a neonatal unit. The physical environment of the neonatal unit is comprised of two main elements:

- Clinical spaces
- Non-clinical spaces

Clinical spaces within the neonatal unit are generally recognised as a source of stress[57,78]. This is not the case for all parents; for some mothers, the physical appearance of their baby left them, at the time, comparatively unconcerned with aspects of the physical environment[96-98].

These negative effects of the clinical environment can to some extent be alleviated by paying attention to ensuring that the non-clinical (parent and family) spaces within the unit provide a 'parent friendly' environment. At present in the UK, Redshaw recognises that the provision of a 'parent friendly' environment varies considerably between units[99]. One of the factors in this variability is that a precise understanding about what constitutes a parent friendly environment is lacking. For some parents it is perfectly possible that the 'high tech' environment of the neonatal unit can be a source of reassurance that their infant is in the best place to receive the best possible treatment and care. Ferketich and Mercer in a study of fathers' role behaviours towards their infants have contended that nurses should provide enjoyable environments for fathers by considering their goals and feelings and consequently help them to negotiate the social system to increase participation[100]. This research clearly implies that a parent friendly environment consists of more than the physical space, its decor and furnishing, and includes intangible elements like ambience and organisational culture.

Emotional responses to the neonatal unit experience

During pregnancy, parents make plans for their unborn child with an expectation of a normal healthy term infant[101-104]. However, the onset of preterm labour and delivery often precipitates a crisis in families and marks a loss of control over events, with a subsequent need to redefine their expectations. During this time, emotions are intense and include[105-115]:

- Feelings of shock
- Confusion
- Abandonment
- Powerlessness
- Anticipatory grief
- Guilt
- Blame seeking

Parents can at times verbalise these concerns by referring to the infant's appearance, likelihood of survival, pain, fears over attachment and separation, but at other times they will indirectly communicate them. There is some evidence to suggest that the mother's health status, her own attitudes and feelings influence her recall of her relationship with her baby. Women who are ill, and experience instrumental deliveries, for example, tend to describe their motherhood experiences in less positive terms[116-118].

Conflict between parents and health care staff concerning the making of decisions about the infants' care and treatment has been reported in a number of studies[119-121], as have a range of strategies to manage them[122-124]. The source of such conflicts can be interpreted in a number of ways; poor communication may be a feature of some, whilst others can be understood in terms of power relationships between parents and staff. These disagreements could represent an attempt by parents to reassert some element of control over the situation they find themselves in. Overall, it seems that the sources of these conflicts seem to relate as much to the organisational culture of the unit under study as to individual staff behaviours that are seemingly working in opposition to how parents perceive they should be.

Men are often characterised as being less emotionally expressive than women are when faced with similar situations[125,126]. When faced with emotionally difficult situations like those following birth and admission, some men respond to this apparent 'public scrutiny' of their emotional experience by adopting stereotypical masculine responses and avoiding overt displays of emotion that they view as unmasculine. While such tensions are evident in everyday practice, they are not well acknowledged within the neonatal literature. They can affect men's relationships with others, particularly their partners, their sense of self and their roles as fathers. Individual differences aside, the overwhelming response of many parents, including fathers, to admission of their infant is one of shock and disconnection from everyday life[127-133].

Whilst the majority of the infants in a neonatal unit are classified as preterm, an important part of the admission profile and work of many neonatal units consists of ill term or near/post-term infants. Few studies have sought to consider the experience and needs of this group of parents alone. Nyström and Axelsson studied mothers separated from their full-term infants following admission to a neonatal unit[134]. It is interesting to note that the experiences of these mothers of full-term infants are very similar to those reported elsewhere by mothers and fathers of preterm infants. Such findings suggest that there are some common components to parental emotional experience in a neonatal unit regardless of the reason for their infant's admission. Whilst acknowledging these needs and experience is important, it is perhaps more important to develop interventions that accentuate the positive whilst minimising the adverse effect associated with admission to a neonatal unit.

Things that help: practical and emotional

The Platt Report[135], has perhaps become one of the most widely recognised and influential reports affecting parents and their children in hospitals. Platt made use of evidence from the work of Bowlby and colleagues[136], such as Robertson's films and earlier writing[137,138], in his report, to bring about dramatic changes in parental access to their children in hospitals. Whilst this report had the greatest impact on children's wards, it also had significant effects upon neonatal care. Institutional changes saw a conceptual move away from parents as visitors towards parents as partners.

A fundamental goal expressed by many neonatal nurses is to facilitate 'family centred care'. The concept is based upon the premise of the family as a system of reciprocal relationships. To provide effective care for an individual within a health care setting it is important also to consider and address the effects upon family members. In this, it implies that service delivery always considers the needs of all family members. Despite the widespread acknowledgement of family centred care as a guiding principle within much paediatric and neonatal nursing care there is limited empirical evidence of either its benefits or its successful application.

Current understanding and application of family centred care reflects a number of different interpretations of what it means and what it constitutes[139–142]. It seems that family centred care and the institutional practices that it brings about exist along a spectrum. These differing understandings and applications within clinical practice affect the experience of care services and may be an important source of tension, complaint and disquiet. Of central concern to many neonatal nurses is the question: how do they deal with what are at times conflicting or exclusive needs, demands and expectations?

For example, in child protection issues the needs of the infant may outweigh the desires or expectations of the family, or one family's needs may conflict with another family's. In these sort of situations nurses can at times tend to fall back upon a patriarchal perspective and take an infant or organisational centred approach which can lead to a marginalisation of parents and a diminishing of their feelings of control and empowerment.

Communication between neonatal nurses and parents can be a considerable source of stress [143–148]. A number of approaches and strategies have been used to enhance the effectiveness of communication between staff and parents; many of these seem to be successful in this aim. Many parents make use of a variety of approaches to gather information to aid their understanding[149–151]. The use of supplemental written and visual materials to aid verbal explanations is routine practice within most neonatal units. The charity BLISS (Baby Life Support Systems) make available a wide range of literature to parents and staff to better promote parents and staff to engage in dialogue and collaboration[152,153].

Counselling is a word often used within health care; it is used to describe a variety of different interventions, techniques and philosophical perspectives. Whilst psychoanalytical approaches have established themselves in some areas of neo-natal practice, they are not widespread. There are a number of national charities (BLISS, for example) and locally focused charities (ADAPT – All Dependent and Preterm infants, for example) who support families by facilitating social communication between parents as well as offering financial support for travel.

Success in managing actual or potential conflicts is enhanced through using interventions that increase parents' understanding of clinically relevant information. This has been demonstrated by Peticuff and Arbeart's evaluation of an 'infant progression chart' and 'parent-professional planning meetings'[154]. The success of techniques to increase parents' knowledge and understanding is unsurprising. Much communication between parents and staff is characterised by information sharing, negotiating and providing emotional support. A major component of communication involves emotional support. Nurse-parent interactions form an important part in enhancing emotional support and positive experiences of the neonatal unit[155–157]. An important element of this emotional support comprises of social talk – 'chatting'. This sort of talk is seemingly an attempt to normalise parents' experiences through culturally based references to the everyday world. It is not something that happens between every parent and every member of staff; if it were to do so staff would be open to accusations of what sociologists refer to as inauthentic. Nevertheless, in spite of these risks social talk can make a significant contribution to parents' assessments of a nurse's competence beyond immediate technical prowess and may form a route through which parents can move from alienation towards familiarity [158, 159].

There is a large body of research, mainly psychological and psychoanalytical, that recognises the adverse effects of separation, particularly upon the mother-child relationship and the development of social bonds, both in general[160–163], and specifically within neonatal units[164–171].

Consequently, through education and socialisation, many neonatal nurses subscribe to a belief that early physical contact with the infant promotes parental attachment. A number of reviewers promote interventions to facilitate early physical and psychological contact with their baby[172–177]. There is some empirical evidence to support the efficacy of such interventions in promoting maternal attachment, reducing abandonment, increasing breast-feeding success, for example, together with a number of specific infant health benefits. Interestingly, the benefits of early physical contact also relate to fathers[178,179]. Sullivan's Australian study and Lundqvist and Jakobsson's Swedish study both report that fathers relayed greater feelings of attachment after holding their infant than before they had done so[180,181]. Concrete experience, rather than abstract notions, at least for fathers, seems to be an important element in developing relationships with their infant.

It is important to recognise that there is a gap between how parents themselves perceive and understand events in the neonatal unit and how staff perceive these same things, as well as issues of emotional attachment and detachment (sometimes identified as professionalism) about these events. Parents' actions and behaviours should not be viewed in isolation as responding to particular stimuli and events but must be interpreted within a cultural framework of shared understandings and assumptions with issues of knowledge, power, relationships and gender coming into play.

Implications for practice

Given the diverse nature of parents, their experiences, needs and desires, together with equal diversity in neonatal nurses and neonatal units, all-purpose interventions are in all likelihood unattainable. Nevertheless, despite these reservations, there is a diverse body of literature and study that suggests that parents want or might benefit from particular approaches to care delivery. These include:

- Neonatal nurses must work with parents to determine a meaningful definition of what constitutes a family friendly environment; elements of domesticity balanced with the messages that a 'high tech' environment convey need to be sought.
- Interventions that aim to increase an individual parent's coping strategies through developing empathy, sensitivity, understanding and developing links to the everyday world beyond the neonatal unit.
- Nursing competence within the neonatal unit is more than about technical skill alone; humanistic qualities feature strongly in parents' assessments of staff competence.
- Staff who have an awareness of their own behaviour and attitudes and the important effect that these may have upon others seem better able to support parents.

Conclusion

Family care makes up a significant part of the neonatal literature. A number of concepts that relate to family care have become established: academically, in practice and in social policy. Whilst physical care and technical care are important elements of neonatal nurse competence, equally important attention needs to be paid towards the emotional care of parents, other and self.

Each parent has a unique experience and perspective upon the care of their baby. Increasingly, neonatal units are faced with a heterogeneous parent population and the variable parent needs and expectations that generates. An individual's stress experience is both reactive and interactive, reflecting and shaping their everyday interaction with others and their self-regulation. Consequently, it is important to observe parents, ask them and others who know them better to decide upon an optimum strategy for promoting parental involvement and social bonding. Sometimes, acknowledging the experience is all that is required, rather than seeking to mitigate its effects.

References

1. Cowan CP, Cowan PA, Heming G, *et al.* (1985) Transitions to parenthood: his, hers and theirs. *Journal of Family Issues*, **6** (4), 451–481.
2. Berman P, Pedersen F (eds) (1987) *Men's transitions to parenthood: Longitudinal Studies of Early Family Experience*. Lawrence Erlbaum, Hillsdale NJ.
3. Draper J (2003) Men's passage to fatherhood: an analysis of the contemporary relevance of transition theory. *Nursing Inquiry*, **10** (1), 66–78.
4. Reeves J (2006) Recklessness, rescue and responsibility: young men tell their stories of the transition to fatherhood. *Practice*, **18** (2), 79–90.
5. Henderson AD, Brouse AJ (1991) The experiences of new fathers during the first 3 weeks of life. *Journal of Advanced Nursing*, **16** (3), 293–298.
6. Reid TL (2000) Maternal identity in preterm birth. *Journal of Child Health Care*, **4** (1), 23–29.
7. Finnbogadóttir H, Crang Svalenius E, Persson EK (2003) Expectant first time fathers' experiences of pregnancy. *Midwifery*, **19** (2), 96–105.
8. Miller T (2007) 'Is this what motherhood is all about?' Weaving experiences and discourse through transition to first-time motherhood. *Gender and Society*, **21** (3), 337–358.
9. BLISS, the premature baby charity (2005) Special Care for Sick Babies – Choice or Chance? The BLISS Baby Report No. 1. http://www.bliss.org.uk (accessed 5 August 2005).
10. Redshaw ME, Hamilton K (2005) *A Survey of Current Neonatal Unit Organisation and Policy*. National Perinatal Epidemiology Unit (NPEU), Oxford.
11. BLISS, the premature baby charity. *Weigh Less, Worth Less? A Study of Neonatal Care in the UK*. The BLISS Baby Report No. 2. http://www.bliss.org.uk (accessed 12 August 2006).
12. BLISS, The premature baby charity. *Too Little, Too Late? Are We Ensuring the Best Start for Babies Born Too Soon?* The BLISS Baby Report No 3. http://www.bliss.org.uk (accessed 2 November 2007).
13. Hille ETM, den Ouden AL, Saigal S, *et al.* (2001) Behavioural problems in children who weigh 1000 g or less at birth in four countries. *Lancet*, **357** (9269), 1641–1643.
14. Davis L, Mohay H, Edwards H (2003) Mothers' involvement in caring for their premature

infants: an historical overview. *Journal of Advanced Nursing*, **42** (6), 578–586.

15. Whitfield MF (2003) Psychosocial effects of intensive care on infants and families after discharge. *Seminars in Neonatology*, **8** (2), 185–193.

16. Wood NS, Costeloe K, Gibson AT, Hennessy EM, Marlow N, Wilkinson AR, for the EPICure Study Group (2005) The EPICure study: associations and antecedents of neurological and developmental disability at 30 months of age following extremely preterm birth. *Archives of Disease in Childhood Fetal and Neonatal Edition*, **90** (1), F134–F140.

17. McLoughlin A, Hillier VF, Robinson MJ (1993) Parental costs of neonatal visiting. *Archives of Disease in Childhood*, **68** (5 Spec No.), 597–599.

18. Bartley M, Power C, Blane D, Davey-Smith G, Shipley M (1994) Birth weight and later socio-economic disadvantage: evidence from the 1958 British cohort study. *BMJ*, **309** (6967), 1457–1459.

19. Cronin C (2003) First time mothers: identifying the needs, perceptions and experiences. *Journal of Clinical Nursing*, **12** (2), 260–267.

20. Manning D, Brewster B, Bundrel P (2005) Social depravation and admission for neonatal care. *Archives of Disease in Childhood Fetal and Neonatal Edition*, **90** (4), F337–F338.

21. Petrou, S (2005) The economic consequences of preterm birth during the first ten years of life in 'The next step forward in reducing the impact of preterm labour' Proceedings of the 2nd international preterm labour congress (2–4/9/04) Montréux Switzerland. *British Journal of Obstetrics and Gynaecology*, **112** (supplement 1), 10–15.

22. Smith LK, Draper ES, Manktelow BN, Dorling JS, Field DJ (2007) Socioeconomic inequalities in very preterm birth rates. *Archives of Disease in Childhood Fetal and Neonatal Edition*, **92** (1), F11–F14.

23. Draper J (2002) 'It's the first scientific evidence': men's experience of pregnancy confirmation. *Journal of Advanced Nursing*, **39** (6), 563–570.

24. Draper J (2002). 'It was a real good show': the ultrasound scan, fathers and the power of visual knowledge. *Sociology of Health and Illness*, **24** (6), 771–795.

25. Bowlby J (1965) *Child Care and the Growth of Love*, 2nd edn. Penguin, Harmondsworth.

26. Bowlby J (1951) *Maternal Care and Mental Health*. World Health Organisation, Geneva.

27. Bowlby J (1975) *Attachment and Loss: Volume 2: Separation: Anxiety and Anger*. Pelican, London.

28. Bowlby J (1984) *Attachment and Loss: Volume 1: Attachment*. 2nd edn. Penguin, Harmondsworth.

29. Bowlby J (2005) *A Secure Base: Clinical Applications of Attachment Theory*. Routledge Classics, London.

30. Klaus MH, Kennell JH (1976) *Maternal-infant Bonding*. CV Mosby Company, St Louis.

31. Klaus MH, Kennell JH (1976) *Maternal-infant Bonding*. CV Mosby Company, St Louis.

32. Klaus MH, Kennell JH (1982) *Parent Infant Bonding*, 2nd edn. CV Mosby Company, St Louis.

33. Robertson J, Robertson J (1989) *Separation and the Very Young*. Free Association Books, London.

34. Daly KJ (1995) Reshaping fatherhood: finding the models. In: Marsiglio W (ed.), *Fatherhood: Contemporary Theory, Research, and Social Policy*. Sage, Thousand Oaks CA. Chapter 2 pp. 21–40.

35. Lewis C (2000) *A Man's Place in the Home: Fathers and Families in the UK*. Family Policy Study Centre and Joseph Rowntree Foundation, London and York.

36. O'Brien M (2005) *Shared Caring: Bringing Fathers into the Frame*. Working Paper Series 18. Equal Opportunities Commission, Manchester.

37. Burgess A (2007) *The Costs and Benefits of Active Fatherhood: Evidence and Insights to Inform the Development of Policy and Practice*. Fathers Direct, London.

38. Bowlby J (1965) *Child Care and the Growth of Love*, 2nd edn. Penguin, Harmondsworth.

39. Bowlby J (2005) *A Secure Base: Clinical Applications of Attachment Theory*. Routledge Classics, London.

40. Klaus MH, Kennell JH (1976) *Maternal-infant Bonding*. CV Mosby Company, St Louis.

41. Klaus MH, Kennell JH (1982) *Parent Infant Bonding*, 2nd edn. CV Mosby Company, St Louis.

42. Cronin C (2003) First time mothers: identifying the needs, perceptions and experiences. *Journal of Clinical Nursing*, **12** (2), 260–267.

43. Miles MS (1990) Parents of critically ill premature infants: sources of stress. *Critical Care Nursing Quarterly*, **12** (3), 69–74.

44. Affonso DD, Hurst I, Mayberry LJ, Haller L, Yost K, Lynch ME (1992) Stressors reported by mothers of hospitalised premature infants. *Neonatal Network*, **11** (6), 63–70.

45. Redshaw ME, Harris A (1995) Maternal perceptions of neonatal care. *Acta Paediatrica*, **84** (6), 593–598.

46. Redshaw ME, Harris A, Ingram JC (1996) *Delivering Neonatal Care: the Neonatal Unit as a Working Environment: a Survey of Neonatal Nursing*. HMSO, London.

47. Redshaw ME (1998) Mothers of babies requiring special care: attitudes and experiences. *Journal of Reproductive and Infant Psychology*, **15** (2), 109–110.

48. Singer LT, Salvator A, Guo S, Collin M, Lilien L, Baley J (1999) Maternal psychological stress after the birth of a very low birth weight infant. *Journal of the American Medical Association*, **281** (9), 799–805.

49. Doering LV, Dracup K, Moser D (1999) Comparison of psychosocial adjustment of mothers and fathers of high-risk infants in the neonatal intensive care unit. *Journal of Perinatology*, **19** (2), 132–137.

50. Doering LV, Moser DK, Dracup K (2000) Correlates of anxiety, hostility, depression and psychosocial adjustment in parents of NICU infants. *Neonatal Network*, **19** (5), 15–23.

51. Fenwick J, Barclay L, Schmied V (2001) Struggling to mother: a consequence of inhibitive nursing interactions in the neonatal nursery. *Journal of Perinatal and Neonatal Nursing*, **15** (2), 49–64.

52. Holditch-Davis D, Miles MS (2000) Mothers' stories about their experiences in the neonatal intensive care unit. *Neonatal Network*, **19** (3), 13–21.

53. Cohen M (2003) *Sent Before My Time: a Child Psychotherapist's View of Life on a Neonatal Intensive Care Unit*. Karnac, London.

54. Holditch-Davis D, Bartlett TR, Blackman AL, Miles MS (2003) Post-traumatic stress symptoms in mothers of premature infants. *Journal of Obstetric, Gynaecological and Neonatal Nursing*, **32** (2), 161–171.

55. Carter JD, Mulder RT, Bartram AF, Darlow BA (2005) Infants in a neonatal intensive care unit: parental response. *Archives of Disease in Childhood Fetal and Neonatal Edition*, **90** (1), F109–F113.

56. Ringland CP (2008) Post-traumatic stress disorder and the NICU graduate mother. *Infant*, **4** (1), 14–17.

57. Carter JD, Mulder RT, Bartram AF, Darlow BA (2005) Infants in a neonatal intensive care unit: parental response. *Archives of Disease in Childhood Fetal and Neonatal Edition*, **90** (1), F109–F113.

58. Henderson AD, Brouse AJ (1991) The experiences of new fathers during the first 3 weeks of life. *Journal of Advanced Nursing*, **16** (3), 293–298.

59. Finnbogadóttir H, Crang Svalenius E, Persson EK (2003) Expectant first time fathers' experiences of pregnancy. *Midwifery*, **19** (2), 96–105.

60. Levy-Shiff R, Hoffman MA, Mogilner S, Levingner S, Mogilner MB (1990) Fathers' hospital visits to their preterm infants as a predictor of father-infant relationships and infant development. *Pediatrics*, **86** (2), 289–293.

61. Vehviläinen-Julkunen K, Liukkonen A (1998) Fathers' experiences of childbirth. *Midwifery*, **14** (1), 10–17.

62. Sullivan JR (1999) Development of father-infant attachment in fathers of preterm infants. *Neonatal Network*, **18** (7), 33–39.

63. Lundqvist P, Jakobsson L (2003) Swedish men's experiences of becoming fathers to their preterm infants. *Neonatal Network*, **22** (6), 25–31.

64. Ferketich SL, Mercer RT (1995) Predictors of role competence for experienced and inexperienced fathers. *Nursing Research*, **44** (2), 89–95.

65. Burgess A (2007) *The Costs and Benefits of Active Fatherhood: Evidence and Insights to Inform the Development of Policy and Practice*. Fathers Direct, London.

66. Bowlby J (1965) *Child Care and the Growth of Love*, 2nd edn. Penguin, Harmondsworth.

67. Bowlby J (2005) *A Secure Base: Clinical Applications of Attachment Theory*. Routledge Classics, London.

68. Levy-Shiff R, Mogilner MB, Sharir H (1989) Mother-father-preterm infant relationship in the hospital preterm nursery. *Child Development*, **60** (1), 96–102.

69. Perehudoff B (1990) Parents' perceptions of environmental stressors in the special care nursery. *Neonatal Network*, **9** (2), 39–44.

70. McHaffie HE (1992) Social support in the neonatal intensive care unit. *Journal of Advanced Nursing*, **17** (3), 279–287.

71. McHaffie HE (1992) Staff perceptions of family needs in neonatal units. *Journal of Clinical Nursing*, **1** (1), 49–50.

72. Redman C (1993) Putting the family back in control: neonatal intensive care units and the emotional needs of families. *Child Health*, **1** (3), 112–116.

73. Shellabarger SG, Thompson TL (1993) The critical times: meeting parental communication needs throughout the NICU experience. *Neonatal Network*, **12** (2), 39–44.

74. Cronin CM, Shapiro CR, Casiro OG, Cheang MS (1995) The impact of very low birth weight infants on the family is long lasting: a matched controlled case study. *Archives of Pediatric Adolescent Medicine*, **149** (2), 151–158.

75. Redshaw ME, Harris A (1995) Maternal perceptions of neonatal care. *Acta Paediatrica*, **84** (6), 593–598.

76. Fenwick J, Barclay L, Schmeid V (2001) Struggling to mother: a consequence of inhibitive nursing interactions in the neonatal nursery. *Journal of Perinatal and Neonatal Nursing*, **15** (2), 49–64.

77. Holditch-Davis D, Miles MS (2000) Mothers' stories about their experiences in the neonatal intensive care unit. *Neonatal Network*, **19** (3), 13–21.

78. Holditch-Davis D, Bartlett TR, Blackman AL, Miles MS (2003) Post-traumatic stress symptoms in mothers of premature infants. *Journal of Obstetric, Gynaecological and Neonatal Nursing*, **32** (2), 161–171.

79. Miles MS, Holditch-Davis D (1997) Parenting the prematurely born child: pathways of influence. *Seminars in Perinatology*, **21** (3), 254–266.

80. Padden T, Glenn S (1997) Maternal experiences of preterm birth and neonatal intensive care. *Journal of Reproductive and Infant Psychology*, **15** (2), 21–40.

81. Shields-Poe D, Pinelli J (1997) Variables associated with parental stress in neonatal intensive care. *Neonatal Network*, **16** (1), 29–37.

82. Bruns DA, McCollum JA (2002) Partnerships between mothers and professional in the NICU: caregiving, information exchange and relationships. *Neonatal Network*, **21** (7), 15–23.

83. Franck LS, Spencer C (2003) Parent visiting and participation in infant care giving activities in a neonatal unit. *Birth*, **30** (1), 31–35.

84. Jackson K, Ternestedt B-M, Schollin J (2003) From alienation to familiarity: experiences of mothers and fathers of preterm infants. *Journal of Advanced Nursing*, **43** (2), 120–129.

85. Morawski Mew A, Holditch-Davis D, Belyea M, Shandor-Miles S, Fishel A (2003) Correlates of depressive symptoms in mothers of preterm infants. *Neonatal Network*, **22** (5), 51–60.

86. Franck CS (2005) Measuring neonatal intensive care unit related parental stress. *Journal of Advanced Nursing*, **49** (6), 608–615.

87. Flacking R, Ewald U, Hedberg Nyqvist K, Starrin B (2006) Trustful bonds: a key to 'becoming a mother' and to reciprocal breastfeeding. Stories of mothers of very preterm infants at a neonatal unit. *Social Science and Medicine*, **62** (1), 70–80.

88. Wigert H, Johansson R, Berg M, Hellström AL (2006) Mothers' experiences of having their newborn child in a neonatal intensive care unit. *Scandinavian Journal of Caring Science*, **20** (1), 35–41.

89. Lam J, Spence K, Halliday R (2007) Parents' perception of nursing support in the neonatal intensive care unit (NICU). *Neonatal Paediatric and Child Health Nursing*, **10** (3), 19–25.

90. Reid T, Bramwell R, Booth N, Weindling AM (2007) A new stressor scale for parents experiencing neonatal intensive care: the NUPS (Neonatal Unit Parental Stress) Scale. *Journal of Infant and Reproductive Psychology*, **25**, 66–82.

91. Fenwick J, Barclay L, Schmeid V (2001) 'Chatting': an important clinical tool in facilitating mothering in neonatal nurseries. *Journal of Advanced Nursing*, **33** (5), 583–593.

92. Nyström K, Axelsson K (2002) Mothers' experience of being separated from their newborns. *Journal of Obstetric, Gynaecological and Neonatal Nursing*, **31** (3), 275–282.

93. Pridham K, Lin C-Y, Brown R (2001) Mothers' evaluation of their care giving for premature and full-term infants through the first year: contributing factors. *Research in Nursing and Health*, **24** (3), 157–169.

94. Raeside L (1997) Perceptions of environmental stressors in the NNU. *British Journal of Nursing*, **6** (16), 914–923.

95. Shaw RJ, Deblois T, Ikuta L, Ginzburg K, Fleisher B, Koopman C (2006) Acute stress disorder among parents of infants in the neonatal intensive care nursery. *Psychosomatics*, **47** (3), 206–212.

96. Redshaw ME, Harris A (1995) Maternal perceptions of neonatal care. *Acta Paediatrica*, **84** (6), 593–598.

97. Redshaw ME (1998) Mothers of babies requiring special care: attitudes and experiences. *Journal of Reproductive and Infant Psychology*, **15** (2), 109–110.

98. Padden T, Glenn S (1997) Maternal experiences of preterm birth and neonatal intensive care. *Journal of Reproductive and Infant Psychology*, **15** (2), 21–40.

99. Redshaw ME (2005) Commentary. *Archives of Disease in Childhood: Fetal and Neonatal Edition*, **90** (1), F96.

100. Ferketich SL, Mercer RT (1995) Predictors of role competence for experienced and inexperienced fathers. *Nursing Research*, **44** (2), 89–95.

101. Draper J (2003) Men's passage to fatherhood: an analysis of the contemporary relevance of transition theory. *Nursing Inquiry*, **10** (1), 66–78.

102. Draper J (2002) 'It's the first scientific evidence': men's experience of pregnancy confirmation. *Journal of Advanced Nursing*, **39** (6), 563–570.

103. Draper J (2002). 'It was a real good show': the ultrasound scan, fathers and the power of visual knowledge. *Sociology of Health and Illness*, **24** (6), 771–795.

104. Sullivan JR (1999) Development of father-infant attachment in fathers of preterm infants. *Neonatal Network*, **18** (7), 33–39.

105. Whitfield MF (2003) Psychosocial effects of intensive care on infants and families after discharge. *Seminars in Neonatology*, **8** (2), 185–193.

106. Burgess A (2007) *The Costs and Benefits of Active Fatherhood: Evidence and Insights to Inform the Development of Policy and Practice*. Fathers Direct, London.

107. Redshaw ME (1998) Mothers of babies requiring special care: attitudes and experiences. *Journal of Reproductive and Infant Psychology*, **15** (2), 109–110.

108. Doering LV, Moser DK, Dracup K (2000) Correlates of anxiety, hostility, depression and psychosocial adjustment in parents of NICU infants. *Neonatal Network*, **19** (5), 15–23.

109. Fenwick J, Barclay L, Schmeid V (2001) Struggling to mother: a consequence of inhibitive nursing interactions in the neonatal nursery. *Journal of Perinatal and Neonatal Nursing*, **15** (2), 49–64.

110. Holditch-Davis D, Miles MS (2000) Mothers' stories about their experiences in the neonatal intensive care unit. *Neonatal Network*, **19** (3), 13–21.

111. Cohen M (2003) *Sent Before My Time: a Child Psychotherapist's View of Life on a Neonatal Intensive Care Unit*. Karnac, London.

112. Holditch-Davis D, Bartlett TR, Blackman AL, Miles MS (2003) Post-traumatic stress symptoms in mothers of premature infants. *Journal of Obstetric, Gynaecological and Neonatal Nursing*, **32** (2), 161–171.

113. Ringland CP (2008) Post-traumatic stress disorder and the NICU graduate mother. *Infant*, **4** (1), 14–17.

114. Wigert H, Johansson R, Berg M, Hellström AL (2006) Mothers' experiences of having their newborn child in a neonatal intensive care unit. *Scandinavian Journal of Caring Science*, **20** (1), 35–41.

115. Shaw RJ, Deblois T, Ikuta L, Ginzburg K, Fleisher B, Koopman C (2006) Acute stress disorder among parents of infants in the neonatal intensive care nursery. *Psychosomatics*, **47** (3), 206–212.

116. Pridham K, Lin C-Y, Brown R (2001) Mothers' evaluation of their care giving for premature and full-term infants through the first year: contributing factors. *Research in Nursing and Health*, **24** (3), 157–169.

117. Oakley A, Richards MPM (1990) Elective delivery attitudes and responses of parents of children. In: Garcia J, Kilpatrick R, Richards MPM (eds) *The Politics of Maternity Care*. Oxford University Press, Oxford. Chapter 10, pp. 183–201.

118. Garcia J, Redshaw M, Fitzsimons B, Keene J (1998) *First Class Delivery: a National Survey of Women's Views of Maternity Care*. Audit Commission, London.

119. Holditch-Davis D, Miles MS (2000) Mothers' stories about their experiences in the neonatal intensive care unit. *Neonatal Network*, **19** (3), 13–21.

120. Fenwick J, Barclay L, Schmeid V (2001) 'Chatting': an important clinical tool in facilitating mothering in neonatal nurseries. *Journal of Advanced Nursing*, **33** (5), 583–593.

121. Alderson P, Hawthorne J, Killen M (2006) Parents' experiences of sharing neonatal information and decisions: consent, cost and risk. *Social Science and Medicine*, **62** (6), 1319–1329.

122. Alderson P, Hawthorne J, Killen M (2006) Parents' experiences of sharing neonatal information and decisions: consent, cost and risk. *Social Science and Medicine*, **62** (6), 1319–1329.

123. Costeloe K, Wilkinson AR (1998) Managing potential conflicts amongst professionals and parents responsible for the care of sick babies. *Seminars in Neonatology*, **3** (4), 323.

124. Peticuff JH, Arbeart KL (2005) Effectiveness of an intervention to improve parent-professional collaboration in neonatal intensive care. *Journal of Perinatal and Neonatal Nursing*, **19** (20), 187–202.

125. Duncombe J, Marsden D (1998) 'Stepford wives' and 'hollow men'? Doing emotion work, doing gender and 'authenticity' in intimate heterosexual relationships. In: Bendelow G, Williams SJ (eds) *Emotions in Social Life*. Routledge, London. Chapter 12, pp. 211–227.

126. Duncombe J, Marsden D (1999) Love and intimacy: the gender division of emotion and 'emotion work': a neglected aspect of sociological discussion of heterosexual relationships. In: Allan G (ed.) *The Sociology of the Family: a Reader*. Blackwell, Oxford. Chapter 4, pp. 91–110.

127. Henderson AD, Brouse AJ (1991) The experiences of new fathers during the first 3 weeks of life. *Journal of Advanced Nursing*, **16** (3), 293–298.

128. Finnbogadóttir H, Crang Svalenius E, Persson EK (2003) Expectant first time fathers' experiences of pregnancy. *Midwifery*, **19** (2), 96–105.

129. Redshaw ME (1998) Mothers of babies requiring special care: attitudes and experiences. *Journal of Reproductive and Infant Psychology*, **15** (2), 109–110.

130. Vehviläinen-Julkunen K, Liukkonen A (1998) Fathers' experiences of childbirth. *Midwifery*, **14** (1), 10–17.

131. Lundqvist P, Jakobsson L (2003) Swedish men's experiences of becoming fathers to their preterm infants. *Neonatal Network*, **22** (6), 25–31.

132. Wigert H, Johansson R, Berg M, Hellström AL (2006) Mothers' experiences of having their newborn child in a neonatal intensive care unit. *Scandinavian Journal of Caring Science*, **20** (1), 35–41.

133. Nyström K, Axelsson K (2002) Mothers' experience of being separated from their newborns. *Journal of Obstetric, Gynaecological and Neonatal Nursing*, **31** (3), 275–282.

134. Nyström K, Axelsson K (2002) Mothers' experience of being separated from their newborns. *Journal of Obstetric, Gynaecological and Neonatal Nursing*, **31** (3), 275–282.

135. Ministry of Health. Chair Platt (1959) *The Welfare of Children in Hospital (The Platt Report)*. Ministry of Health, London.

136. Bowlby J (1951) *Maternal Care and Mental Health*. World Health Organisation, Geneva.

137. Robertson J, Robertson J (1989) *Separation and the Very Young*. Free Association Books, London.

138. Robertson J (1970) *Young Children in Hospital*, 2nd edn. Tavistock Press, London.

139. Darbyshire P (1994) *Living With a Sick Child in Hospital: the Experiences of Parents and Nurses*. Chapman and Hall, London.

140. Plaas KM (1994) The evolution of parental roles in the NICU. *Neonatal Network*, **13** (6), 31–33.

141. Hutchfield K (1999) Family-centred care: a concept analysis. *Journal of Advanced Nursing*, **29** (5), 1178–1187.

142. Melling SE (2000) Mothers' and fathers' experience of family centred care in a hospital setting (MPhil. Thesis). Coventry University, Coventry.

143. Affonso DD, Hurst I, Mayberry LJ, Haller L, Yost K, Lynch ME (1992) Stressors reported by mothers of hospitalised premature infants. *Neonatal Network*, **11** (6), 63–70.

144. Redshaw ME (1998) Mothers of babies requiring special care: attitudes and experiences. *Journal of Reproductive and Infant Psychology*, **15** (2), 109–110.

145. Fenwick J, Barclay L, Schmied V (2001) Struggling to mother: a consequence of inhibitive nursing interactions in the neonatal nursery. *Journal of Perinatal and Neonatal Nursing*, **15** (2), 49–64.

146. Holditch-Davis D, Miles MS (2000) Mothers' stories about their experiences in the neonatal intensive care unit. *Neonatal Network*, **19** (3), 13–21.

147. Alderson P, Hawthorne J, Killen M (2006) Parents' experiences of sharing neonatal information and decisions: consent, cost and risk. *Social Science and Medicine*, **62** (6), 1319–1329.

148. Costeloe K, Wilkinson AR (1998) Managing potential conflicts amongst professionals and parents responsible for the care of sick babies. *Seminars in Neonatology*, **3** (4), 323.

149. Bruns DA, McCollum JA (2002) Partnerships between mothers and professional in the NICU: caregiving, information exchange and relationships. *Neonatal Network*, **21** (7), 15–23.

150. Alderson P, Hawthorne J, Killen M (2006) Parents' experiences of sharing neonatal information and decisions: consent, cost and risk. *Social Science and Medicine*, **62** (6), 1319–1329.

151. Brazy JE, Anderson BMH, Becker PT, Becker M (2001) How parents of premature infants gather information and obtain support. *Neonatal Network*, **20** (2), 41–48.

152. BLISS, the premature baby charity. *Ventilation and Chronic Lung Disease – Your Questions Answered.* http://www.bliss.org.uk (accessed 12 August 2006).

153. BLISS, the premature baby charity. *Parent Information Guide.* http://www.bliss.org.uk (accessed 25 November 2007).

154. Peticuff JH, Arbeart KL (2005) Effectiveness of an intervention to improve parent-professional collaboration in neonatal intensive care. *Journal of Perinatal and Neonatal Nursing*, **19** (20), 187–202.

155. Fenwick J, Barclay L, Schmeid V (2001) Struggling to mother: a consequence of inhibitive nursing interactions in the neonatal nursery. *Journal of Perinatal and Neonatal Nursing*, **15** (2), 49–64.

156. Fenwick J, Barclay L, Schmeid V (2001) 'Chatting': an important clinical tool in facilitating mothering in neonatal nurseries. *Journal of Advanced Nursing*, **33** (5), 583–593.

157. Cescutti-Butler L, Galvin K (2003) Parents' perceptions of staff competency in a neonatal intensive care unit. *Journal of Clinical Nursing*, **12** (5), 752–761.

158. Jackson K, Ternestedt B-M, Schollin J (2003) From alienation to familiarity: experiences of mothers and fathers of preterm infants. *Journal of Advanced Nursing*, **43** (2), 120–129.

159. Cescutti-Butler L, Galvin K (2003) Parents' perceptions of staff competency in a neonatal intensive care unit. *Journal of Clinical Nursing*, **12** (5), 752–761.

160. Bowlby J (1965) *Child Care and the Growth of Love*, 2nd edn. Penguin, Harmondsworth.

161. Bowlby J (1951) *Maternal Care and Mental Health*. World Health Organisation, Geneva.

162. Robertson J, Robertson J (1989) *Separation and the Very Young*. Free Association Books, London.

163. Duncombe J, Marsden D (1999) Love and intimacy: the gender division of emotion and 'emotion work': a neglected aspect of sociological discussion of heterosexual relationships. In: Allan G (ed.) *The Sociology of the Family: a Reader*. Blackwell, Oxford. Chapter 4, pp. 91–110.

164. Whitfield MF (2003) Psychosocial effects of intensive care on infants and families after discharge. *Seminars in Neonatology*, **8** (2), 185–193.

165. Cohen M (2003) *Sent Before My Time: a Child Psychotherapist's View of Life on a Neonatal Intensive Care Unit*. Karnac, London.

166. Sullivan JR (1999) Development of father-infant attachment in fathers of preterm infants. *Neonatal Network*, **18** (7), 33–39.

167. Ferketich SL, Mercer RT (1995) Predictors of role competence for experienced and inexperienced fathers. *Nursing Research*, **44** (2), 89–95.

168. Richards MPM (1978) Possible effects of early separation on later development of children: a review. In: Brindlecombe FSW, Richards MPM, Roberton NRC (eds), *Separation and Special Care Baby Units: Clinics in Developmental Medicine (68)*. Heineman, London. pp.12–32.

169. Bialoskurski M, Cox CL, Hayes JA (1999) The nature of attachment in a neonatal intensive care unit. *Journal of Perinatal and Neonatal Nursing*, **13** (1), 66–77.

170. Cox CL, Bialoskurski M (2001). Neonatal intensive care: communication and attachment. *British Journal of Nursing*, **10** (10), 668–676.

171. Adamson-Macedo EN (2004) Separation: the stresses on parents and babies. *Newborn News* (Spring, 6–7).

172. Klaus MH, Kennell JH (1976) *Maternal-infant Bonding*. CV Mosby Company, St Louis.

173. Klaus MH, Kennell JH (1982) *Parent Infant Bonding*, 2nd edn. CV Mosby Company, St Louis.

174. Miles MS (1990) Parents of critically ill premature infants: sources of stress. *Critical Care Nursing Quarterly*, **12** (3), 69–74.

175. Raeside L (1997) Perceptions of environmental stressors in the NNU. *British Journal of Nursing*, **6** (16), 914–923.

176. Bond C (1999) Positive touch and massage in the neonatal unit: a means of reducing stress levels. *Journal of Neonatal Nursing*, **5** (5), 16–20.

177. Bond C (2002) Positive touch and massage in the neonatal unit: a British approach. *Seminars in Neonatology*, **7** (6), 477–486.

178. Vehviläinen-Julkunen K, Liukkonen A (1998) Fathers' experiences of childbirth. *Midwifery*, **14** (1), 10–17.

179. Lundqvist P, Jakobsson L (2003) Swedish men's experiences of becoming fathers to their preterm infants. *Neonatal Network*, **22** (6), 25–31.

180. Sullivan JR (1999) Development of father-infant attachment in fathers of preterm infants. *Neonatal Network*, **18** (7), 33–39.

181. Lundqvist P, Jakobsson L (2003) Swedish men's experiences of becoming fathers to their preterm infants. *Neonatal Network*, **22** (6), 25–31.

Chapter 5

THE SMALL BABY

Maggie Meeks and Jonathan Cusack

Learning outcomes

After reading this chapter the reader will be expected to be able to:

- Compare and contrast the terms *intrauterine growth restriction (IUGR)* and *small for gestational age (SGA)*

- Summarise the causes of intrauterine growth restriction

- Explain the medical complications of an infant with IUGR

- List some of the complications of prematurity

- Provide a rationale for the nursing care given when a preterm infant is stabilised

- Explain the term retinopathy of prematurity and how it is assessed

---

Introduction

The significant advances in perinatal care that have occurred since the 1980s have led to an increase in survival rates for very small and preterm babies. This chapter will begin with some definitions of each specific group before briefly reviewing some of the relevant embryology and the implications for their nursing care. The groups that will be discussed are:

- Small for gestational age (SGA) infants
- *In utero* growth restricted infants (IUGR)
- Preterm infants

Definitions

The terms small for gestational age (SGA) and intrauterine growth restriction (IUGR) are often confused and it is important to be clear that they have different meanings. These terms are defined below:

- *Small for gestational age (SGA)* is used to describe infants with a birthweight below the third centile (some definitions describe below the tenth centile) when plotted on a standardised growth chart. This definition will include 3% of infants that are appropriately grown and therefore *do not* have intrauterine growth retardation (see Table 5.1). A further consideration is that the most commonly used growth charts (for example Tanner and Whitehouse 1966) refer to data collected from white Caucasian children in 'developed' countries. There is a strong argument for using specific growth charts for each sub-population based on race and even medical history (e.g. trisomy 21) to prevent over investigation of normal small individuals[1,2].

- *Intrauterine growth retardation* describes those infants that have not reached their *predicted* potential for growth *in utero* because of maternal, placental or foetal factors and most of these will be small for gestational age, but this is not always the case. For example, it is possible to see an infant whose birthweight lies on the fiftieth centile that has suffered *in utero* growth retardation and is therefore appropriately grown for age (AGA) using the SGA definition[3].

- *Prematurity* refers to an infant born before 37 weeks gestation. The term extreme prematurity is often used to describe infant of 26 weeks gestation and below since the anatomy and physiology of an infant at 24–26 weeks differs significantly to that of an infant at 34–36 weeks[4].

An alternative classification that is often used in epidemiological studies is that objectively based on birthweight as described in the International Classification of Diseases 9:

- Low birthweight   less than 2500 g
- Very low birthweight   less than 1500 g
- Extremely low birthweight less than 1000 g

This is a useful definition and there is evidence that birthweight follows a normal distribution for each gestation[5]. However, it must be remembered that in this definition the term low birthweight may be used to describe an infant that is small for gestational age, growth restricted, premature or all three.

Table 5.1 Physiological differences between the preterm baby and the growth restricted one.

Characteristic	Preterm baby	Growth restricted
Vernix	Copious	Little or more
Skin	Red and shiny	Dry and baggy
Face	Smooth, doll-like	Wizened, mature
Abdomen	Protruding	Flat
Posture	Hypotonic	Active
Skull	Soft, bones movable	Firmer
Cord	Thick and fleshy	Thin
Cry	Feeble	Normal

A brief review of embryology

An understanding of the way that the human body is formed (embryology) is helpful when thinking about a number of neonatal conditions, including congenital malformations (see Chapter 10).

Immediately following fertilisation there is a period of rapid cell division and a ball of cells called a blastocyst is formed. The blastocyst implants into the wall of the uterus around six days after fertilisation and part of the blastocyst, the trophoblast, develops into the early placenta. By the third week of development, the embryo has developed into three layers, which are described below:

- Endoderm: this gives rise to the lining of the gut, the respiratory tract and other organs such as the thyroid gland
- Mesoderm: this goes on to form cartilage, bone, muscle and organs such as the heart and the kidney
- Ectoderm: this will eventually form into the brain and spinal cord, the epidermis, hair and teeth

Embryonic period

The period from the third to the ninth week is known as the embryonic period and many vital organs are formed during this period. Any disruptions to this normal developmental sequence can produce serious malformations in the baby. It is important to remember that many women do not even know they are pregnant during this time, and therefore prospective parents should be advised about their lifestyle with regards to smoking, alcohol, drug use and starting folate supplements, even before they start trying for a baby (see Chapter 2).

There are a number of important areas of embryology which give specific insight into congenital defects, such as neural tube defects and congenital heart defects:

Neural tube defects
Over the first five weeks the neural tube forms and will eventually develop into the brain and

spinal cord. Disruption of the folding of the neural tube can lead to neural tube defects such as spina bifida, which literally translated means 'spine split in two' or a defect of the vertebral arch. The least severe is spina bifida occulta (affecting the bone only) and an example of a more severe type is meningomyelocele, where the spinal cord and meninges are exposed. This can cause neurological problems in the areas of the body supplied by the nerves coming off the spinal cord below the lesion. Spina bifida can also cause a disruption of the flow of cerebrospinal fluid around the brain and spinal cord, and is commonly associated with hydrocephalus (a fluid filled enlargement of the ventricles within the brain) (see Chapter 14).

Congenital heart defects

The primitive heart is formed from two endocardial tubes which fold to produce the structures of the mature heart. The heart first beats at around 22 days of age. Problems with the way the heart folds and the vessels separate can lead to structural changes in the heart and congenital malformations of the heart account for 25% of all congenital malformations. Examples include septal defects and transposition of the great vessels (see Chapter 11).

Abnormalities of head and neck

At the end of the fourth week a number of arches and pouches form around the future head and neck region. These are known as the branchial arches and pharyngeal pouches. They go on to form the muscles of the head and neck, the inner ear, and some of the organs in the neck, the thyroid and parathyroid glands and the thymus.

Problems with development of the branchial arches can lead to head and neck problems in the baby, such as the Pierre Robin sequence, where babies have a very small, poorly formed lower jaw.

Gastrointestinal conditions

The development of the respiratory and gastrointestinal systems is closely linked and problems with their formation can lead to conditions such as tracheo-oesophageal fistula and oesophageal atresia (see Figure 5.1). These are discussed further in Chapters 8 and 9.

The commonest type of tracheo-oesophageal fistula (TOF) is that shown in oesophageal atresia and TOF to the lower part of oesophagus (a). The least common are what is known as the 'H' type (c).

Between the sixth and the tenth weeks of development the intestine grows rapidly and herniates into the umbilical cord, before rotating in a counterclockwise direction and returning into the abdomen. Problems with this physiological herniation can lead to conditions such as exomphalos major, where the gut remains out of the abdomen in the umbilical cord, or malrotation of the gut, where the counterclockwise rotation does not occur, so that the intestine is not fixed securely within the abdomen. Exomphalos is often accompanied by other congenital abnormalities and malrotation in itself may result in volvulus, which is a surgical emergency.

In contrast to exomphalos, a separate condition, gastroschisis, occurs when there is a failure

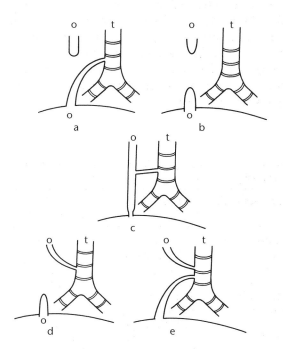

Figure 5.1　Types of tracheo-oesophageal atresia.

of the lateral folds of the abdominal wall to fuse properly. This leads to a defect in the abdominal wall and peritoneum that allows the abdominal contents to herniate out without any protective peritoneal covering. Gastroschisis is usually an isolated abnormality (see Chapter 9).

Foetal period

The period from the ninth week to term is known as the foetal period. During this time, the organ systems that have been formed grow and develop and from the twenty-fourth week to term the foetus gains weight rapidly. Any problems occurring at this stage will often cause *functional* defects rather than *structural* defects in the baby. These can be considered as the problems of the preterm infant and will be discussed under the section on prematurity in this chapter, as well as in more detail in other chapters.

The foetal circulation

An understanding of the foetal circulation is needed when considering foetal development. The foetal circulation is different from the adult circulation, because the foetus does not need to perfuse the lungs (see Chapter 3).

There are three main shunts that act to bypass areas where blood is not needed *in utero*:

- The ductus venosus bypasses the liver
- The foramen ovale connects the two atria, and allows blood to flow from the right atrium to the left atrium, so bypassing the lungs
- The ductus arteriosus connects the pulmonary artery to the aorta, so that any blood heading towards the lungs in the pulmonary artery is diverted to the aorta and the systemic circulation.

Implications for practice

Major organ development takes place often before the prospective mother is aware that she is pregnant; it is important therefore that couples consider lifestyle changes before trying for a baby.

Intrauterine growth retardation

As mentioned above, SGA refers to any infant whose growth is below the third centile and IUGR refers to those infants that have a pathological reason for being small or failing to realise their growth potential. There is a significant relationship between the severity of growth restriction and risk of death[6], which should be considered in order to counsel the parents honestly and appropriately.

The term IUGR is itself often subdivided in to symmetrical and asymmetrical growth restriction. Symmetrical IUGR describes the symmetrical restriction in head circumference, length and height and is associated with intrinsic foetal conditions such as genetic abnormalities or severe early onset foetal hypoxia secondary to maternal or placental factors. These infants are likely to remain small in adult life. Asymmetrical IUGR is used to describe the situation where the head circumference is preserved because the foetus has compensated by diverting blood to the organs that need it most, such as the brain. This is associated with poor placental function and these infants may show catch up growth following delivery[7]. Detailed antenatal scan and assessment of foetal well-being are therefore very important in evaluating foetal growth.

Implications for practice

When discussing asymmetrical IUGR with parents emphasis should be placed on the preservation of brain growth and that body weight will catch up.

The causes of IUGR can be classified into maternal, placental and foetal and these are discussed briefly below.

Maternal causes

Maternal causes for IUGR refer to factors within the mother and the commonest of these worldwide is malnutrition[8]. Unfortunately poor nutrition remains common in developed countries, especially in lower socioeconomic groups. The three main other causes are:

- Maternal illness: those that result in chronic hypoxia are especially important. These include cardiovascular diseases, e.g. congenital heart disease, severe anaemia, hypertension, as well as respiratory and renal diseases.
- Recreational drugs:
  - These include smoking, which can cause chronic hypoxia of the foetus[9–11]. The risk is directly proportional to the number of cigarettes smoked and if a mother is unable to give up completely, a reduction in the number of cigarettes smoked will reduce her infant's risk.
  - It is now advised that alcohol should be completely avoided during pregnancy as growth restriction and congenital anomalies are associated with exposure of the foetus to alcohol at critical stages of development (Department of Health, *The Pregnancy Book 2007*). Although small amounts of alcohol are thought to be safe this has not been confirmed[12,13].
- Prescription medication: there are a number of prescription drugs e.g. anticonvulsants that increase the risk of growth restriction or congenital anomalies within the foetus and preconception counselling should be sought where possible[14].

Placental causes

The term *placental* as a cause of IUGR should be used specifically in cases of poor placental function where there has been no relevant maternal pre-pregnancy disease. This includes:

- Pregnancy induced hypertension: this describes all women in whom hypertension is induced by pregnancy and includes pre-eclampsia
- Vascular placental events: the placenta may be affected by thrombosis or infarction and this is associated with the presence of maternal

anti-phospholipids or anti-cardiolipin antibodies – the anti-phospholipid syndrome
- Multiple pregnancy: the sharing of the placental vascular supply may lead to the blood flow of one of the foetuses being compromised

Foetal causes

In the obstetric evaluation of a foetus with poor growth or the neonatal evaluation of an infant with IUGR it should be remembered that the infant may have a congenital problem contributing to the growth failure. The two commonest reasons for this are chromosomal abnormalities and congenital infection.

Chromosomal abnormalities

These include:

- Trisomy 21 (Down's syndrome)
- Trisomy 18 (Edwards' syndrome)
- Trisomy 13 (Patau syndrome)

These are often screened for during pregnancy using nuchal thickness fold screening and maternal blood tests. They are definitively diagnosed by looking at the foetal chromosomes following chorionic villus sampling or amniocentesis and these tests should be offered if there was concern about poor foetal growth early in pregnancy. Additional chromosomal abnormalities can also cause IUGR and these would be investigated in specific cases, e.g. chromosome 22 deletion in congenital heart disease.

Congenital infections

Congenital infections which cause poor foetal growth include toxoplasmosis, rubella and cytomegalovirus (CMV), of which the last is the most common. These can be diagnosed by evaluation of the maternal immune response to the specific infection using blood tests. There are no current treatments although treatment to reduce the viral load in CMV (in a similar way to in HIV) is currently being evaluated[15,16].

Implications for practice

As well as categorising by weight it is important to clinically assess the newborn infant to ascertain whether it is small for gestational age or exhibiting signs of intrauterine retardation. The causes of IUGR should be considered and the consequences of IUGR predicted and managed appropriately (e.g. hypoglycaemia, hypothermia, polycythaemia).

Nursing care of the term infant with IUGR

Introduction

Most babies that are born at term with IUGR can be cared for on the post-natal ward or 'transitional care' unit and do not need admitting to the neonatal intensive care unit. It is, however, important to evaluate these infants fully and clinically both for the potential congenital causes of IUGR and for the possible complications of IUGR.

Problems at delivery

These babies may have experienced a compromised placental blood flow with chronic hypoxia and their lack of fat and glycogen stores will certainly mean that they are more vulnerable to foetal distress during the normal transient periods of hypoxia seen during labour than AGA term infants. The implication of this is that they may require both experienced obstetric and neonatal staff to be available during labour and at delivery.

Initial clinical evaluation

Babies with IUGR should be examined and their head circumference and weight plotted on their growth chart. They should be carefully assessed for evidence of any underlying 'foetal' cause of their IUGR, such as chromosomal problems, or congenital infection as well as the clinical severity of their growth restriction (e.g. fat stores).

Post-natal problems

Temperature control

All newborn babies have an increased surface area to volume ratio compared to adults and this affects their ability to conserve heat (see Chapter 6). This effect is exaggerated in small babies and they can become cold very quickly. In addition, babies with IUGR may have less fat stores, further impairing their ability to conserve heat. It is therefore important that the infant is adequately dried at delivery and dressed, including a hat. The infant may need additional support from an overhead heater or heated mattress.

Energy stores/glucose homeostasis

Babies with IUGR have very little fat, and few glycogen energy stores. They are therefore more likely to become hypoglycaemic and require early feeding. Small babies should be fed early and frequently, and their feeding closely monitored. Small for gestational age babies should be considered for routine prefeed blood glucose screening but this is particularly appropriate for those that are IUGR.

Polycythaemia

IUGR may be secondary to chronic hypoxia *in utero* and even chronic mild hypoxia will result in an increase in red blood cell production (this is an identical mechanism to that used by athletes training at high altitude). Babies with IUGR are therefore more likely to have polycythaemia. If the infant looks very red (plethoric), their haematocrit should be measured. Babies with a high haematocrit may require a partial exchange transfusion, particularly if symptomatic; however, a recent systematic review has questioned the need for partial exchange transfusions[17]. See Chapter 17.

Preterm infants

Introduction

Prematurity has been defined above as infants born at less than 37 weeks gestation and there are a number of causes. These include infection (chorioamnionitis, e.g. Group B streptococci, CMV), antepartum haemorrhage, cervical incompetence, intrauterine growth restriction, maternal smoking and hypertension, but in many cases there is a spontaneous onset of labour with no identifiable cause[18].

Over the last decade, there has been an increase in the survival rates for preterm infants. The Epicure Study was a large cohort study looking at survival and disability rates for all babies between 20 and 25 weeks gestation, born during a ten-month period in 1995[19]. This looked at the survival rates of babies born before 26 weeks gestation and provides the best UK data about the outcome of these babies. It showed an overall survival rate of 39%, with 44% survival in the 25-week gestation babies. The Epicure Group have continued to follow up their cohort of babies, and a second cohort is currently being recruited. Charts have also been published to predict the survival chances for infants of different gestations, according to weight rather than gestation[20]. The information from the Epicure studies and from these outcome charts is exceptionally useful when counselling parents antenatally but data from one's own unit should be used to supplement this where available.

Preterm or extreme preterm

For practical purposes, preterm infants can be divided into at least two groups, those less than 26 weeks and those greater than 26 weeks. These groups differ in a number of ways, which can be summarised by saying that infants less than 26 weeks gestation have organ systems that are significantly less mature and more susceptible to the complications of prematurity. These complications include:

- Loss of heat and water through an immature skin barrier
- Poorly developed lungs requiring respiratory support, and surfactant administration
- Hypotension in the first few days requiring inotropic support
- Immature brain at high risk of intraventricular haemorrhage
- Immature gut at high risk of necrotising enterocolitis
- Increased risk of retinopathy of prematurity

Babies of greater than 26 weeks can have similar problems, but with an increased maturity the incidence decreases. Surfactant production, for example, begins to increase at 24 weeks and more mature babies are less likely to get infantile respiratory distress syndrome and to need mechanical ventilation and surfactant administration.

These complications are summarised in Table 5.2 below and will be discussed in more detail in the relevant chapters.

Clearly preterm babies have very different nursing needs to term babies and these problems are elaborated below along with the implications for their nursing management.

Early care: management of extremely preterm infants in the first few hours

The birth of a preterm or compromised infant cannot always be predicted, which is why neonatal units should be staffed and have the available resources to manage these infants at short notice. Local protocols should be in place to ensure that management of the preterm infant is transferred as seamlessly as possible from the antenatal care of the obstetric and midwifery team to the neonatal team. Ideally, the parents will have met a senior member of the neonatal team prior to the delivery and issues around the resuscitation and stabilisation of the infant will have been discussed. Unfortunately preterm deliveries are often unexpected and this is a frightening experience for the parents and family involved. There may not be time to talk calmly with the parents to outline important issues around resuscitation, neonatal intensive care and neonatal outcome but the importance of establishing empathic communication cannot be overemphasised even when the practicalities of resuscitation may be at the forefront of the professional's mind.

Temperature

It is important that the delivery is attended by staff skilled in the resuscitation of the preterm and that more senior staff are present at high-risk preterm deliveries. This was supported by

Table 5.2 Brief overview of neonatal complications of extreme preterm and preterm infants.

	Babies of < 26 weeks	Babies of > 26 weeks
Weight	Usually extremely low birthweight	May be very low, or low birthweight
Skin	Very immature and likely to lose heat and water	Increasingly thicker and provides a better barrier to water loss (see Chapter 6)
Lungs	Likely to be immature and surfactant deficient – most babies will need respiratory support and surfactant administration	More mature– babies are less likely to need respiratory support
Cardiovascular	Many babies will be hypotensive and will need inotropic support; patent ductus arteriosus (PDA) is common	Less likely to need inotropes; clinically significant PDA is less common
Brain	Immature brain – risk of intraventricular haemorrhage and periventricular leucomalacia (see later)	More mature – risk of intracranial haemorrhage is less
Gut	Immature gut – tend to be slow to establish feeds; higher risk of necrotising enterocolitis	Usually quicker to establish feeds; risk of NEC is less and occurs earlier in neonatal course

recommendations from the CESDI 27/28 Project. This was a two- year enquiry conducted in 1998–2000 into the quality of care provided for infants between 27 and 28 weeks gestation. The outcome of this study was that a number of recommendations were made; one of these was that there were suitable senior practitioners present at high-risk preterm deliveries[21]. The CESDI report also highlighted the importance of temperature control; babies that were hypothermic on admission to the neonatal unit had an increased mortality. This issue has become less of a problem with the placement of preterm infants into a plastic bag from the shoulders down. Vohra *et al.* showed that preterm babies placed directly into a plastic bag and under a radiant heater without drying, at delivery had better temperature control than those who were dried and wrapped[22]. This is because the air immediately around the infant becomes saturated with water, and heat loss through evaporation is minimised. It remains important to dry the head and place a hat on the infant. Many units have now adapted this policy and the plastic bag can be left in place until the infant is inside a humidified incubator.

Surfactant
Babies of less than 28 weeks are likely to need surfactant, and studies have shown that prophylactic surfactant use is associated with decreased mortality. Surfactant should be given early to babies of less than 30 weeks (prophylactically) as this improves outcome when compared to 'rescue' surfactant[23,24]. Most units do aim to give the surfactant as early as possible, often on

> ### Implications for practice
>
> Priority should be given to keeping the newly born preterm infant warm with the use of a plastic bag or rapid drying and wrapping with warm towels and the use of a hat.

the delivery suite, for very preterm infants. There is some animal evidence that surfactant may be beneficial if it is given before the first breath on the delivery suite[25].

Once the infant has been stabilised on the delivery suite, they should be transferred to the NICU for further care.

The first 24 hours on NNU

Respiratory support

Many preterm infants will require respiratory support which will range from ambient incubator oxygen to intubation and ventilation (see Chapter 8).

Fluid balance

The preterm infant should be nursed in a double walled incubator with high humidity, as water loss through the skin will be high in the first few days. Once venous access has been established, maintenance fluids are commenced and obsessive attention to fluid balance should be encouraged, particularly over the first 72 hours. This includes daily weighing, monitoring of urine output, recording of the amount of blood removed for blood tests and the volume of flushes inserted, as well as regular measuring of creatinine and electrolytes. Those infants with RDS will have an increase in their urine output (a diuresis) at between 24 to 48 hours of age and this is associated with an improvement in their respiratory illness. It is important not to give excessive water or sodium before this diuresis has taken place (see Chapters 6 and 7).

Practical procedure and access

Preterm babies do not tolerate any form of handling well, and once on the neonatal unit, the aim should be to perform the necessary practical procedures as quickly and smoothly as possible. Venous access is a priority and in infants requiring significant cardiac or respiratory support arterial access should also be gained. The insertion of umbilical artery and venous catheters using a strict aseptic technique is a common procedure undertaken in these infants within the first hour of life (the so-called Golden Hour). Umbilical venous catheters are useful for the administration of drugs and fluids, and umbilical artery catheters can be used for blood sampling and invasive blood pressure monitoring. The infant will often require the administration of medications in the first hour, which may include antibiotics and vitamin K.

Monitoring

Observations including heart rate, oxygen saturations, blood pressure, blood glucose, ventilator settings and blood gases should be regularly recorded. Pulse oximetry is essential to avoid rapid changes in oxygenation. The heart rate and blood pressure can be recorded from an indwelling arterial line, which reduces the need for topical electrodes applied to the infant's delicate skin. Transcutaneous monitoring of oxygen and carbon dioxide levels is particularly useful for the extreme preterm infant as it minimises blood sampling.

Emotional support

The delivery of a preterm infant is very stressful for the parents, and staff can help relieve some of the anxiety by providing a photograph and explaining what is happening to their infant as soon as possible.

Analgesia

During their stay on the neonatal unit, preterm babies will undergo many different procedures, which may include capillary and venous blood sampling, IV line insertion, umbilical line insertion, percutaneous central line insertion, intubation and placing of chest drains. It must always be remembered that these procedures are painful, and appropriate analgesia and comfort care should be offered. A number of pain scoring tools exist. These look at physiological changes and facial expressions, and are helpful in monitoring the response to analgesia[26]. These are more accurate than the commonly used clinical cues that are used in neonatal nursing practice[27].

Non-pharmacological methods, such as positioning and swaddling the infant can help during procedures, and positive touch can be comforting. There is increasing evidence that oral sucrose, and topical amethocaine gel are beneficial in reducing neonatal pain scores[28]. Local anaesthesia is helpful in chest drain insertion, and opiate infusions should be used for particularly painful procedures.

Administration of medications

Vitamin K is usually given shortly after birth to prevent haemorrhagic disease of the newborn. This is given intramuscularly, but most other medications are given intravenously because of more reliable pharmacokinetics. Most preterm babies receive antibiotics at some point during their time on the neonatal unit. The combination of antibiotics will depend on local guidelines.

Cardiovascular support

Many sick babies will receive inotropes. These should ideally be given via a central vein (UVC or percutaneous long line) as they can cause serious extravasation injuries because of their 'vasoconstricting' effect. Most inotropes work by stimulating the adrenoreceptors but different inotropes act on different adrenoreceptors. There are two subclasses of adrenoreceptors: alpha receptors are found particularly in the peripheral blood vessels and beta adrenoreceptors are found in the heart (beta 1) and in the airways (beta 2). Stimulating beta 1 receptors will increase the heart rate and stroke volume of the heart, and stimulating alpha receptors will cause peripheral vasoconstriction, and increase peripheral vascular resistance. Both of these actions will increase the blood pressure (see Chapter 11).

Nutrition

Nutrition is critically important in all VLBW babies. Nutrition can be delivered enterally (expressed breast milk) or parenterally (total parenteral nutrition or TPN). Enteral feeds (ideally expressed breast milk) should be commenced as soon as the infant is able to tolerate them as this will aid colonisation of the gastrointestinal tract with healthy bacteria (see Chapter 12).

Many infants, especially those born extremely preterm will require a period of parenteral nutrition while enteral feeds are being increased. This is given into a central vein unless there are significant problems with access, as extravasation of TPN into a peripheral vein can cause severe tissue injury.

Infection

Meticulous care when inserting and handling central lines is imperative. Particular care should be taken to ensure good aseptic technique is followed whenever accessing a central line. Staphylococcal infections are a serious problem on neonatal units, and percutaneous lines are often a source of this infection (see Chapter 16).

Clinical risk

Staff should take particular care when preparing intravenous drugs for tiny babies. Doses should be meticulously checked, paying particular attention to the units used. It is very easy to confuse milligrams and micrograms when working out doses.

Similarly, infusions should always be double checked for accuracy, as errors in prescribing and administering these are common. Many neonatal drugs are drawn up from adult vials, and one study showed that in up to a third of drug dose errors, the drug dose is incorrect by a factor of ten, due to errors in calculating the dose and dilution[29].

Positioning and handling

Preterm babies are mildly hypotonic when compared to term infants and should be encouraged to maintain a flexed posture. Containment and providing boundaries may also be beneficial. Careful positioning of the infant and regular changes of position will help to minimise joint contractures and subsequent neuromuscular problems as well as prevent pressure sores[30]. Prone positioning is often used and can help improve gas exchange for ventilated infants[31], but care must be taken to observe the infant carefully (see Chapter 18).

Once the infant is more stable, they can spend some time with their parents, experiencing 'kangaroo care'. This can help with bonding, and has been shown to be safe for preterm babies. Kangaroo care supports nurturing behaviour that can help growth and development[32]. Ventilated infants can be nursed using kangaroo care, and parents often appreciate this close contact with their child.

Implications for practice

In nursing the extreme preterm it is important to be aware of the complications of prematurity, which include poor temperature and fluid regulation and cardiorespiratory immaturity as well as the complications of intensive care such as excessive inappropriate handling, pain and infection.

Problems of the preterm infant

Most of the problems of prematurity are covered in specific chapters within this book. Those that are not specifically covered are summarised below:

Retinopathy of prematurity

Retinopathy of prematurity (ROP) is an eye condition that affects preterm babies and is defined as an abnormal vasoproliferative response affecting the immature retina. The normal pattern of the development of blood vessels within the retina is for vascularisation to begin at the optic nerve at around 16 weeks gestation and extend outwards in both directions towards the periphery. The current theory for the development of ROP is that there are two phases; an initial hyperoxia phase[33,34], followed by a hypoxia phase and a vascular derived endothelial growth factor (VEGF) is thought to play a central role in stimulating the abnormal vascularisation. Late supplemental oxygen does not exacerbate pre-threshold disease[35].

The incidence of ROP varies with gestation and birthweight and it is more common in the very small babies. ROP occurs in about half of all babies with a birthweight of < 1700 g[36–39] and is classified according to the stage of ROP, the retinal zones affected, the extent of the disease and whether there is plus disease. The stages are according to the International Classification of ROP[40]:

Stage 1: there is a line of clear demarcation seen on the retina
Stage 2: a vascular ridge is formed

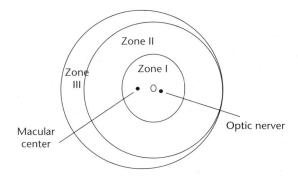

Figure 5.2 Classification zones of the retina used in ROP. Classification of ROP by zone and extent (a) The zones around the optic nerve (b) The use of a clock face to delineate the extent of ROP (e.g. from 12 o'clock to 3 o'clock)

Stage 3: the abnormally proliferating vessels appear to grow forwards into the vitreous of the eye
Stage 4: the retina is partially detached
Stage 5: the retina is completely detached

The area of the eye affected by ROP is subclassified according to circumferential zones around the optic nerve and areas corresponding to a clock face (see Figure 5.2).

The final term that is commonly used is 'plus' disease which refers to how tortuous the vessels are.

Infants of less than 32 weeks should be screened by an ophthalmologist who is experienced in examining the eyes of preterm infants and they should then be screened regularly from 30–32 weeks until term, or until the retina is fully developed. The neonatal nurse should administer dilating drops prior to the examination, and be available to assist the ophthalmologist and comfort the infant.

Treatment of ROP is indicated in stage 3 disease or plus disease and particularly when zone 1 or the posterior portion of zone 2 are involved. Cryotherapy or laser treatments are available. These work by causing tiny scars on the retina that stop the blood vessels dividing and prevents the retina from detaching. Treatment reduces the rate of visual loss by about 50% (CRYO-ROP group 2001). Laser treatment often takes a few

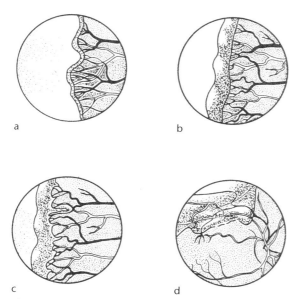

Figure 5.3 Showing the stages of retinopathy (adapted from Bernbaum and Hoffman-Williamson, 1991). (a) Stage 1: demarcation line between vascularised and avascularised retina. (b) Stage 2: ridge at the edge of the avascularised retina. (c) Stage 3: ridge with extraretinal proliferation. (d) Stage 4 and 5: peripheral and total retinal detachment. Total detachment is shown.

hours, and many babies return to the neonatal unit ventilated. It must be remembered that infants undergoing laser treatment are likely to have been the smallest sickest infants and any surgery is a major procedure. Particular attention should also be taken to make sure that the infant has adequate analgesia post-operatively.

Unfortunately ROP is often diagnosed at a time when the infant is improving from a cardiorespiratory point of view, and parents often feel that the diagnosis is a significant 'setback'. It is important to discuss ROP screening early, especially in high-risk babies, to adequately prepare parents. Babies with ROP have an increased risk of other visual problems in later life, and will require long-term ophthalmology follow-up.

Hearing problems in preterm babies
In the UK about 1 in 1500 babies are born with a permanent deafness[41], and many others may have a serious hearing impairment. Prematurity,

IUGR[42], hypoxia and the use of ototoxic drugs such as gentamicin and frusemide increase the risk of hearing impairment. In view of this a newborn screening programme was introduced in the UK in 2002. Screening involves the use of oto-acoustic emissions (OAE), where a small earpiece is placed in the ear and a click is produced. This stimulates the cochlear and a sound wave is produced in response. This test is quick, painless and accurate. If there is doubt then a second type of test, the automated auditory brainstem response, can be performed and this measures the brain's response to the click, with a sensor placed on the baby's head[43].

Because preterm babies fall into a high-risk group, many hospitals offer both screening tests to all babies that have been admitted to a neonatal unit.

Long-term outcomes
The great majority of babies admitted to neonatal intensive care units survive and have normal neurological outcomes without handicap. The situation is more guarded with the tiniest of babies. The Epicure study showed that in the UK survival rates were around 55% in babies born at 25 weeks gestation[44]. When these babies were followed up at six years 14% had severe disability, 10% had moderate disability, 29% had moderate impairment and 46% were normal[45]. These babies continue to be followed up and are being studied using neuropsychological and behavioural assessments.

It is important that parents are accurately counselled about potential neurological problems and that the importance of long-term neurodevelopmental follow-up is highlighted.

Conclusion

Extremely preterm and very low birthweight babies are now treated in highly technical intensive care units, providing great challenges and great rewards, for the nurses caring for them. The care given to these babies is evolving, and there is a drive towards more evidence-based practice. The nursing care of these babies is continually developing, and increasing attention is being paid to the developmental care of these high-risk infants.

References

1. Cronk C, Crocker AC, Pueschel SM, *et al.* (1988) Growth charts for children with Down syndrome: 1 month to 18 years of age. *Pediatrics*, **81** (1), 102–110.
2. Styles ME, Cole TJ, Dennis J, Preece MA (2002) New cross sectional stature, weight, and head circumference references for Down's syndrome in the UK and Republic of Ireland. *Arch Dis Child*, **87** (2), 104–108.
3. Bakketeig LS (1998) Current growth standards, definitions, diagnosis and classification of foetal growth retardation. *Eur J Clin Nutr*, **52** (Suppl. 1), S1–S4.
4. Vavasseur C, Foran A, Murphy JF (2007) Consensus statements on the borderlands of neonatal viability: from uncertainty to grey areas. *Ir Med J*, **100** (8), 561–564.
5. Vergara G, Carpentieri M, Colavita C (2002) Birthweight centiles in preterm infants. A new approach. *Minerva Pediatr*, **54** (3), 221–225.
6. Kamoji VM, Dorling JS, Manktelow Bradley N, Draper E, Field D (2006) Extremely growth-retarded infants: is there a viability centile? *Pediatrics*, **118** (2), 758–763.
7. Ranke MB (2002) Catch-up growth: new lessons for the clinician. *J Pediatr Endocrinol Metab*, **15** (Suppl 5), 1257–1266.
8. Ergaz Z, Avgil M, Ornoy A (2005) Intrauterine growth restriction-etiology and consequences: what do we know about the human situation and experimental animal models? *Reprod Toxicol*, **20** (3), 301–322.
9. Editorial (1979) Smoking and intrauterine growth. *Lancet*, **1** (8115), 536–537.
10. Hammoud AO, Bujold E, Sorokin Y, Schild C, Krapp M, Baumann P (2005) Smoking in pregnancy revisited: findings from a large population-based study. *Am J Obstet Gynecol*, **192** (6), 1856–1862; discussion 1862–1863.
11. Delpisheh A, Kelly Y, Rizwan S, Brabin BJ (2006) Socio-economic status, smoking during pregnancy and birth outcomes: an analysis of cross-sectional community studies in Liverpool (1993–2001). *J Child Health Care*, **10** (2), 140–148.
12. Henderson J, Gray R, Brocklehurst P (2007) Systematic review of effects of low-moderate prenatal alcohol exposure on pregnancy outcome. *BJOG*, **114** (3), 243–252.
13. Bagheri MM, Burd L, Martsolf JT, Klug MG (1998) Foetal alcohol syndrome: maternal and neonatal characteristics. *J Perinat Med*, **26** (4), 263–269.
14. Morrow J, Russell A, Guthrie E, *et al.* (2006) Malformation risks of antiepileptic drugs in pregnancy: a prospective study from the UK Epilepsy and Pregnancy Register. *J Neurol Neurosurg Psychiatry*, **77** (2), 193–198.
15. Adler SP, Nigro G, Pereira L (2007) Recent advances in the prevention and treatment of congenital cytomegalovirus infections. *Semin Perinatol*, **31** (1), 10–18.
16. Jacquemard F, Yamamoto M, Costa JM, *et al.* (2007) Maternal administration of valaciclovir in symptomatic intrauterine cytomegalovirus infection. *BJOG*, **114** (9), 1113–1121.
17. Dempsey EM, Barrington K (2006) Short and long term outcomes following partial exchange transfusion in the polycythaemic newborn: a systematic review. *Arch Dis Child Foetal Neonatal Ed*, **91** (1), F2F6.
18. Tucker J, Parry G, Fowlie PW, McGuire W (2004) Organisation and delivery of perinatal services. *BMJ*, **329** (7468), 730–732.
19. Costeloe K Hennessy E, Gibson AT, Marlow N, Wilkinson AR (2000) The EPICure study: outcomes to discharge from hospital for infants born at the threshold of viability. *Pediatrics*, **106** (4), 659–671.
20. Draper ES, Manktelow B, Field DJ, James D (1999) Prediction of survival for preterm births by weight and gestational age: retrospective population based study. *BMJ*, **319** (7217), 1093–1097.
21. Acolet D, Elbourne D, McIntosh, N, *et al.* (2005) Project 27/28: inquiry into quality of neonatal care and its effect on the survival of infants who were born at 27 and 28 weeks in England, Wales, and Northern Ireland. *Pediatrics*, **116**, 1457–1465.
22. Vohra S, Frent G, Campbell V, Abbott M, Whyte R (1999) Effect of polyethylene occlusive skin wrapping on heat loss in very low birth weight infants at delivery: a randomized trial. *J Pediatr*, **134** (5), 547–551.
23. Soll RF (2000) Prophylactic synthetic surfactant for preventing morbidity and mortality in

preterm infants. *Cochrane Database Syst Rev* (2), CD001079.

24. Soll RF (2000) Prophylactic natural surfactant extract for preventing morbidity and mortality in preterm infants. *Cochrane Database Syst Rev* (2), CD000511.

25. Bjorklund LJ, Vilstrup CT, Larsson A, Svenningsen NW, Werner O (1996) Changes in lung volume and static expiratory pressure-volume diagram after surfactant rescue treatment of neonates with established respiratory distress syndrome. *Am J Respir Crit Care Med*, **154** (4 Pt 1), 918–923.

26. Blauer T, Gerstmann D (1998) A simultaneous comparison of three neonatal pain scales during common NICU procedures. *Clin J Pain*, **14** (1), 39–47.

27. Fuller B, Thomson M, Conner DA, Scanlan J (1996) Relationship of cues to assessed infant pain level. *Clin Nurs Res*, **5** (1), 43–66.

28. Anand KJ, Hall RW, Desai N, *et al.* (2004) Effects of morphine analgesia in ventilated preterm neonates: primary outcomes from the NEOPAIN randomised trial. *Lancet*, **363**, 1673–1682.

29. Chappell K, Newman C (2004) Potential ten-fold drug overdoses on a neonatal unit. *Arch Dis Child Foetal Neonatal Ed*, **89** (6), F483–F484.

30. Hallsworth M (1995) Positioning the pre-term infant. *Paediatr Nurs*, **7** (1), 18–20.

31. Kurlak LO, Ruggins NR, Stephenson TJ (1994) Effect of nursing position on incidence, type, and duration of clinically significant apnoea in preterm infants. *Arch Dis Child Foetal Neonatal Ed*, **71** (1), F16–F19.

32. Dodd VL (2005) Implications of kangaroo care for growth and development in preterm infants. *J Obstet Gynecol Neonatal Nurs*, **34** (2), 218–232.

33. Coe K, Butler M, Reavis N, *et al.* (2006) Special Premie Oxygen Targeting (SPOT): a program to decrease the incidence of blindness in infants with retinopathy of prematurity. *J Nurs Care Qual*, **21** (3), 230–235.

34. Saugstad OD (2006) Oxygen and retinopathy of prematurity. *J Perinatol*, **26** (Suppl. 1), S46–S50; discussion S63–S64.

35. The STOP-ROP Multicenter Study Group (2000) Supplemental Therapeutic Oxygen for Pre-threshold Retinopathy of Prematurity (STOP-ROP),

a randomized, controlled trial. I: primary outcomes. *Pediatrics*, **105** (2), 295–310.

36. Fielder AR, Shaw DE, Robinson J, Ng YK (1992) Natural history of retinopathy of prematurity: a prospective study. *Eye*, **6** (Pt 3), 233–242.

37. Vyas J, Field D, Draper ES, *et al.* (2000) Severe retinopathy of prematurity and its association with different rates of survival in infants of less than 1251 g birth weight. *Arch Dis Child Foetal Neonatal Ed*, **82** (2), F145–F149.

38. Haines, L, Fielder AR, Baker H, Wilkinson AR (2005) UK population based study of severe retinopathy of prematurity: screening, treatment, and outcome. *Arch Dis Child Foetal Neonatal Ed*, **90** (3), F240–F244.

39. Stephenson T, Wright S, O'Connor A, *et al.* (2007) Children born weighing less than 1701 g: visual and cognitive outcomes at 11–14 years. *Arch Dis Child Foetal Neonatal Ed*, **92** (4), F265–F270.

40. International Committee for the Classification of Retinopathy of Prematurity (2005) The International Classification of Retinopathy of Prematurity revisited. *Arch Ophthalmol*, **123** (7), 991–999.

41. Stewart IF (1977) Newborn infant hearing screening – a five year pilot project. *J Otolaryng*, **6** (6), 477–481.

42. Jiang ZD, Brosi DM, Wilkinson AR (2001) Hearing impairment in preterm very low birthweight babies detected at term by brain-stem auditory evoked responses. *Acta Paediatr*, **90** (12), 1411–1415.

43. Kennedy CR (1999) Controlled trial of universal neonatal screening for early identification of permanent childhood hearing impairment: coverage, positive predictive value, effect on mothers and incremental yield. Wessex Universal Neonatal Screening Trial Group. *Acta Paediatr Suppl*, **88** (432), 73–75.

44. Costeloe K Hennessy E, Gibson AT, Marlow N, Wilkinson AR (2000) The EPICure study: outcomes to discharge from hospital for infants born at the threshold of viability. *Pediatrics*, **106** (4), 659–671.

45. Marlow N, Wolke D, Bracewell MA, Samara M (2005) Neurological and developmental disability at six years of age after extremely preterm birth. *N Engl J Med*, **352** (1), 9–19.

Chapter 6
THERMOREGULATION

Maggie Hallsworth

Learning outcomes

After reading this chapter the reader will be expected to be able to:

- Describe the four main mechanisms of heat loss/gain

- Compare and contrast the problems of maintaining an infant's temperature on a busy labour ward with a home delivery

- Describe the main challenges of thermoregulation on a neonatal unit

- Explain how physiological maturity of an infant relates to thermal stability

- Solve common problems of thermal instability

- Demonstrate in practice the clinical skills of maintaining a thermoneutral environment

---

Introduction

Temperature control in the foetus is controlled by the mother but once delivered the infant must initiate thermal control. The physiological capacity to initiate thermal control may be compromised, depending on the maturity of the infant and also the circumstances at the time of delivery, irrespective of the infant's gestation. The point of delivery is where the newborn infant is at greatest risk of thermal instability but it may also occur at any point during the time that he/she remains small or sick. It is therefore crucial that those people involved in the care of newborn infants develop their knowledge and skills to ensure a suitable thermoneutral environment is provided for the infant at all times.

Thermoregulation

The thermoneutral environment may be described as the environmental temperature at which minimal oxygen consumption and energy expenditure occur in order for an infant to maintain a normal temperature[1]. As the temperature rises or falls outside of this thermoneutral range oxygen consumption and energy expenditure will be increased. A normal core temperature of 36.5°C is the temperature where heat production and heat loss should be balanced. Thermoregulation may be described as the individual's ability to balance heat loss and heat gain to maintain the body temperature within this normal range[2].

Implications for practice

The environment into which the infant is delivered and later nursed should therefore be that which will minimise excessive heat loss/heat gain. This is a thermoneutral environment.

Anatomy and embryology relating to temperature control

Temperature control is regulated by the hypothalamus, the development of which begins in the fourth to fifth week of gestation[3], maturing by the thirty-fifth week of gestation. The hypothalamus also regulates the pituitary hormones, including the thyroid stimulating hormone which stimulates the release of thyroxine. This also contributes to the maintenance of body temperature[4].

Skin

The skin is the main organ responsible for heat loss in the newborn. It is a large organ in the newborn infant, comprising 13% of body weight compared to 3% in an adult[5]. The skin has numerous functions which include:

- Thermoregulation
- Fat storage and insulation
- Excretion
- Protection
- Tactile stimulation

The ability to perform these functions is limited in newborn and preterm infants, and may be further reduced by the effects of neonatal intensive care. Preterm infants particularly will be at risk of skin damage as a result of neonatal intensive care procedures. This may include the percutaneous absorption of chemicals, viruses or drugs, including oxygen and fluid and electrolyte imbalance from trans-epidermal fluid losses.

The skin consists of three layers: the epidermis, the dermis and the subcutaneous layer.

Epidermis

The epidermis is comprised of two layers: the stratum corneum and the basal layer. The stratum corneum is formed from lipids and protein and the cells are keratinised and continually replaced by cells from the basal layers as the surface layers are worn away. At 26 weeks the epidermis is only 2–3 cells thick, which make it a poorly functioning barrier that can easily be stripped and damaged. By 34 weeks gestation the stratum corneum is well developed[6]. Whatever the gestation at delivery, skin maturation takes place following transfer from the intrauterine environment to the post-natal, but in the very preterm infant this process can take from 2–4 weeks to complete[7].

Dermis

The dermis is a layer of collagen and elastin fibres consisting of nerves, blood vessels and hair follicles and the sensations to heat, touch and pain originate here. With increasing prematurity there is less collagen and elastin present and the layer is prone to oedema. This may impede blood flow to the epidermis by compression of the smallest blood vessels and in severe cases result in tissue damage.

Subcutaneous layer

The subcutaneous layer is composed of fatty connective tissue which provides heat insulation and may also act as a calorie reserve. It is laid down primarily during the last trimester of pregnancy[8].

The skin of a term infant is covered in vernix caseosa, a cheesy substance deposited during the last month of pregnancy as protection from the effects of the amniotic fluid. They also have a relatively alkaline skin pH which will fall during the first 3–4 days to that of an acid mantle, whereas with premature infants this process may take longer. An acid mantle has been shown to be protective against some pathogens and micro-organisms[9].

Implications for practice

The skin of a preterm infant is thin and easily damaged and may remain relatively alkalotic. It therefore forms a limited mechanical and immunological barrier as well as providing poor insulation, which is why care must be taken when handling the infant to prevent further skin breakdown.

Mechanisms of heat loss/gain

There are four main ways in which heat may be lost or gained from the body and these are:

- Conduction
- Convection
- Radiation
- Evaporation

Infants will be at risk of a combination of the four mechanisms of heat loss, with some groups being more vulnerable than others. The methods will be discussed individually.

Conduction

Conduction is when heat is transferred between two solid objects placed together. See Figure 6.1. This may be from the infant to the cold surface upon which it is placed, for example a cold towel at delivery, a cold X-ray plate, or cold weighing scales. The greater the temperature difference between the two objects the faster the heat loss will occur. This highlights the need to pre-warm all surfaces upon which the infant may be placed, as well as all objects which may come into contact with the infant, including stethoscopes and carers' hands, and to provide an insulating layer on scales, X-ray plates, and any surfaces upon which the infant may be placed. The newborn's head represents a large surface area in relation to the body so applying a bonnet at delivery will contribute to reducing heat loss. Kangaroo care, the practice of placing the naked infant against the mother or father's naked chest, is an excellent method of promoting positive conductive heat transfer[10].

Implications for practice

All solid objects which will come into contact with a newborn infant should be prewarmed.

Convection

Convection is when heat is lost from currents of cool air. See Figure 6.2.

In practice, convection occurs because of draughts from open windows, doors, air conditioning, or open incubator portholes. These losses may be accelerated in the delivery room when the room temperature has been set with the labouring mother in mind. The recommendations are for a room temperature of 25–28°C as the delivery room temperature for a premature birth[11]. Additionally, by keeping the sides of the resuscitaire up during resuscitation and extended procedures, draughts will be further reduced. More recent studies promote the use at delivery

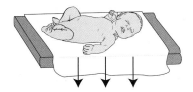

Conduction

Direct heat loss to solid surfaces with which they are in contact

Figure 6.1 Schematic representation of heat loss by conduction. Reproduced from Lissauer and Fanaroff, *Neonatology at a Glance* (2006), by kind permission of Blackwell Publishing Ltd.

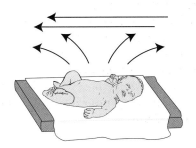

Convection

Heat is lost to currents of air

Figure 6.2 Schematic representation of heat loss by convection. Reproduced from Lissauer and Fanaroff, *Neonatology at a Glance* (2006), by kind permission of Blackwell Publishing Ltd.

of plastic wrappings for very low birthweight and premature infants, as a means of reducing both convective and evaporative heat losses. The recommendations are that the infant is placed directly into the bag without drying, whilst leaving the face uncovered[12, 13].

Implications for practice

Ensure that all room windows and doors are shut and resuscitaire sides are up during resuscitation. Keep incubator portholes closed.

Evaporation

Evaporative heat loss refers to the evaporation of fluid and consequent cooling of a surface. See Figure 6.3.

This method of heat loss occurs predominantly when the newborn has wet skin, especially immediately after delivery. It also occurs within their lungs via the evaporation of water from their expired respiratory gases. These losses are defined as insensible losses in comparison to the 'sensible' losses of urine and faeces[14]. Preterm infants who have poorly developed skin will be at particular risk of insensible heat loss, as will infants with the surgical condition gastroschisis (the abdominal contents are exposed and not protected by a skin covering). The use of a plastic wrapping as previously described will be of particular benefit in reducing insensible heat and fluid loss in those defined as at significant risk. In most other infants a prewarmed towel should be used to quickly dry the infant, including the head, before discarding this towel and wrapping the infant in a further warmed towel[15]. By providing warmed and humidified respiratory gases if needed, insensible losses will be further reduced. Infants who are born with a birthweight below 1500 g and gestation less than 30 weeks will also require humidity into the incubator for the first 1–2 weeks post-delivery whilst maturation of their skin takes place[16].

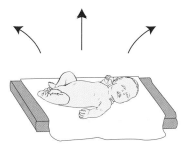

Evaporation

Heat loss when water evaporates from skin or breath

Figure 6.3 Schematic representation of heat loss by evaporation. Reproduced from Lissauer and Fanaroff, *Neonatology at a Glance* (2006), by kind permission of Blackwell Publishing Ltd.

Implications for practice

At delivery ensure that an infant is dried thoroughly before wrapping in a prewarmed dry towel.

Preterm infants should be placed in a plastic bag with their face uncovered and a hat on and will require incubator humidity as well as humidified oxygen if respiratory support is required.

Radiation

This is when heat is lost from two surfaces that are not in contact, e.g. from the warm surface (usually the infant) to the colder surroundings. See Figure 6.4. The greater the exposure of the infant to the cold surroundings the greater the heat loss. A neonatal nursery should therefore be maintained at 26–28°C and double walled incubators used[10]. Most infants are delivered onto resuscitaires which provide easy access to the infant and use a radiant heat mode to maintain the temperature. It is important to ensure the heat can get to the infant by ensuring that the health care providers do not impede its passage, especially during lengthy and prolonged resuscitations.

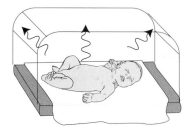

Radiation

Heat loss via electromagnetic waves
from skin to surrounding surfaces

Figure 6.4 Schematic representation of heat loss
by radiation. Reproduced from Lissauer and Fanaroff,
Neonatology at a Glance (2006), by kind permission of
Blackwell Publishing Ltd.

Implications for practice

Resuscitaires and incubators should be placed
away from cold windows and objects.
 Ensure health care providers do not obstruct
the radiant heat source of the resuscitaire during
resuscitation following delivery.

Hypothermia

Hypothermia is a preventable condition which
presents challenges to health care providers at
the delivery of any newborn infant, and subsequently on the neonatal unit:

- Mild (36–36.4°C)
- Moderate (32.0–35.9°C)
- Severe (below 32°C).

All newborn infants are vulnerable, but especially those who are born prematurely or sick,
and preterm and low birthweight infants may
have particular difficulties with the transition at
birth[17]. This is due to immature or absent ther-
moregulatory mechanisms in combination with
a large surface area and increased heat loss. The
importance of hypothermia is that it can have
adverse effects on the infant's health, which
include reduced surfactant production, increased
oxygen consumption and depletion of calories[18].

Maintaining the infants in a thermoneutral
environment will reduce these risks.

Infant response to cold stress

When an infant becomes cold, several reactions
take place in an attempt to increase heat production and decrease heat loss. An increase in heat
production can be classified as shivering and
non-shivering thermogenesis. Newborn infants
have a limited ability to shiver and if sick may
not have the physical capacity to increase heat
production by muscle activity (moving, crying,
etc.). Non-shivering thermogenesis refers to the
release of norepinephrine and thyroxine and
the metabolism of brown adipose tissue (BAT).
Brown adipose tissue is a specialised tissue laid
down in increasing amounts throughout gestation, especially during the last trimester of pregnancy. Preterm infants have limited stores of BAT,
depending on their gestational age, and they will
therefore have a limited ability to generate heat
by non-shivering thermogenesis. BAT is located
around the neck, between the scapulae, and down
the sternum, around the thoracic vessels and the
kidneys[19]. It is therefore centrally placed where
it is easily accessible. Norepinephrine release
from the sympathetic nervous system stimulates
the nerve endings in the BAT cells to metabolise
this specialised fat, resulting in the production of
heat and energy. BAT cells produce more energy
than any other body cells but oxygen and glucose
are both required for its metabolism. Thyroxine
release increases the rate of glucose oxidation,
thus increasing metabolic rate[4]. Infants who are
hypoglycaemic and/or hypoxic will therefore be
unable to mount these reactions.

Implications for practice

Preterm infants and term infants that are unwell,
hypoxic or hypoglycaemic have a limited
capacity for shivering and non-shivering thermogenesis. Particular care to optimising the
thermoneutral environment should be paid to
these infants.

Effects of hypothermia

Temperature control is under the influence of the hypothalamus of the brain and hypothermia stimulates the release of norepinephrine. The release of norepinephrine not only stimulates the metabolism of BAT but also has other widespread effects. These include systemic vasoconstriction, which occurs in a further effort to maintain core temperature by diverting flow of blood from the peripheries and pulmonary vasoconstriction. The pulmonary vasoconstriction increases pulmonary vascular resistance and may lead to right-to-left shunting of blood through the ductus arteriosus and/or foramen ovale. This right-to-left shunting will divert blood away from the lungs, causing hypoxaemia, which will in turn worsen the pulmonary vasoconstriction. As a consequence of the combination of right-to-left shunting and systemic peripheral vasoconstriction there is a reduction of oxygen availability to the tissues. When these effects are prolonged, the body will convert to anaerobic metabolism, with the production of lactic acid and the development of a metabolic acidosis[21]. The infant who is already compromised with respiratory distress and /or hypoglycaemia may therefore be further compromised by the hypothermia. The preterm infant is particularly vulnerable to hypothermia and its effects due to reduced or absent BAT, limited ability to move, flex and shiver to retain heat. Longer term effects of hypothermia include hypoglycaemia, increased early weight loss and slow or delayed weight gain. Surfactant production will be affected should the infant's temperature fall below 35°C, increasing the infant's potentially compromised respiratory status[22].

Implications for practice

Pulmonary hypertension and metabolic acidosis may occur secondary to hypothermia.

Rewarming the hypothermic infant

Work currently being undertaken on the use of hypothermia as a means of reducing apoptosis (cell destruction) and brain damage following hypoxic ischaemic encephalopathy suggests that rewarming should be at 0.5°C/hour[23,24]. Such work supports gradual rewarming of cold infants due to the risk of complications such as apnoea, hypotension and seizures.

Hyperthermia

A core temperature above 37.5°C is classed as hyperthermic[25]. The infant may appear red and warm to touch. Term infants will attempt to lose heat by vasodilation of surface capillaries and by sweating, but infants less than 36 weeks gestation have a limited ability to do this. Further signs of hyperthermia may include irritability, hypotonia, tachycardia and tachypnoea and the later sign of apnoea. Oxygen consumption and metabolic rate will both be affected by pyrexia in what may already be a compromised infant. The infant who is hyperthermic will therefore require close monitoring to quickly recognise the complications of high temperature. Vasodilation may result in hypotension and excess fluid loss leading to dehydration; strict fluid balance should therefore be recommended. The infant may develop seizures, signs of which may be subtle and are discussed in the chapter on neurology.

Hyperthermia may occur as a result of the environment being too hot, particularly if the cot or incubator is lying in direct sunlight, with phototherapy, by over swaddling the infant, or as a result of a combination of these factors. Pyrexia may be an initial sign of an infant who is septic and it should not therefore be assumed that it is due to environmental factors; it may also occur as a side effect of certain medications, e.g. prostin E2. The initial management of the infant who is pyrexial would be to remove external heat source and/or remove excessive blankets, reducing the incubator temperature initially by 0.5–1°C whilst maintaining continuous temperature monitoring and gradually continue until normothermia is achieved. Non-environmental causes of the pyrexia should be considered and treated.

Maintenance of thermal stability on the neonatal unit

On the neonatal unit the neonatal nurse has a wide variety of warming devices to facilitate the maintenance of each infant's thermoneutral environment. The exact way in which this is done will to a large extent depend on the clinical condition and gestational age of the infant.

Radiant warmers

These provide infra-red heat to the infant's skin using the radiation method of heat conduction. They are particularly useful in the delivery suite and most resuscitaires are equipped with a radiant warmer to allow easy access to the infant by the carers. The more modern radiant warmers are equipped with a servo device (servo is a term used to describe the task of feedback control and in this instance refers to the infant's temperature feeding back to the strength of the radiant warmer). They may also be of benefit on the neonatal unit during times when extensive procedures and continued access to the infant are required. A disadvantage of radiant warmers is that they do increase metabolic rates due to the increase in evaporative and convective heat loss, and this should be taken into account when calculating daily fluid requirements[26]. Radiant warmers should therefore be used with caution in very low birthweight and premature infants.

Incubators

These are widely used on the neonatal unit, and are available in a multitude of designs, providing a wide variety of options. An additional advantage of incubators is that the infant may also be protected from excess noise, light and disturbance. Modern incubators are double walled and provide the facility to administer servo controlled oxygen, humidity and air or skin temperature. Some also allow the infant to be weighed, further reducing the need to expose the infant to the cooling effects of the outside. Use of the servo control mode has been shown to reduce infant mortality in the low birthweight group when compared to air temperature mode[27]. When used in servo temperature mode, the sensor should be placed with insulated temperature patches on the exposed right upper outer quadrant of the abdomen to facilitate accurate temperature measurement[28]. The use of humidity into the incubator is of particular benefit for the extreme premature and low birthweight infants as a means of reducing trans-epidermal water loss (TEWL) and reducing the risks of electrolyte disturbances in this group of infants. Previously, a micro-environment may have been achieved by the use of bubble wrap, making observation of the infant more difficult and with the additional risk of variation in TEWL when the wrap was removed for caregiving and procedures. The integral humidification system provides a uniform environment for the infant, reducing these risks. Recommendations are that infants under 30 weeks' gestation and 1 kg in weight will require humidity for 8–10 days until maturation of the stratum corneum.

Water filled mattresses

These are useful when caring for healthy newborns who have difficulty in maintaining a normal temperature. The water filled mattress needs to be maintained at a sufficiently high temperature to prevent conductive heat loss[29,30]. They provide easy access to the infant by both the health care providers and, more importantly, the parents. A disadvantage of this access is that it may facilitate unnecessary handling which may impact on heat loss from the infant. There may also be an increased exposure to nosocomial infections which may impact on general well-being and weight gain.

Skin to skin care (kangaroo care)

This provides another method of maintaining the infant's temperature. The infant is naked except for a nappy and hat and is placed upright against the parent's bare chest and covered with a blanket. This method facilitates not only a thermoneutral environment but also close contact and bonding with the infant, resulting in reduced weight loss and length of hospital stay[31,32].

Implications for practice

It is recommended that the environmental temperature of the neonatal unit is maintained at 26–28°C.

In addition, there are methods (such as kangaroo care) and equipment (radiant warmers, incubators, transwarmers) that facilitate the provision of a thermoneutral micro-environment for the newborn infant).

Monitoring temperature

This may be achieved by a variety of methods, but in general the non-invasive route is utilised for neonatal care[33]. Sick infants should have continuous monitoring of core or near core temperature with the additional facility to monitor peripheral temperature. A wide gap between the core and peripheral temperatures (> 2–3°C) is abnormal and may be a helpful adjunct in assessing hypovolaemia, cold stress and early sepsis[34].

Conclusion

An infant's thermal balance may frequently be precarious due to a variety of reasons, but particularly so when he is sick and/or premature. Thermoregulation is therefore a vital component of the care of sick and premature infants, providing a challenge to the health care professionals involved. Knowledge of the anatomy and embryology and the responses by different gestational age infants is essential, as is knowledge of the four different methods of heat loss and the types and use of equipment used in temperature control. The neonatal nurse is required to achieve an appropriate thermoneutral environment for the infant at all times during the infant's stay on the neonatal unit. At times achieving this may be more difficult – during an extensive resuscitation, or prolonged procedures, for example. Meticulous attention to detail and continuous temperature monitoring for the very sick infant will facilitate this.

References

1. Roncoli M, Medoff-Cooper B (1992) Thermoregulation in low-birth-weight infants. *NAACOGS Clin Issu Perinat Womens Health Nurs*, **3** (1), 25–33.
2. Thomas K (1994) Thermoregulation in neonates. *Neonatal Netw*, **13** (2), 15–22.
3. Moore KL (1988) *Essentials of Human Embryology*. Blackwell Scientific, Oxford.
4. Tortora GJ (ed.) (1990) *Principles of Anatomy & Physiology*, 6th edn. Harper & Row, London.
5. Merenstein GB, Gardner SL (eds) (2002) *Handbook of Neonatal Intensive Care*, 5th edn. Mosby, London.
6. Yeo H (ed.) (1998) *Nursing the Neonate*, 1st edn. Blackwell Science, Oxford.
7. Kalia YN, Nonato LB, Lind CH, Guy RH (1998) Development of skin barrier function in premature infants. *J Invest Dermatol*, **111** (2), 320–326.
8. Houska-Lund CD, Durand DJ (2002) Skin and skin care. In: Gardner M (ed.) *Handbook of Neonatal Intensive Care*. Mosby, London.
9. Merenstein GB, Gardner SL (eds) (2002) *Handbook of Neonatal Intensive Care*, 5th edn. Mosby, London.
10. Ludington-Hoe SM, Thompson C, Swinth JY, Hadeed AJ, Anderson GC (2004) Randomized controlled trial of kangaroo care: cardiorespiratory and thermal effects on healthy preterm infants. *Neonatal Netw*, **23** (3), 39–48.

11. WHO: Dept of Reproductive Health & Research (RHR) (1997) *Thermal Protection of the Newborn: a Practical Guide* (WHO/RHT/MSM/97.2). WHO, Geneva.

12. Vohra S, Roberts R, Zhang B, Janes M, Schmidtet B (2004) Heat Loss Prevention (HeLP) in the delivery room: A randomized controlled trial of polyethylene occlusive skin wrapping in very preterm infants. *J Pediatr*, **145** (6), 750–753.

13. Lenclen R, Mazraani M, Jugie M, *et al.* (2002) Use of a polyethylene bag: a way to improve the thermal environment of the premature newborn at the delivery room. *Arch Pediatr*, **9** (3), 238–244.

14. Karlsen K (2006) *The STABLE Programme Learner Manual 2006*, Module 2 Temperature. Utah USA (www.stableprogram.org).

15. Resuscitation Council (2006) *Neonatal Life Support Manual*. Resuscitation Council, London.

16. Lund C, Kuller J, Lane A, Lott JW, Raines DA (1999) Neonatal skin care: the scientific basis for practice. *Neonatal Netw*, **18** (4), 15–27.

17. Boxwell G (ed.) (2005) *Neonatal Intensive Care Nursing*. Routledge, London and New York.

18. Karlsen K (2006) *The STABLE Programme Learner Manual 2006*, Module 2 Temperature. Utah USA (www.stableprogram.org).

19. Boxwell G (ed.) (2005) *Neonatal Intensive Care Nursing*. Routledge, London and New York.

20. Tortora GJ (ed.) (1990) *Principles of Anatomy & Physiology*, 6th edn. Harper & Row, London.

21. Blackburn ST (2003) *Thermoregulation*, in *Maternal, Foetal, and Neonatal Physiology: a Clinical Perspective*. Sanders, St Louis.

22. Hackman PS (2001) Recognizing and understanding the cold-stressed term infant. *Neonatal Netw*, **20** (8), 35–41.

23. Azzopardi D, Robertson NJ, Cowan FM, Rutherford MA, Rampling M, Edwards AD (2000) Pilot study of treatment with whole body hypothermia for neonatal encephalopathy. *Pediatrics*, **106** (4), 684–694.

24. Loughead MK, Loughead JL, Reinhart MJ (1997) Incidence and physiologic characteristics of hypothermia in the very low birth weight infant. *Pediatr Nurs*, **23** (1), 11–15.

25. Roberts RS, Rennie JM (eds) (1999) *Textbook of Neonatology*, 3rd edn. Churchill Livingstone, New York.

26. Flenady VJ, Woodgate PG (2003) Radiant warmers versus incubators for regulating body temperature in newborn infants. *Cochrane Database Syst Rev* (4), CD000435.

27. Sinclair JC (2002) Servo-control for maintaining abdominal skin temperature at 36C in low birth weight infants. *Cochrane Database Syst Rev* (1), CD001074.

28. Woods WB, Murray J (2002) Heat balance. In: Merenstein GB, Gardner SL (eds) *Handbook of Neonatal Intensive Care*. Mosby, St Louis.

29. Boxwell G (ed.) (2005) *Neonatal Intensive Care Nursing*. Routledge, London and New York.

30. Ellis J (2005) Neonatal hypothermia. *Journal of Neonatal Nursing*, **11**, 76–82.

31. Browne JV (2004) Early relationship environments: physiology of skin-to-skin contact for parents and their preterm infants. *Clin Perinatol*, **31** (2), 287–298, vii.

32. Chwo MJ, Anderson GC, Good M, Dowling DA, Shiau SH, Chu DM (2002) A randomized controlled trial of early kangaroo care for preterm infants: effects on temperature, weight, behavior, and acuity. *J Nurs Res*, **10** (2), 129–142.

33. Sganga A, Wallace R, Kiehl E, Irving T, Witter LA (2000) A comparison of four methods of normal newborn temperature measurement. *MCN Am J Matern Child Nurs*, **25** (2), 76–79.

34. McIntosh NW, Wilmhurst A, Hailey J (1995) Experiences with Thermal Monitoring, Influences of Neonatal Care and How it Should be Monitored. Okken A, Koch J (eds). Springer, Berlin.

Chapter 7

FLUIDS, ELECTROLYTES AND GLUCOSE

Elaine Boyle

Learning outcomes

After reading this chapter, the reader will be expected to be able to:

- Explain some of the important factors that affect the physiology of fluid and electrolyte balance in:
  - Term infants
  - Preterm infants
- Explain some of the important factors that affect the physiology of glucose metabolism in:
  - Term infants
  - Preterm infants
- Describe the nursing management of fluid balance in a preterm infant of < 28 weeks gestation following delivery
- Define hypoglycaemia and develop a management plan for:
  - an asymptomatic term infant
  - a symptomatic term infant
- Define hyperglycaemia and describe management of a preterm infant with hyperglycaemia

---

Introduction

This chapter aims to provide a clear summary of the important features of fluid, electrolyte and glucose metabolism that need to be considered in the term and preterm neonate. The first section concentrates on fluid and electrolytes and will begin with a review of the physiology, followed by the application of this knowledge to common situations in clinical practice. It begins with a discussion of fluid and sodium physiology. These two areas are discussed together because they are very closely linked and the correct interpretation of serum sodium results requires knowledge of fluid balance within the infant. The second section concentrates on glucose metabolism and is constructed in a similar way so that an understanding of the physiology can be applied to common clinical situations. In the final section some case studies are presented and management strategies are suggested.

Fluid and sodium balance

Physiology

Water accounts for approximately 75% of the body weight of a baby born at term and an even larger portion of a preterm baby[1]. It is clear, therefore, that maintenance of fluid balance is an extremely important part of early care of all newborn babies, but particularly those born prematurely. The foetus has to undergo physiological changes for successful transition from the intrauterine environment to the outside world and some of these changes will affect fluid balance (see Chapter 3). In addition, effects of immaturity, acute disease processes or underlying pathology and their treatments conspire to make management of fluids and electrolytes more challenging.

Term infants

Total body water is divided into two compartments – intracellular fluid (ICF) and extracellular fluid (ECF):

- Intracellular fluid is fluid that is contained within cell membranes.
- Extracellular fluid comprises all other fluid in the body, including that within the lymphatic and vascular systems and the interstitial fluid that is filtered from the blood and bathes the cells within the tissues.

Both ICF and ECF contain electrolytes; potassium is the major intracellular electrolyte and sodium is mainly extracellular. It is often helpful to consider water and electrolytes completely separately since although they are closely associated they are influenced by a wide variety of different factors.

The size of the extracellular compartment decreases with increasing gestational and postnatal age, falling from approximately 40% at term to around 20% by the age of ten years[2]. Neonates start life with an excess of total body water, which is mainly extracellular. After birth, the ECF space contracts in response to the production of atrial natriuretic peptide during cardiopulmonary adaptation to the extrauterine environment. The glomerular filtration rate, which is very low *in utero*, also increases sharply, producing a rise in urine output.

This diuresis ceases when the ECF volume has decreased to normal. In term babies a weight loss in the first week of life of 5–10% is normal and reflects the rapid loss of this fluid[3]. Healthy mature babies can adjust to varying intakes of water during first few days of life by increasing or decreasing urinary excretion; however, they require a minimum intake that will cover urinary and insensible losses[4].

Sodium is the main electrolyte in ECF and sodium loss accompanies the initial diuresis (this is what natriuretic as in 'atrial natriuretic' really means) and the baby is in negative sodium balance at this time. Sodium is essential for optimum growth and development and so the early state of negative sodium balance must change after the first few days of life to one of sodium retention. Human breast milk or an equivalent formula provides just enough sodium to maintain normal growth and avoid hyponatraemia in the healthy term baby. Kidney function changes and develops considerably during early life; renal tubular function is mainly responsible for regulation of sodium metabolism but is not fully developed at birth. Adults are able to alter their sodium excretion rapidly in response to changes in intake. This is not the case for babies who, in comparison with adults, have a low capacity to excrete excess sodium and are therefore at risk of hypernatraemia if excessive sodium is administered.

Implications for practice

Following delivery, term infants are initially in negative sodium and water balance as a result of the release of atrial natriuretic peptide and a weight loss of 5–10% is normal.

Subsequently, a positive sodium and water balance is necessary for growth and sodium is an essential component of breast or formula milk.

Hypoxic ischaemic insults

In infants who have experienced a significant hypoxic ischaemic insult either due to severe placental insufficiency or difficulties at or around the time of delivery, the effects of this may compromise the function of all organs, including the kidneys. This can often lead to a poor urine output in the first few days of life, which usually, though not always, resolves thereafter. In this early stage, these infants have a limited capacity to deal with fluid and pass very little urine. Restriction of the fluid intake to volumes less than those normally given to a term baby will avoid the associated problems caused by 'fluid overload'. It is common to limit the fluids given to a volume equalling the likely insensible losses, plus the volume of urine passed. Following this phase, the urine output can increase markedly as renal function recovers. Close monitoring of the urine output and serum sodium levels will be needed to guide management and ensure that input matches requirements. This is important as, if the input is not increased in line with the urine output, hypovolaemia will occur, which can then lead to a decrease in renal perfusion and pre-renal failure.

Preterm infants

In the healthy preterm baby, the course of post-natal adaptation is similar to that of a baby born at term. For sick or very preterm infants, the maintenance of fluid balance is a much more complex process and becomes increasingly so with decreasing gestational age.

Insensible losses are the principal mechanism of fluid loss in the preterm baby. Skin immaturity and a large surface area to weight ratio mean that babies readily lose water by the trans-epidermal route. For the most preterm, those under 28 weeks of gestation, these losses will be around fifteen times more than those of a term baby[5,6]. In practice, a preterm infant can lose up to 200 ml/kg/day from this route if humidity is not provided. Although the skin begins to mature within a few days of birth, the large losses during these first crucial days can lead to significant fluid and electrolyte imbalance. Babies born before 36 weeks of gestation are not capable of sweating and therefore do not excrete sodium in this way – the fluid loss is predominantly water. The ability to sweat develops over the first two weeks of post-natal life[7]. High evaporative fluid losses through the skin also mean significant loss of heat (see Chapter 6) and it is known that damaged skin will lose even more heat than intact skin.

In preterm infants with respiratory distress syndrome (RDS), the contraction of the ECF compartment and physiological diuresis is delayed[8]. In the natural history of the condition, the diuresis heralds the onset of recovery from RDS. The loss of ECF is precipitated by atrial natriuretic peptide during cardiopulmonary adaptation rather than renal maturation and no benefit has been shown in the use of diuretic therapy to enhance diuresis in RDS[9]. In infants whose mothers have received treatment with antenatal steroids and in those given surfactant replacement therapy, the natural progression of RDS is altered such that diuresis often occurs a little earlier. As in term babies, both fluid and sodium balance are negative at this time of adaptation.

Implications for practice

In preterm infants with clinical evidence of respiratory distress syndrome the physiological natriuresis and diuresis (sodium and water loss) secondary to the release of atrial natriuretic hormone occurs once the RDS is beginning to resolve.

Preterm infants are poor at controlling their sodium balance in response to intake of salt and water. Antenatal corticosteroids accelerate renal maturation[10], but further post-natal development of renal tubular reabsorption is necessary for efficient sodium regulation. In the first days of life, preterm babies are at high risk of hypernatraemia if given inappropriate early supplementation of sodium or if fluids are excessively restricted[11]. Hypernatraemia and weight gain secondary to inappropriate sodium supplementation and water retention has been associated with an increased risk of chronic lung disease. During the diuresis phase they then become particularly susceptible to hyponatraemia because of the kidneys' limited capacity for conservation of sodium. Hyponatraemia is accompanied by high rates of urinary sodium excretion. Studies have shown that replacement of the sodium by supplements at this stage can allow maintenance of sodium balance even in very low birthweight infants[12,13]. Mechanisms of sodium regulation are not sufficiently matured until between 32 and 34 weeks of gestation and most preterm infants will require supplementation until this time. An inadequate intake will lead to ongoing depletion of sodium with poor weight gain and growth.

Potassium balance

Potassium is the main intracellular cation. Serum potassium concentrations rise in the first 24 to 72 hours of life in preterm infants, even if no extra potassium is being given. This increase seems to be the result of potassium moving from the intracellular to extracellular space. As the kidneys mature, the level then falls as potassium is excreted in the urine.

Hyperkalaemia

Spuriously high levels of potassium are seen quite commonly in the newborn. This occurs because of haemolysis of the blood sample that can occur if samples are difficult to obtain, particularly in capillary heel stick samples where the heel has been squeezed and the blood does not flow freely. However, it is very important not to assume that this has occurred and to ensure that a further sample is checked to prove that the level is normal, as true hyperkalaemia can be life-threatening.

True hyperkalaemia (> 6.5 mEq/L) is caused either by decreased removal or increased load of potassium. The most common cause of decreased removal of potassium is renal failure.

A less common, but important, cause is adrenal failure, as in congenital adrenal hyperplasia. Preterm infants sometimes have high levels in the first few days of life. An increased load of potassium in the blood can build up in haemolysis, bleeding, such as intraventricular haemorrhage or other haematoma, or as a result of large blood transfusion. Acidosis will also affect levels of potassium as it causes potassium to shift out of the cells. Neonates can tolerate relatively high levels of potassium before becoming symptomatic, so it is important to carefully monitor levels with blood tests to avoid symptoms. The main adverse effect of hyperkalaemia is to produce cardiac arrhythmias, initially indicated by changes in the electrocardiogram (ECG), principally in the T waves, which become tall and peaked. ECG abnormality is a late sign and requires urgent treatment. Any potassium supplementation should be discontinued immediately. Drug treatments include infusion of glucose and insulin or calcium gluconate. In renal failure, it is important to discontinue and monitor levels of any drugs that are potentially toxic to the kidneys, such as gentamicin.

Hypokalaemia

Hypokalaemia is defined as a potassium level of less than 3.5 mEq/L. It may be due either to impaired renal function causing loss of potassium in the urine or to inadequate intake. In neonates it most commonly occurs as a result of chronic use of diuretics or inadequate replacement of nasogastric losses. Hypokalaemia can be avoided by monitoring and ensuring adequate supplementation as necessary if levels are falling. Very low levels of potassium will lead to cardiac rhythm abnormalities, with the ECG showing flattening of the T waves or prolongation of the QT interval. Severe hypokalaemia should be treated by slow replacement of potassium by infusion. If replacement is too rapid, life-threatening cardiac dysfunction may occur.

Application to clinical practice

Minimise fluid and heat loss

Maintenance of temperature and the avoidance of trans-epidermal fluid loss are important right from the moment of delivery. For term babies, radiant heaters should be available in delivery rooms. Combined with drying and covering a baby, this will probably suffice in most cases. For preterm babies who are at greater risk, many neonatal units have now adopted the policy of placing the wet newborn infant into a plastic bag before stabilising under a radiant heater. This has been shown to improve temperature control and reduce the likelihood of babies becoming hypothermic[14,15]. Fluid loss is also minimised with this technique. Modern incubators and the ability to provide high humidification will also decrease trans-epidermal water loss. In the smallest infants, humidity should be between 80–90% (see also Chapter 6).

Skin care

In preterm infants with fragile skin, the use of adhesive tapes and non-essential monitoring devices should be avoided. Similarly, invasive skin-breaking procedures should be kept to a minimum.

Monitoring of fluid and electrolyte balance

Measurement of fluid intake and output is crucial to allow effective fluid management, particularly in preterm babies. Urine output must be monitored as accurately as possible; this will necessitate the use of an indwelling urinary catheter in the sickest babies. This is especially important as premature babies enter the diuretic phase of respiratory distress syndrome, in order for fluid input to be tailored to match the increasing output. An output of approximately 1 ml/kg/hour is considered to be satisfactory. An abrupt and unexpected reduction in urine output

should be noted early in order to determine the cause.

Monitoring of weight can provide a good guide to fluid balance and a daily weight is recommended in the first few days of life if this can be achieved with minimal disruption to the baby, as is the case with most modern incubators. Immediate weight gain or no loss in weight is indicative of fluid retention. The initial weight loss should be followed by weight gain.

Implications for practice

Daily weights are an important guide to fluid balance in the preterm infant during the first few days following delivery or at times of critical illness.

Measurement of sodium will help to guide fluid management. A rising sodium level is likely to be an indicator of fluid depletion, whereas low sodium, particularly in the first few days of life before significant diuresis occurs, is likely to reflect fluid retention.

Fluid composition

Most healthy term and near term infants will be able to maintain appropriate fluid and electrolyte balance from breast or formula feeds without intervention. There are no fixed rules for the administration of fluids in sick and preterm infants and clinicians should be guided by the individual baby's clinical condition. However, suggestions for general guidance and composition of fluids can be made (see Chapter 12).

In unwell or preterm babies, milk intake will initially be small; fluid and nutrition requirements will be provided intravenously. A reasonable rule of thumb for intravenous fluid volumes is to provide 30–60 ml/kg/day plus extra for estimated insensible losses. Dextrose 10% is a suitable choice of fluid initially, but the glucose concentration can be increased or decreased in response to changing blood glucose levels. Maintenance requirements of potassium (2 mmol/kg/day) may be added to the fluid from day two onward. In preterm infants, sodium supplementation should be delayed until weight loss has been achieved and this should be then tailored to individual requirements based on measurement of serum sodium and fluid balance. Once serum electrolyte levels have stabilised, frequency of measurements can be reduced. Nutritional requirements must also be taken into account. For most infants, it will be appropriate to begin giving parenteral nutrition from the first or second days after birth to promote optimal growth.

Glucose metabolism

Term infants

Glucose represents around 80% of the energy available to the foetus before birth. Foetal glucose levels are maintained a little lower than those of the mother, allowing passive diffusion down a concentration gradient from mother to foetus via the placenta[16]. The glucose is supplied as a continuous infusion of approximately 4–6 mg/kg/min, which is enough to maintain normoglycaemia in a healthy term foetus. Normally, the foetus itself does not produce any glucose, but can generate a limited response to a large rise in maternal glucose levels by secreting insulin. Under extreme circumstances such as severe placental insufficiency and intrauterine growth restriction, foetal regulation of blood glucose may fail, leading to intrauterine hypoglycaemia[17].

Glycogen deposition in the liver begins in early pregnancy and increases until term in preparation for the provision of glucose during labour and early post-natal life. After birth, the baby must adapt to extra-uterine life when the supply of glucose from the placenta ceases. First, this requires the endogenous production of glucose until the establishment of feeding and the use of other nutrients including fat. Hormonal

responses lead to breakdown of glycogen, fat and protein and the production of ketone bodies. Studies have shown that, in the fasting newborn infant, glucose can only provide around 70% of the energy required for the high metabolic needs of the brain[18]. At this time, the liver is the only source of glucose production; ketone bodies and lactate are important as alternative fuels. The efficient use of these alternative fuels probably assists the baby in remaining well and asymptomatic, despite frequent transient falls in blood glucose levels in very early life.

Blood glucose levels fall sharply immediately after delivery, reaching the lowest point at approximately one hour of age[19]. However, few term infants experience extremely low levels or symptoms of hypoglycaemia[20]. After the first two or three hours of life, levels begin to rise and usually stabilise by 24 hours. Concentrations after this are principally dependent on feeding practices[21,22]. Initially, exclusively breast-fed babies tend to have lower blood glucose concentrations than those receiving formula; however, their levels of ketone bodies are higher. By the end of the first week of life, both breast and formula fed babies exhibit similar glucose responses to feeding, although the ketone body levels remain higher in those who are breast-fed.

Implications for practice

Ketone bodies as well as glucose are an important source of fuel for the newborn infant. Ketone body levels remain higher in infants that are breast-fed.

Preterm infants

Preterm infants do not have extensive glycogen or fat stores and appear to be less able than infants born at term to adapt rapidly to the changes that occur at birth. Glucose levels decrease more after birth in the preterm infant, which suggests that they are less able to cope with the sudden cessation of the constant glucose supply from the placenta[23]. Some research studies have suggested that enzyme mechanisms necessary for glucose production may be less well developed than at term[24]. However, others have shown that preterm infants can produce glucose as early as 25–26 weeks of gestation[25], so the degree to which preterm infants are able to produce their own glucose remains uncertain. It is known that preterm infants have lower ketone body concentrations than their term counterparts and are therefore less able to benefit from this alternative fuel[26]. This may make them more susceptible to the potential risks of hypoglycaemia.

Hypoglycaemia

Definition

The definition of hypoglycaemia remains controversial[27–29]. A number of studies have sought to determine the level at which brain injury is likely to occur due to insufficient glucose for adequate brain metabolism. The signs and symptoms that are thought to be associated with low glucose levels are by no means specific for hypoglycaemia alone, making it difficult clinically to identify those who are at risk of brain damage. Relatively limited knowledge of neonatal physiological responses to hypoglycaemia, particularly in preterm infants does not allow the definition of a 'safe' range on this basis. Neurodevelopmental follow-up studies suggested that 18-month outcomes were poorer in infants who had experienced glucose levels of below 2.6 mmol/L[30]. Specific associations with occipital lobe damage and visual development have been reported, especially in infants with hyperinsulinism[31,32]. It is likely, however, that the duration of exposure to hypoglycaemia may be as important as the absolute glucose level. Published definitions are very variable in the absence of any firm evidence of a critical level below which neurological impairment is certain. Most neonatal units adopt a pragmatic

approach, aiming to allow a margin of safety; for a 'symptomatic' baby, it is recommended that glucose levels are maintained above 2.5 mmol/L. For infants who are assessed to be 'at risk', but are asymptomatic, a glucose level of < 2.0 mmol/L should be actively managed and for infants who are known to have hyperinsulinism, a higher level (3.5 mmol/L) should be maintained as these infants have very little capacity to utilise alternative fuels if glucose levels fall[33].

Implications for practice

It is important to be aware of the glucose content of infusions:
10% dextrose means 100 g (100,000 mg) glucose per litre (1000 ml) = 100 mg per ml
20% dextrose means 200 g (200,000 mg) glucose per litre = 200 mg per ml

Symptoms of hypoglycaemia

Most infants with hypoglycaemia will be asymptomatic. Symptoms that do arise from severe hypoglycaemia reflect either central nervous system (CNS) excitation or CNS depression. It is important to be aware of both of these aspects. Signs of excitation are jitteriness, high-pitched crying and seizures. CNS depression leads to drowsiness and lethargy, poor feeding and in extreme cases, to apnoeic episodes. Whilst these symptoms can all be indicative of other pathologies, it is crucial to consider hypoglycaemia as the cause, since it is eminently treatable by increasing the glucose intake, but if left untreated, may lead to neurological impairment.

Causes of hypoglycaemia

The causes of hypoglycaemia can be considered as those due to hyperinsulinism or those due to other metabolic or endocrine abnormalities. The glucose requirements of the infant can help to differentiate between these two; infants in whom there is hyperinsulinism will require large amounts of glucose to maintain normoglycaemia (see below) while infants in whom there is no hyperinsulinaemia will remain normoglycaemic on glucose infusions of 4–8 mg/kg/minute.

Infants of diabetic mothers

Suggestions have been made to explain the high frequency with which hypoglycaemia is seen in infants of women with diabetes. It was believed for many years that it was entirely due to poorly controlled maternal hyperglycaemia leading to foetal hyperglycaemia. Subsequent hyperinsulinism was felt to be due to over stimulation of the foetal pancreas. However, it is now known that hypoglycaemia can occur even in babies of women whose glucose control during pregnancy has been good and it has now been suggested that excellent control of maternal glucose during labour may be important in reducing neonatal hypoglycaemia[34]. In fact, a number of factors are probably involved in the causation of hypoglycaemia in this group. Hypoglycaemia usually occurs in infants of diabetic mothers during the first eight hours, but may extend for up to 48 hours after birth.

Hyperinsulinism

Babies that have a persistent and excessively high glucose requirement may have hyperinsulinism. The threshold that is generally used to indicate this is a glucose infusion of 12 mg/kg/minute or more. The diagnosis of hyperinsulinism is made by demonstrating inappropriately high insulin levels in the baby's blood relative to the glucose levels.

Transient hyperinsulinism is sometimes observed in infants of diabetic mothers, babies with Beckwith-Weidemann syndrome, severe intrauterine growth restriction or following perinatal hypoxic-ischaemic insults. Occasionally, no underlying cause is found. In these babies, as long as the glucose supply given is sufficient in the first few days of life, the condition will resolve. In contrast, persistent and severe hyperinsulinism is rare, but can lead to neurological impairment.

Implications for practice

A simple way of classifying the cause of hypoglycaemia is:
- Too little fuel: these infants will respond quickly to physiological levels of intravenous glucose
- Too much insulin (hyperinsulinsim): these infants will require significant delivery of glucose to maintain normoglycaemia

---

Other causes of hypoglycaemia

There are other rare causes of neonatal hypoglycaemia. Such babies will require special investigations to rule out inborn errors of metabolism and endocrine problems. It is vital that these investigations are carried out at a time when the baby is hypoglycaemic. Samples taken when the glucose level is normal will not produce reliable results. Possible metabolic causes of intractable hypoglycaemia include fatty acid oxidation disorders, glucose-6-phosphatase deficiency, galactosaemia and others. Some endocrine causes are hypopituitarism, growth hormone deficiency and adrenal disorders. Septo-optic dysplasia is a disorder in which optic nerve hypoplasia is associated with midline brain abnormalities including abnormalities of the pituitary gland. An ophthalmologist should examine infants in whom a diagnosis of severe and/or symptomatic hypoglycaemia is made and an MRI brain should be considered.

Hyperglycaemia

Definition

Neonatal hyperglycaemia is much less common than hypoglycaemia and occurs only rarely in healthy babies born at term. In contrast, it occurs more frequently in infants born prematurely and in particular those born before 28 weeks of gestation. Hyperglycaemia is usually defined as a blood glucose level of > 7 mmol/L, though no normative values have been specifically proposed for intravenously fed preterm infants.

Symptoms

In infants with high blood glucose levels, the potential exists for the development of an osmotic diuresis with associated weight loss and dehydration; glucose can often be detected in the urine, which provides an indirect indication of this. Increased mortality and neurological impairment have been seen in infants following hyperglycaemia[35].

Causes

There is only a very limited understanding of the mechanisms involved in hyperglycaemia in preterm infants. It is likely to be related to incomplete production of insulin in immature infants. Processing of insulin is also poor at early gestations until some weeks after delivery, sometimes referred to as insulin resistance[36]. In addition, although administration of intravenous glucose by infusion will suppress endogenous glucose production in older children and adults, there is evidence that this is not the case in preterm neonates.

Unexpected hyperglycaemia in an infant in whom an appropriate amount of glucose is being given should prompt consideration of the presence of sepsis. Severe systemic infection can be associated with hyperglycaemia that is profound enough to require treatment with insulin until the sepsis is under control. It can also be observed as a transient response to stress such as that associated with surgery.

Management

It appears that critically ill adults with hyperglycaemia benefit from treatment with continuous insulin infusion[37]. However, recommendations for treatment of hyperglycaemia in premature babies must be made with caution, given the limited evidence available and ongoing research may help to provide more definitive answers to this question. At present, a pragmatic approach is often adopted in neonatal units, with treatment with insulin usually being started when blood glucose rises to a persistently high level of 12–15 mmol/L over a number of hours. Episodes of hyperglycaemia often resolve spontaneously. For those in whom treatment is started, continuation of insulin is usually only required for one or two days but will depend on the assessment by the responsible clinician.

Blood glucose monitoring

How?

Accurate and rapid blood glucose measurement is crucial to effective glycaemic control in the neonatal period. Devices suitable for near-patient testing of whole blood are convenient and are frequently used. Unfortunately, none of these devices can be relied upon for accurate measurement of blood glucose levels that are significantly below or above the normal range in the neonatal population. Measurement of plasma or serum glucose concentrations in a laboratory is preferable and less subject to variability. Arterial blood glucose levels are usually a little higher than venous levels and capillary samples provide intermediate measurements, but the differences between methods are not clinically significant.

Which babies?

Measurement of blood glucose in any infant who is less than three hours of age is inappropriate. The concentration at this time will simply reflect the normal fall in glucose concentration following delivery and is of little, if any, value. The glucose level will rise in all babies, regardless of feed intake, and measurement after this time is much more useful for distinguishing normal from abnormal babies.

Routine measurement of blood glucose during the first 48 hours of life in healthy, asymptomatic term born infants is not necessary. In this population, low levels are likely to represent the course of normal post-natal adaptation rather than pathology, particularly in breast-fed infants.

Any infant who is sick should have blood glucose levels measured, since hypoglycaemia may be a symptom of serious neonatal illness. In others, the disease process may promote hyperglycaemia.

Infants who are at risk of hypoglycaemia, (including preterm, growth restricted, septic, polycythaemic infants, those with known syndromes prone to hypoglycaemia and infants of diabetic mothers) will require monitoring, but there is no evidence to suggest, even in this group, that monitoring in the first two hours of life is beneficial. It is usual, in such babies, to measure levels at a time when they might be expected to be at the lowest point, with the most appropriate time being immediately before a feed. If near-patient testing is used, abnormal values should be confirmed with formal laboratory measurement where possible.

Case studies and suggested management strategies

Case studies

The following case studies illustrate commonly occurring scenarios and highlight areas in which management of fluid balance or glucose is important. Try to think about how fluids for these babies should be managed before referring to the suggested management plans. Remember that these scenarios provide only a general guide and that individual babies will require individual management depending on the clinical condition and underlying problems.

(1) An extremely preterm infant

A baby boy is delivered at 26 weeks of gestation. What are the important things to consider for this baby (1) at delivery; (2) on admission to the neonatal unit; (3) during the first few days of life? The baby's birth weight is 740 g.

(2) An infant following a perinatal hypoxic-ischaemic insult ('perinatal asphyxia')

A baby girl at term is born following a difficult delivery with shoulder dystocia. The baby required extensive resuscitation at birth and the cord pH level was low, indicating that there had been a significant hypoxic-ischaemic insult. The baby is intubated, ventilated and transferred to the neonatal unit.

(3) An asymptomatic infant with hypoglycaemia

A term infant weighing 3.6 kg, born by caesarean section is 20 hours old. His mother's pregnancy was uncomplicated. He is being breast-fed, but his mother has been feeling unwell post-operatively and the baby does not seem to be feeding very well. His blood glucose is measured using a bedside monitoring device and is found to be 1.8 mmol/L. This is confirmed on a sample measured in the laboratory. The baby looks otherwise well and is alert and responsive when he is awake.

(4) A baby with symptoms of hypoglycaemia

A term infant whose mother had gestational diabetes was born by normal delivery and is now eight hours old. He is being breast-fed, but does not seem to be feeding very well. The baby is very sleepy and reluctant to feed. He has also been noted to be rather jittery at times. His blood glucose has been measured on two occasions before feeds and has been around 2.0 mm0l/L on each occasion. He has been put to the breast more regularly, but is still slow to feed and his glucose level has not improved.

Suggested management strategies

(1) The extremely preterm infant

Place the baby into a plastic bag at delivery and ensure that a hat is put on to minimise heat and fluid loss. On admission to the neonatal unit, he should be transferred quickly to a pre-warmed incubator with high (80–100%) humidity. It is important not to lose the benefit of this humidity by trying to minimise the number of times and length of time that the incubator is opened for procedures. The baby will require monitoring and venous access, but avoid applying more monitoring devices or adhesive tape than is clinically necessary, as his skin will be very fragile. Once venous access is established, an infusion of dextrose 10% should be set up. A suitable starting volume for a baby of this size and gestation is 100 ml/kg/day. This will ensure adequate input to cover urinary and insensible losses.

The baby is likely to have respiratory distress syndrome and so the expected early diuresis may be delayed. He should be weighed daily and have regular monitoring of serum sodium levels. Until the urine output increases and the weight starts to fall, the baby should not have any sodium supplements added to the infusion. A low or normal sodium occurring before this in the first few days of life indicates that it is not yet time to start increasing fluid volumes. It is important to continue to watch the sodium levels carefully once the urine output increases – a rapid increase in serum sodium may mean that the fluid input is not 'keeping up with' the baby's losses. Tiny babies can very quickly become dehydrated at this time and the sodium level will often be the first indicator. Nutrition is crucial in extremely preterm babies. This baby's maintenance fluid should be changed to parenteral nutrition containing dextrose 10% as early as possible.

Measurement of the baby's blood and urine glucose levels should be performed regularly. In an extremely preterm baby, hyperglycaemia is more likely to occur than hypoglycaemia. If levels rise to persistently above 12 mmol/L and there is a significant amount of glucose detected in the urine, then treatment with insulin may be considered.

Towards the end of the first week of life, if the baby's course is not complicated by other illness, his electrolytes and fluid requirement should stabilise. For many babies, this requirement will be a maintenance volume of around 150 ml/kg/day, later increasing in line with nutritional demands that are indicated by the rate of weight gain.

(2) The infant following a perinatal hypoxic-ischaemic insult ('perinatal asphyxia')
We can anticipate that this baby is likely to have some degree of renal impairment as a result of her hypoxic ischaemic insult. Her urine output will probably be very low or she may pass no urine initially. Her fluid requirements should be limited from the start to just cover her urine output and insensible losses. An estimate of the appropriate volume is 40 ml/kg/day. She will have a requirement for glucose, so a suitable fluid to give is dextrose 10%. Some babies with this condition become hypoglycaemic because of the small amounts of fluid (and therefore glucose) being administered. Blood glucose levels should be monitored regularly and if significant hypoglycaemia is persistent, the glucose concentration should be increased to correct this, rather than the volume of fluid. Renal impairment is confirmed by monitoring the baby's urea, creatinine and electrolytes. The urine output is likely to remain low and the renal function abnormal for some days before gradually improving. When diuresis begins, it is appropriate to cautiously increase fluids with the increasing urine output and weight loss. Hopefully, the renal function will gradually continue to improve and become normal and the baby's condition will stabilise, allowing fluid management to be more liberal and the introduction of feeding as in other mature babies.

(3) The asymptomatic hypoglycaemic infant
This baby has no significant risk factors for hypoglycaemia and is an appropriate size for a term baby. It is likely that his low blood glucose level relates to a poor intake of milk since birth. Since his mother has been unwell

since surgery, her milk supply may be slow to establish. He is not displaying symptoms, but it is sensible to prevent him from deteriorating until symptoms are present. He is able to feed by mouth and the glucose level is not sufficiently low to require immediate treatment with intravenous fluids. The hypoglycaemia will probably resolve simply with an adequate intake of milk, but if increasing breast-feeds is not possible, this can be by some other method using either expressed breast milk or a suitable formula. Many breast-feeding mothers prefer their babies to be given cup feeds rather than bottles in such circumstances, while breast-feeding is established. Feeding via nasogastric tube may be necessary in some cases. An intake of 60–80 ml/kg/day should be ensured. This can be increased if the glucose fails to rise and the baby is able to take more.

(4) The symptomatic hypoglycaemic infant

This is a baby who is at high risk of significant hypoglycaemia, due to his mother's diabetes. He is clearly feeding poorly and has started to show symptoms that are compatible with hypoglycaemia. An accurate measurement of blood glucose confirms that this may be the cause of his symptoms. Attempts to increase feed frequency by breast have not been successful. As with the asymptomatic baby, it is appropriate to ensure adequate intake of milk by breast, cup or nasogastric tube. If this fails to produce improvement or is not tolerated, the baby will require intravenous dextrose. If the glucose level has fallen further, to below 1.0 mmol/L, an initial bolus of 2–3 ml/kg will usually correct this, and should be followed by an infusion. A continuous infusion of dextrose 10% at a volume of 120 ml/kg/day will provide a glucose intake of 8 mg/kg/minute (see below). This is sufficient for many babies, but if the hypoglycaemia is unresponsive, the concentration can be increased to dextrose 15% (12 mg/kg/minute). Infusions of dextrose at a concentration above 12.5% are better to be given via central venous catheters.

Calculation of glucose delivery

120 ml/kg/day of 10% dextrose
120 ml contains 120 × 100mg = 12000 mg (see above)
The infant is therefore getting 12000 mg/kg/day
= 12000/24 mg/kg/hr = 500 mg/kg/hr
= 500/60mg/kg/min = 8 mg/kg/min

Once the glucose levels have stabilised, the concentration of dextrose can be gradually reduced and milk feeds gradually reintroduced or increased. Rapid discontinuation of intravenous fluids should be avoided, as this will induce 'rebound' hypoglycaemia. If hypoglycaemia persists in this baby, despite adequate infusion of high concentrations of dextrose, there is likely to be an underlying cause. This will require further investigation and blood should be obtained during a hypoglycaemic episode for the necessary tests to exclude metabolic and endocrine disorders.

Conclusion

An understanding of the physiology of fluid, electrolyte and glucose requirements of well term and preterm infants can facilitate an understanding of their requirements in a variety of clinical situations. Knowledge in these areas, together with attention to detail in the clinical scenario can significantly improve their clinical management.

References

1. Friis-Hansen B (1961) Body water compartments in children: changes during growth and related changes in body composition. *Pediatrics*, **28**, 169–181 (accession number 13702099).
2. Friis-Hansen B (1961) Body water compartments in children: changes during growth and related changes in body composition. *Pediatrics*, **28**, 169–181 (accession number 13702099).

3. Modi N, Hutton JL (1990) The influence of post-natal respiratory adaptation on sodium handling in preterm neonates. *Early Hum Dev*, **21** (1), 11–20.

4. Aperia A, Herin P, Lundin S, Melin P, Zetterstrom R (1984) Regulation of renal water excretion in newborn full-term infants. *Acta Paediatr Scand*, **73** (6), 717–721.

5. Hammarlund K, Sedin G (1979) Transepidermal water loss in newborn infants. III. Relation to gestational age. *Acta Paediatr Scand*, **68** (6), 795–801.

6. Hammarlund K, Sedin G, Stromberg B (1983) Transepidermal water loss in newborn infants. VIII. Relation to gestational age and post-natal age in appropriate and small for gestational age infants. *Acta Paediatr Scand*, **72** (5), 721–728.

7. Harpin VA, Rutter N (1982) Sweating in preterm babies. *J Pediatr*, **100** (4), 614–619.

8. Modi N, Hutton JL (1990) The influence of post-natal respiratory adaptation on sodium handling in preterm neonates. *Early Hum Dev*, **21** (1), 11–20.

9. Brion LP, Soll RF (2001) Diuretics for respiratory distress syndrome in preterm infants. *Cochrane Database Syst Rev* (2), CD001454.

10. Modi N (1998) Hyponatraemia in the newborn. *Arch Dis Child Foetal Neonatal Ed*, **78** (2), F81–F84.

11. Shaffer SG, Meade VM (1989) Sodium balance and extracellular volume regulation in very low birth weight infants. *J Pediatr*, **115** (2), 285–290.

12. Al-Dahhan J, Haycock GB, Nichol B, Chantler C, Stimmler L (1984) Sodium homeostasis in term and preterm neonates, III. Effect of salt supplementation. *Arch Dis Child*, **59** (10), 945–950.

13. Ekblad H, Kero P, Takala J, Korvenranta H, Valimaki I (1987) Water, sodium and acid-base balance in premature infants: therapeutical aspects. *Acta Paediatr Scand*, **76** (1), 47–53.

14. Knobel RB, Wimmer JE, Jr, Holbert D (2005) Heat loss prevention for preterm infants in the delivery room. *J Perinatol*, **25** (5), 304–308.

15. McCall EM, Alderdice FA, Halliday HL, Jenkins JG, Vohra S (2005) Interventions to prevent hypothermia at birth in preterm and/or low birth-weight babies. *Cochrane Database Syst Rev* (1) CD004210.

16. Bozzetti P, Ferrari MM, Marconi AM, *et al.* (1988) The relationship of maternal and foetal glucose concentrations in the human from midgestation until term. *Metabolism*, **37** (4), 358–363.

17. Rozance P, Limesand SW, Zerbe GO, Hay WW Jr (2007) Chronic foetal hypoglycemia inhibits the later steps of stimulus-secretion coupling in pancreatic beta-cells. *Am J Physiol Endocrinol Metab*, **292** (5), E1256–E1264.

18. Denne SC, Kalhan SC (1986) Glucose carbon recycling and oxidation in human newborns. *Am J Physiol*, 251 (1 Pt 1), E71–E77.

19. Srinivasan G, Pildes R, Cattamanchi G, Voora S, Lilien LD (1986) Plasma glucose values in normal neonates: a new look. *J Pediatr*, **109** (1), 114–117.

20. Hoseth E, Joergensen A, Ebbensen F, Moeller M (2000) Blood glucose levels in a population of healthy, breast fed, term infants of appropriate size for gestational age. *Arch Dis Child Foetal Neonatal Ed*, **83** (2), F117–F119.

21. Hawdon JM, Ward Platt MP, Aynsley-Green A (1992) Patterns of metabolic adaptation for preterm and term infants in the first neonatal week. *Arch Dis Child*, **67** (4 Spec No.), 357–365.

22. Diwakar KK, Sasidhar MV (2002) Plasma glucose levels in term infants who are appropriate size for gestation and exclusively breast fed. *Arch Dis Child Foetal Neonatal Ed*, **87** (1), F46–F48.

23. van Kempen AA, Romijn JA, Ruiter AF, *et al.* (2003) Alanine administration does not stimulate gluconeogenesis in preterm infants. *Metabolism*, **52** (8), 945–949.

24. van Kempen AA, Romijn JA, Ruiter AF, *et al.* (2003) Alanine administration does not stimulate gluconeogenesis in preterm infants. *Metabolism*, **52** (8), 945–949.

25. Sunehag A, Ewald U, Gustafsson J (1996) Extremely preterm infants (< 28 weeks) are capable of gluconeogenesis from glycerol on their first day of life. *Pediatr Res*, **40** (4), 553–557.

26. Hawdon JM, Ward Platt MP, Aynsley-Green A (1992) Patterns of metabolic adaptation for preterm and term infants in the first neonatal week. *Arch Dis Child*, **67** (4 Spec No.), 357–365.

27. Koh TH, Eyre JA, Aynsley-Green A (1988) Neonatal hypoglycaemia – the controversy regarding definition. *Arch Dis Child*, **63** (11), 1386–1388.

28. Koh TH, Vong SK (1996) Definition of neonatal hypoglycaemia: is there a change? *J Paediatr Child Health*, **32** (4), 302–305.

29. Cornblath M, Hawdon JM, Williams A, *et al.* (2000) Controversies regarding definition of neonatal hypoglycemia: suggested operational thresholds. *Pediatrics*, **105** (5), 1141–1145.

30. Lucas A, Morley R, Cole TJ (1988) Adverse neurodevelopmental outcome of moderate neonatal hypoglycaemia. *BMJ*, **297** (6659), 1304–1308.

31. Alkalay AL, Sarnat HB, Flores-Sarnat L, Simmons CF (2005) Neurologic aspects of neonatal hypoglycemia. *Isr Med Assoc J*, **7** (3), 188–192.

32. Filan PM, Inder TE, Cameron FJ, Kean MJ, Hunt RW (2006) Neonatal hypoglycemia and occipital cerebral injury. *J Pediatr*, **148** (4), 552–555.

33. Ward Platt M, Deshpande S (2005) Metabolic adaptation at birth. *Semin Foetal Neonatal Med*, **10** (4), 341–350.

34. Taylor R, Lee C, Kyne-Grzebalski D, Marshall SM, Davison JM (2002) Clinical outcomes of pregnancy in women with type I diabetes (1). *Obstet Gynecol*, **99** (4), 537–541.

35. Pildes REST, Pyati SP (1986) Hypoglycemia and hyperglycemia in tiny infants. *Clin Perinatol*, **13** (2), 351–375.

36. Mitanchez-Mokhtari D, Lahlou N, Kieffer F, Magny JF, Roger M, Voyer M (2004) Both relative insulin resistance and defective islet beta-cell processing of proinsulin are responsible for transient hyperglycemia in extremely preterm infants. *Pediatrics*, 113 (3 Pt 1), 537–541.

37. van den Berghe G, Wouters P, Weekers F, *et al.* (2001) Intensive insulin therapy in the critically ill patients. *N Engl J Med*, **345** (19), 1359–1367.

Chapter 8

RESPIRATORY DIFFICULTIES AND VENTILATORY SUPPORT

Venkatesh Kairamkonda

Learning outcomes

After reading this chapter the reader will be expected to be able to:

- Describe the stages of lung development

- Describe the functions of surfactant and the factors that influence surfactant production

- Identify common respiratory diseases in the neonatal unit

- Describe the diagnosis and management of chronic lung disease

- Explain some of the standard and more recent modalities of ventilation

- Recognise common blood gas abnormalities and understand the implications for practice

---

Introduction

Respiratory difficulties are the most common presenting complaint in both preterm and term neonates in the neonatal intensive care unit and are associated with significant morbidity and mortality. The first part of this chapter looks at some fundamental principles of embryology, anatomy and physiology as well as the common neonatal respiratory diseases. The second part will cover ventilation principles and strategies used in the neonatal intensive care.

Pulmonary embryology

This section is a brief overview of human lung development and physiology which will aid in the understanding of the pathophysiology of neonatal lung problems. The primordial lung bud appears on day 26 of gestation as a ventral epithelial outgrowth from the foregut (Figure 8.1). Each epithelial branch that is formed divides into two (dichotomous branching) and penetrates into the lung mesenchyme in a caudal (foot) direction.

Lung development may be divided into the following five phases[1]. A summary of the stages of lung development is provided in Figure 8.1 (shown later in this chapter).

Phase 1
Embryonic period: formation of proximal airways (4 to 6 weeks)
During this phase the airways develop to the level of the bronchopulmonary segments. The right and left main bronchi are the first to appear, followed by the five lobar bronchi

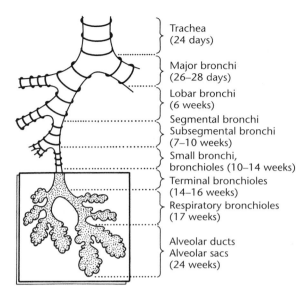

Trachea
(24 days)

Major bronchi
(26–28 days)

Lobar bronchi
(6 weeks)

Segmental bronchi
Subsegmental bronchi
(7–10 weeks)

Small bronchi,
bronchioles (10–14 weeks)

Terminal bronchioles
(14–16 weeks)

Respiratory bronchioles
(17 weeks)

Alveolar ducts
Alveolar sacs
(24 weeks)

Figure 8.1 A summary of the stages of lung development.

(two on the left and three on the right) and finally the ten segmental bronchi on each side.

Phase 2
Glandular period: formation of conducting airways (7 to 16 weeks)
During this phase the dichotomous branching continues to the level of the acinus (gas exchange unit) and cartilage begins to appear in the trachea, developing peripherally and reaching the last bronchi at term. The pleural membranes and pulmonary lymphatics also begin to develop. By the end of the glandular phase a total of about 20 generations of conducting airways have developed and the last eight generations are called bronchioles. Also during this phase there is differentiation of cartilage and the respiratory epithelial cells.

Phase 3
Canalicular period: formation of acini (17 to 27 weeks)
At 17 weeks the first intra-acinar respiratory bronchioles have developed by dichotomous branching from the terminal bronchioles. There are two or three generations of respiratory bronchioles which contribute to the acinus.

Two separate capillary networks develop within the lung: The capillaries that develop from pulmonary arteries drain into the pulmonary veins to form a network around the alveoli for gas exchange to occur. This is in contrast to the bronchial circulation that functions to maintain the oxygen and nutrient supply to the lung tissue itself. At 19 to 20 weeks apposition of the capillary endothelial cells and the alveolar-lining epithelial cells occurs, with sporadic points of fusion of their respective basement membranes. From that time the total area of the alveolar-blood barrier increases exponentially.

Phase 4
Saccular period: expansion of the gas-exchanging sites (28 to 35 weeks)
At 28 weeks, the appearance of secondary ridges begins the division of primary saccules into sub-saccules or primitive alveoli, which have a flattened epithelium and a double-capillary network. The interstitium becomes less prominent and saccular and sub-saccular development accelerates greatly, contributing to the increase in lung volume and surface area.

Phase 5
Alveolar period: expansion of surface area (36 weeks to three years post-term)
The formation of alveoli is accomplished by further thinning of the interstitium and the appearance of a single capillary network, in which one capillary bulges into both the alveoli with which it is associated. There are about 50 million alveoli at term, reaching 300 million by approximately three years of age, thereafter all components grow proportionately until adulthood[2].

Implications for practice

- The lungs of preterm infants born between 24 to 30 weeks gestation are at a very important stage, due to alveolar and capillary development.
- The lung of a normal term baby has one-fifth of the final number of alveoli and extreme preterm infants have no alveoli at all.

Table 8.1 Factors influencing surfactant production.

Factors associated with an increase in surfactant production and *decreased* risk of RDS	Factors associated with a decrease in surfactant production and/or *increased* risk of RDS
Maternal factors • Maternal steroids (used in preterm deliveries) [3] • Narcotic/cocaine use • Pregnancy induced hypertension • Increased thyroid hormone • Prolonged rupture of membranes **Foetal/infant factors** • Intrauterine growth restriction • Twin gestation	**Maternal factors** • Maternal diabetes • Chorioamnionitis **Foetal/infant factors** • Hypoxia/acidosis • Hypothermia • Meconium • Congenital abnormality of surfactant production (e.g. surfactant protein B deficiency)

Foetal lung

Foetal lung fluid

Foetal lung fluid first appears during the second trimester and is approximately 30 ml/kg at term. The composition of this fluid is different from amniotic fluid and plasma especially due to high chloride levels of 157 mmol/l (plasma contains 90–110 mmol/l).

Surfactant synthesis

Surfactant is produced in the type II pneumocytes of the alveoli and stored in its lameller bodies. The lipoprotein mixture of surfactant helps lower the surface tension and increase lung compliance, thereby preventing alveolar collapse following expiration. Type II pneumocytes appear in the human lung at about 20 weeks of gestation and surfactant production progressively increases until 30–34 weeks, when the lungs are mature and the baby is less likely to develop respiratory distress syndrome when delivered. Surfactant once released has a half-life of about ten hours. Some is washed up the bronchial tree, some ingested by lung macrophages, and some broken down by enzymes. However, the majority is taken up by the type II pneumocytes and recycled. Hypothermia, hypoxia and acidosis inhibit surfactant production and spreading within the lungs. Additionally, the rate of surfactant breakdown is increased when breathing pure oxygen and by over ventilation.

Table 8.1 (also Table 3.1 in Chapter 3) summarises factors that affect surfactant production.

Implications for practice

- Surfactant appears in the lung after 20 weeks and is present in adequate amounts at 30–34 weeks gestation, which means that respiratory distress secondary to surfactant deficiency is less likely after this gestation.
- Cold, acidosis and hypoxia rapidly decreases the amount of surfactant in pharyngeal aspirates.

Surfactant composition

Surfactant is composed of 90% lipid and 10% protein. About 85% of the lipid is phospholipid, and the remainder consists of neutral lipid, cholesterol and sphingomyelin. The major phospholipids are phosphotidylcholine (lecithin), phosphotidylglycerol and phosphotidylinositol. There are four main surfactant proteins: namely SP-A, SP-B, SP-C and SP-D. SP-B and SP-C play an important role in the surface tension lowering properties of the surfactant complex. Congenital deficiency of surfactant protein B is a lethal disorder affecting mature newborns who present as if they had 'idiopathic respiratory distress syndrome' (this is discussed later).

Post-natal adaption

This has already been described in Chapter 3 but will be summarised again here. At the time of delivery, the foetal lungs contain about 30 ml/kg of fluid. Shortly before birth the production of foetal lung fluid is reduced, lung cells switch from secretion to absorption, and the lung interstitium rapidly removes fluid via lymphatics and lung capillaries. The newborn at birth is stimulated by the cold environment and the clamping of the cord to take its first breaths and generates an opening pressure of 20 to 30 cm H_2O. This pressure is enough to overcome the surface tension of the alveoli as well as the elastic recoil and resistance of the lungs and chest wall to achieve initial aeration of the lungs and force the remaining lung fluid into the lung lymphatics.

Implications for practice

Foetal lung fluid is produced throughout the second half of pregnancy and must be cleared rapidly from the lungs for normal gas exchange to start.

Lung physiology

Control of respiration

Spontaneous unconscious respiration is controlled by the respiratory centre that lies within the brainstem. This centre stimulates contraction of the diaphragm, intercostal and subcostal muscles, which causes expansion of the thoracic cage. This generates negative intra-thoracic pressure that results in air being sucked in through an unobstructed upper airway. This can be termed negative pressure ventilation and is in complete contrast to the common methods of artificial ventilation that use the generation of positive intra-thoracic pressure. Normal inspiration is therefore the active phase and expiration is largely passive, except when there are increased exercise demands when it becomes more forceful or active. The respiratory centre itself responds to messages from chemoreceptors that respond to the level of CO_2 (carbon dioxide) and O_2 (oxygen) within the blood.

Mechanics of respiration

Understanding the exact mechanics of normal respiration as well as ventilation requires an understanding of some terms that are commonly used and these are defined below.

Compliance

- This refers to how easily the chest will move with normal pressure ventilation and is written using a formula:

  compliance = volume/pressure

- This formula suggests that if a large pressure is needed to cause a specific volume of movement then the compliance of the lungs and chest is lower than if a smaller pressure is needed.
- Lungs that are poorly compliant are commonly referred to as 'stiff' lungs.

Resistance

- This term is used to describe the frictional resistance to flow caused by the air/oxygen rubbing against the walls of bronchi, ventilator circuit, endotracheal tube etc.
- There are two main types of flow; laminar or turbulent. Laminar flow is smooth and has a low resistance, while turbulent flow describes a gas that swirls around and has a higher resistance.
- Airway calibre is by far the most important factor affecting the type of flow; halving the airway diameter increases airway resistance by a factor of 16.
- High flow rates, narrow tubes, kinks and bifurcations all increase the likelihood of turbulent flow.

Work of breathing

- This term is used to describe the work or force to expand the lung against its visco-elastic

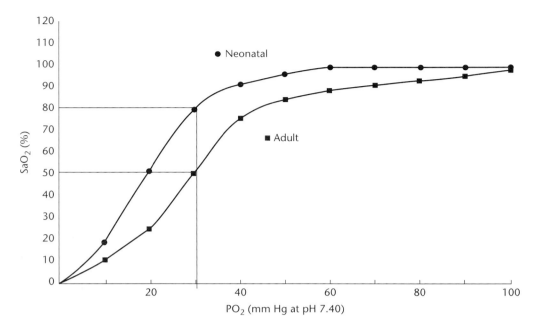

Figure 8.2 Oxygen dissociation curve.

(lung and chest wall) and frictional (air-flow resistance) properties.

- This measure is one of many useful indicators to evaluate for successful extubation of infants from ventilators.

Minute ventilation

- This term describes the volume of gas ventilated in one minute and expressed as: minute ventilation = (tidal volume × number of breaths) per minute

- It is a useful measure to consider when adjusting ventilator parameters in response to blood gas and transcutaneous CO_2 and PO_2 levels.

Physiology of gas exchange

In order for effective gas exchange to occur there must be a close relationship between the gas within the alveoli and the red blood cells within the pulmonary capillary network, as well as a physiological method for exchanging oxygen molecules (and carbon dioxide). One of the complications that can affect the efficiency of

gas exchange is what is known as a ventilation (V)/perfusion (Q) mismatch. This can occur in the following situations:

- There are areas of the lung in which the alveoli are well aerated but there is a no effective capillary perfusion:
  ○ This may be because of blood taking a short cut (shunting) that means that some pulmonary capillaries next to alveoli are not filled with blood
  ○ This can also happen if there is a clot or embolus blocking the route to the capillary network; this is uncommon
- There may be areas of the lung which are not well aerated although the blood flow through the capillary network is completely normal. This is common and occurs because of areas of collapse or consolidation within the lungs.

If there is good ventilation and perfusion the oxygen should be able to move from the alveoli into the capillaries and the efficiency of this transport across the fused capillary/alveolar membrane is influenced by a variety of factors that affect the position of the oxygen dissociation curve. This has already been referred to in Chapter 3 but is expanded on within this chapter.

The position of the adult oxygen-haemoglobin dissociation curve is controlled by pH (acid-base balance), temperature, the intracellular concentration of 2,3-DiPhosphoGlycerate (2,3-DPG) and the interaction between these three factors. 2,3-DPG decreases the affinity of haemoglobin for oxygen.

The oxygen dissociation curve (see Figure 8.2) will move to the right and allow the haemoglobin to release oxygen under the following conditions:

- Increase 2,3 DPG
- A decrease in pH or increase in CO_2
- A rise in temperature

The oxygen dissociation curve (see Figure 8.2) will move to the left to allow the haemoglobin to receive oxygen under the following conditions:

- Decrease 2,3, DPG
- An increase in pH or decrease in CO2
- A decrease in temperature

The blood of the neonate has a left-sided oxyhaemoglobin dissociation curve because the cells contain foetal haemoglobin (Hb F) which reacts poorly with 2,3-DPG (the gamma chain present in foetal haemoglobin does not bind to 2,3 DPG). This means that during the first weeks of life the haemoglobin of a neonate has no problems with the uptake of oxygen from the lungs but may find it more difficult to release oxygen into the tissues.

Implications for practice

Foetal blood has a high affinity for oxygen and is reluctant to release oxygen to the tissues, especially in hypothermia, hypoxia and over ventilation.

Respiratory problems in the newborn

Newborn infants often present with non-specific signs and symptoms and it is therefore important to examine them systematically in order to identify specific differential diagnoses.

The signs and symptoms of respiratory difficulty include:

- Grunting (moaning): forced expiration against a closed glottis
- Head bobbing, nasal flare, and intercostal, subcostal and sternal recessions
- Tachypnoea > 60 breaths/minute
- Gasping breathing
- Slow or shallow breathing
- Apnoea

It is important to be aware that respiratory difficulty can also be a sign of congenital heart disease. In addition, tachypnoea is common in spontaneously breathing infants with a metabolic

Table 8.2 The respiratory diseases of the preterm and term infant that present early after birth.

Preterm	Term > preterm
Respiratory distress syndrome	Transient tachypneoa of the newborn
Massive pulmonary haemorrhage	Meconium aspiration syndrome
Pneumonia (group B streptococcal disease)	Pneumonia (group B streptococcal disease)
Persistent pulmonary hypertension of the newborn	Pneumothorax or pneumomediastinum
	Congenital lung malformation, e.g. CCAM
	Congenital diaphragmatic hernia
	Congenital heart disease e.g. transposition of the great arteries
	Persistent pulmonary hypertension of the newborn
	Feed aspiration
	Upper airway obstruction

Table 8.3 The respiratory diseases of the preterm and term infants that may have a delayed presentation.

Aetiology of respiratory illness after four hours of birth	
Preterm	**Term > preterm**
Pneumonia	Pneumonia
Late-onset lung diseases of the VLBW infants (Wilson-Mikity syndrome and chronic pulmonary insufficiency of prematurity)	Congenital heart disease, e.g. duct dependent congenital heart disease or large VSD
	Congenital malformation
	Acidaemia associated with inborn error of metabolism

acidosis as they attempt to clear CO_2 in order to return the pH to normal (compensation).

Some diseases that present with respiratory symptoms and signs will present immediately after birth and these are listed in Table 8.2 These should be compared to those in Table 8.3, which may present slightly later in view of the natural history of the disease.

Idiopathic respiratory distress syndrome (hyaline membrane disease)

The historical terminology of hyaline membrane disease refers to a pathological diagnosis of surfactant deficient lung disease and the more correct terminology is idiopathic respiratory distress syndrome. This occurs due to insufficient and/or inefficient surfactant and the main aetiologies are:

- Prematurity < 34 weeks
- Perinatal asphyxia
- Maternal diabetes

Main causes of respiratory distress syndrome
Prematurity
Gestational age is the major determinant of respiratory distress syndrome (RDS) since surfactant does not appear in the lungs until the second trimester and not in large amounts until the third trimester. However, not all premature infants will develop the disease and it can also occur at term, especially in infants of diabetic mothers.

Perinatal asphyxia
Infants with hypoxic ischaemic encephalopathy may have respiratory distress due to hypoxaemia and acidaemia, reducing surfactant synthesis.

Maternal diabetes
The respiratory distress seen in infants of mothers with diabetes occurs secondary to a delay in surfactant maturation, in particular the appearance of phosphotidylglycerol.

Prevention of RDS
The incidence and the severity of neonatal RDS may be reduced by antenatal administration of steroids to the mother and prophylactic administration of surfactant to the baby at resuscitation[4]. The benefits of antenatal steroids are maximum if they have been administered at least four hours before delivery and ideally not longer than 14 days before delivery[5-7]. However, repeated doses of antenatal steroids are not recommended and there is concern that this practice may have detrimental effects on the developing neonatal brain[8]. The benefits of antenatal steroids include maturation of immature lung structure and the initiation of surfactant apoprotein synthesis. The avoidance of prematurity, hypothermia, acidosis and hypoxia will also decrease the severity of the RDS.

Clinical signs of RDS
Surfactant deficient lung disease presents within the first four hours after birth with the following signs and symptoms:

- Respiratory rate more than 60/minute
- Respiratory distress
- Nasal flare, intercostal, sternal and subcostal recession
- Grunting: this is forced expiration against a partially closed glottis to maintain expiration pressure or PEEP

Radiological signs of RDS

The chest X-ray (see Figure 8.3) changes do not appear until a few hours of age and include:

- Increased lung expansion with flattened diaphragms
- Homogenous reticulogranular (ground glass) pattern due to alveolar collapse
- 'Air bronchograms' that extend to the lung periphery; this refers to air filled bronchi superimposed on the background of alveoli collapse. It is normal to see air bronchograms within the first third of the lung field but extension to the periphery suggests lung disease.

Implications for practice

Preterm infants < 34 weeks gestation are those most at risk of respiratory distress syndrome, but good attention to perinatal care (antenatal steroids, early surfactant, thermoregulation) can reduce this risk.

Surfactant therapy

History

Exogenous surfactant has now been in use for over a decade and it has had a dramatic impact on the incidence and severity of RDS. The administration of surfactant has been demonstrated to reduce neonatal mortality secondary to RDS by about 40% and the administration of antenatal steroids as well as post-natal surfactant have been shown to have independent effects on mortality and morbidity[9, 10]. Surfactant treatment in isolation has not been demonstrated to have an effect against complications such as chronic lung disease (CLD). There is some evidence to suggest that elective intubation and administration of surfactant with the first breath may reduce this serious complication in the preterm infant[11,12]. The complications of surfactant use include the development of clinically significant PDA (this makes theoretical sense since the administration of surfactant will drop the pulmonary blood pressure and allow

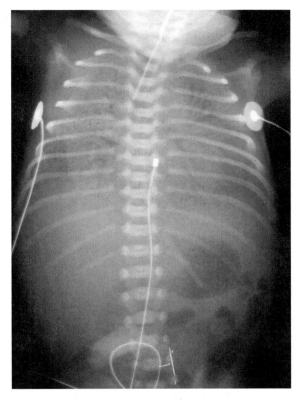

Figure 8.3 This chest X-ray demonstrates the features of RDS (also note sub-optimal position of endotracheal tube tip).

the development of a left to right shunt (see Chapter 11) and increase the risk of pulmonary haemorrhage[13].

Indications and administration

Surfactant administration should be considered in all preterm infants that require ventilation at birth and initial intubation and ventilation should be considered in preterm infants < 1.5 kg or 28 weeks gestation even if they show moderate respiratory effort to allow for this to occur. The first dose of surfactant should be given as soon as the infant has been intubated and this should be done on the delivery suite[14]. There are two main types of surfactant; those derived from animal sources and those that are artificial. Systematic reviews favour prophylactic natural surfactant versus rescue artificial surfactant

Table 8.4 A summary of the commonly used surfactants in the UK.

Surfactants used in clinical trials and available in the UK		
Surfactant (manufacturer)	Animal source	Dose in mg/kg
Beractant/Survanta (Abbott)	Cow	100 (4 ml)
Curosurf (CHEISI)	Pig	100 (1.25 ml)
Exosurf/Colfosceril palmitate (Glaxo)	Artificial	5 ml/kg

and the commonly used surfactants are listed in Table 8.4[15]. Current recommendations are for two doses to be given within 12 hours; if the baby remains ill further doses can be given and in infants with surfactant protein B deficiency multiple doses may be required until the diagnosis has been confirmed.

Management of infants with respiratory distress syndrome

Delivery room

A dedicated experienced neonatal team should attend those deliveries in which respiratory concern has been predicted. Routine intubation and early surfactant administration should be considered in all extreme preterm deliveries (<26 weeks) and in the moderately preterm who do not quickly establish regular respiration. Prophylactic surfactant is better than rescue and there is increasing evidence that early prophylactic is better than late prophylactic[16]. The use of immediate CPAP following delivery can be considered in infants that do establish spontaneous regular respiration[17–19].

Intensive care

The mainstay of treatment is to provide the appropriate oxygenation and ventilatory support, monitoring and supplementary intensive care support until the infant starts to synthesise his/her own surfactant (usually 2–3 days). Ventilatory support will be discussed in detail in the second half of this chapter.

Monitoring is an important aspect of all neonatal intensive care. In most cases an umbilical arterial line will have been inserted to optimise the monitoring of blood pressure. This will also allow blood tests to be easily taken as well as allowing access to blood in order to perform regular blood gases and other blood investigations.

Some of the important elements of monitoring are summarised below:

- Core-peripheral temperature difference: a difference of >2°C may point to perfusion problems
- Invasive and non-invasive monitoring:
  - Arterial PaO_2, $PaCO_2$, pH, base deficit: continuous or intermittent arterial PaO_2 monitoring from indwelling peripheral or umbilical arterial lines
  - transcutaneous PO_2 (TcPo2), PCO_2 (TcCO$_2$) and oximetry (SpO_2) should also be used if available as this reduces the need for blood collection and also gives a trend over time to identify ventilatory problems such as endotracheal tube (ETT) block
  - Preductal (right hand) and postductal SpO_2 monitoring will help in the early diagnosis of pulmonary hypertension due to blood shunting right to left across the PDA
  - Targeted oxygen saturation monitoring as per local guidelines to prevent oxygen induced lung damage and retinopathy of prematurity
- Blood pressure: continuous recording from indwelling arterial catheter to maintain a mean arterial pressure that ensures adequate organ perfusion (see Chapter 11)
- Urine ouput: a urine output of > 1 ml/kg/hour suggests adequate renal perfusion
- Respiratory activity: to assess work of breathing; this is the respiratory rate and suprasternal, sternal, intercostal and subcostal recessions

The following are examples of the supplementary intensive care that will also be required:

- Ensure vitamin K has been given
- Maintain in a thermoneutral environment (see Chapter 6)
- Maintain electrolyte and renal homeostasis (see Chapter 7)
- Avoid hypoxemia, hyperoxia and acidemia
- Maintain adequate nutrition either via nasogastric tube or as total parenteral nutrition (see Chapter 12)
- Antibiotics should be prescribed and administered as RDS cannot be distinguished clinically and radiologically from Group B streptococcal infection

Implications for practice

- Monitoring of vital signs is a crucial part of care.
- Nursing staff have a responsibility to maintain their clinical knowledge and skills so that subtle changes are quickly recognised and responded to.

SP-B deficiency

Congenital deficiency of surfactant protein B is a rare, lethal, autosomal recessive disorder affecting mature newborns. The affected infants present soon after birth with clinical and radiological findings similar to 'idiopathic respiratory distress syndrome'. However, while respiratory distress syndrome improves with surfactant replacement therapy and supportive care, SP-B deficiency progresses to severe respiratory failure that is refractory to all treatment modalities.

Chronic lung disease/bronchopulmonary dysplasia

Chronic lung disease (CLD) or bronchopulmonary dysplasia, first described in 1967[20], usually evolves following treatment for respiratory distress syndrome (RDS). The incidence of CLD is rising and this is likely to be due to the increasing survival of extremely preterm and low birthweight infants. CLD is a major cause of long-term pulmonary sequelae such as bronchial obstruction and hyper-responsiveness in early childhood that may persist until schoolage or adulthood.

Diagnosis of CLD

There are different diagnostic criteria for CLD which are largely based on a single clinical criterion, the need for prolonged oxygen therapy, which serves as a marker for chronic respiratory failure. The most widely used definitions of CLD are the need for continuous supplemental oxygen beyond 36 weeks post-menstrual age or the need for oxygen at 28 days of life. The National Institute of Child Health and Human Development (NICHD) criteria further classify CLD in < 32 weeks infants into[21]:

- Mild CLD: oxygen requirement at 28 days but no oxygen requirement at corrected gestational age of 36 weeks
- Moderate CLD: oxygen requirement of < 30% at corrected gestational age of 36 weeks
- Severe CLD: oxygen requirement of > 30% or the use of positive pressure ventilation at corrected gestational age of 36 weeks

Epidemiology of CLD

Recently, two types of CLD have been recognised: namely 'classical' or 'old' CLD and 'atypical' or 'new' CLD. Atypical CLD refers to the CLD that develops in infants that went into air shortly after birth or had a minimal oxygen requirement but subsequently developed prolonged oxygen dependence[22,23]. The incidence of atypical CLD is also increasing and has been reported to be 31–41% of CLD, depending on the clinical criteria used[24]. There has also been a change in the pathology of CLD, with the severe airway injury and fibrosis that characterised 'classical CLD' (Figure 8.4) being replaced by arrested lung development and alveolar hypoplasia of 'atypical' CLD.

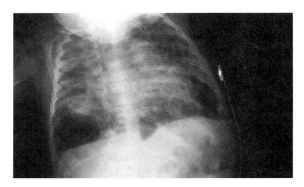

Figure 8.4 Chest radiograph demonstrating hyper-inflation, interstitial changes, and generalised emphysema characteristic of severe CLD.

Aetiology of CLD

Many factors are thought to play a part in the aetiology of CLD, including genetic susceptibility. The main predisposing risks include:

- Ventilator induced lung injury (VILI): complications associated with assisted mechanical ventilation such as barotrauma and volutrauma
- Biotrauma: antenatal, (chronic chorioamnionitis) perinatal and post-natal infections, including those caused by staphylococcus epidermidis
- Oxygen trauma: oxygen free radicals and anti-oxidant imbalance
- Fluid and nutrition:
  - Patent ductus arteriosus and fluid overload
  - Malnutrition

Prevention of CLD

Specific preventive therapy is not available. Post-natal steroids and/or surfactant do not prevent CLD but CPAP at delivery, 'gentle' ventilation, targeted oxygen saturations, the avoidance of calorie and protein malnutrition, careful fluid balance and the avoidance of infection, probably do.

Treatment of CLD

Treatment at 7–10 days with systemic corticosteroids is currently the most effective therapy, but may increase the risk of cerebral palsy[25–27]. Long-term treatment with diuretics, inhaled steroids or bronchodilators are not of proven benefit. The aim of treatment is to improve respiratory morbidity and prevent the development of pulmonary hypertension. At present the mainstay of long-term treatment is home oxygen therapy and respiratory follow-up with good nutritional support, but other areas continue to be investigated, such as the use of nitric oxide.

Prognosis

Infants surviving with severe CLD have a higher risk of death, are at increased risk of life-threatening respiratory infections such as respiratory syncytial virus, may have abnormal pulmonary function testing into late childhood, and are at increased risk for neurodevelopmental sequelae, compared with infants with mild or no CLD.

Implications for practice

Chronic lung disease (CLD) is defined as those requiring oxygen at 28 days and/or 36 weeks CGA.
Infants with CLD:
- Require careful nursing as these infants may easily become tired and stressed.
- May require an increase in calories due to increased work of breathing.

Wilson-Mikity syndrome

Wilson-Mikity syndrome was first described in 1960 in a group of preterm very low birth-weight infants who had minimal or absent early respiratory distress but later developed clinical and radiological picture of CLD. Some experts believe that this condition is no different to 'new' CLD[28].

Other respiratory problems

Transient tachypnoea of the newborn (TTN)

This condition affects mainly mature infants, but it does occur in those born prematurely. It is attributed to delayed clearing of the foetal lung liquid after the onset of respiration and is more common in infants delivered by caesarean section before the onset of labour. As a result, the Royal College of Obstetricians and Gynaecologists recommend that elective caesarean section should be performed no earlier than 39 weeks gestation because of the increased frequency of TTN at lower gestations[29,30].

TTN presents immediately from birth and the management consists of respiratory support in the form of oxygen or CPAP. A CXR may help differentiate TTN from RDS or pneumonia as the lung fields appear 'wet' and fluid can be seen occupying the horizontal fissure of the right lung. However, in view of the risk of infection antibiotics are usually commenced. The symptoms usually resolve within 24 hours and certainly by 2–3 days.

Persistent pulmonary hypertension of the newborn (PPHN)

Persistent pulmonary hypertension of the newborn occurs when the pulmonary vascular resistance fails to decrease after birth despite lung expansion. It has also been referred to as persistent foetal circulation because the venous blood is shunted right to left into the systemic circulation in a similar to way to *in utero* (through the foramen oval and patent ductus arteriosus). This leads to systemic hypoxaemia and tissue hypoxia. In addition, a large mechanical load is placed on the right heart to continue to pump blood to both the pulmonary and systemic high resistance circuits. With high vascular resistance and the subsequent hypoxemia, myocardial performance may become extremely compromised, resulting in right heart dilation, tricuspid insufficiency and right heart failure.

This disorder can be classified into three forms depending on the likely aetiology of the pulmonary hypertension:

- *PPHN associated with pulmonary parenchymal disease*, such as hyaline membrane disease or meconium aspiration syndrome
- *PPHN with radiographically normal lungs* and no evidence of parenchymal disease, such as perinatal hypoxia

- *PPHN associated with hypoplasia of the lungs*, such as diaphragmatic hernia associated with an anatomic reduction in capillary number

Diagnosis of PPHN

The infant presents clinically with cyanosis and tachypnoea and other signs and symptoms reflecting the underlying aetiology of the PPHN. An oxygen tension gradient may be noted between the preductal arterial circulation (i.e. right upper extremity) and the postductal arterial circulation (i.e. lower extremities) especially with a large right-to-left shunt through a patent ductus arteriosus. However, this gradient may not be present if substantial shunting is present at the level of the foramen ovale. Systemic hypotension is a late finding, usually resulting from both heart failure and persistent hypoxemia. A CXR may show signs of the underlying aetiology as well as oligaemic lung fields secondary to poor pulmonary blood flow because of the high pulmonary pressures. Oxygenation is one of the main challenges and arterial gases should be closely monitored.

Echocardiography will confirm the diagnosis by excluding congenital cyanotic heart disease and demonstrating elevated pulmonary arterial pressures which are higher than systemic arterial pressures.

Treatment of PPHN

The initial management of PPHN is conservative, paying particular attention to the cardiovascular and respiratory systems with the aim of maintaining all physiological variables within the normal range. The priority of management is in three main areas:

- Ventilation: the mainstay of treatment is to improve alveolar oxygenation. Oxygen is a very potent pulmonary vasodilator and therefore supplemental oxygen improves pulmonary blood flow and corrects arterial hypoxemia. High mean airway pressures may be required. These should be weaned slowly once the infant begins to recover.
- Minimise pulmonary vasoconstriction: minimal handling, adequate sedation and paralysis

help to minimise pulmonary hypertensive crises. Routine suctioning of the endotracheal tube should be avoided as this can precipitate pulmonary vasoconstriction.

- Maintain systemic blood pressure and perfusion: maintenance of systemic blood pressure by use of inotropes and fluid volume helps to minimise right to left shunting across foetal circulation and also improves myocardial contractility.

Inhaled Nitric Oxide (iNO) has a specific role as a pulmonary vasodilator in PPHN and serious consideration should be given to the transfer of an infant with PPHN to a unit where iNO is available. Although the lowest effective initial dose for iNO in term newborns with PPHN has not been determined, available evidence supports the starting dose at 20 ppm. Additionally, sustained improvement in oxygenation after four hours of treatment has been demonstrated for doses of less than 10 ppm. Although brief doses of 40 to 80 ppm appear to be safe, sustained treatment with 80 ppm should be avoided due to increased risk of methemoglobinaemia[31].

The infant should have regular blood tests for methaemoglobin while receiving iNO and once clinically stable the iNO should be weaned slowly. Extracorporeal membrane oxygenation (ECMO) support should be considered in any clinical situation where the PPHN is thought to be reversible. This treatment is also likely to require transport of the infant to a centre where ECMO is provided.

Meconium aspiration syndrome (MAS)

Meconium in the amniotic fluid can be detected in 10% of all labours at term (15% to 20% after 41 weeks gestation). The incidence of MAS seems to be decreasing from 5.8% to 1.5% of meconium stained infants > 37 weeks due to changing obstetric practises[32]. MAS mainly affects term and post-term infants and rarely occurs in preterm infants less than 34 weeks. *In utero* meconium passage results from neural stimulation of a mature gastrointestinal tract and usually results from a response to foetal hypoxic stress. Aspiration of this meconium antenatally or perinatally occurs secondary to a further hypoxia stimuli and infant gasps. Following delivery the aspiration of meconium can cause:

- Airway obstruction:
  - Complete obstruction of an airway will cause atelectasis distal to the site of obstruction
  - Partial obstruction causes air trapping and hyperdistention of the alveoli due to a ball-valve effect in which inspiration sucks air in, which is trapped during expiration because of the physiological narrowing of the airways that occurs during expiration
- Air leaks: the gas that is trapped, hyperinflating the lung, may rupture into the pleura (pneumothorax), mediastinum (pneumomediastinum), or pericardium (pneumopericardium)
- Chemical pneumonitis: meconium is a chemical irritant and can cause chemical pneumonitis, and the presence of inhaled organic material predisposes to bacterial infection
- Surfactant dysfunction: the meconium denatures surfactant on the alveolar surface causing atelectasis
- PPHN: secondary PPHN develops due to pulmonary atelectasis and right to left ductal and/or foramen ovale shunting

Management of meconium aspiration
The routine suctioning of the nose and mouth at the perineum after delivery of the head does not prevent MAS as aspiration of meconium is predominantly an antenatal event[33,34]. Vigorous suction of the airway at birth is only indicated if the baby is floppy, in order to clear the airway prior to ventilation.

Many infants with MAS require ventilation and some may also require treatment with iNO due to severe PPHN. In addition, there have been good results from the management of these infants using ECMO and this should be seriously considered in infants with an oxygen index of > 20.

Prognosis of meconium aspiration syndrome

The prognosis of these infants depends upon the underlying cause but respiratory outcome has markedly improved with early referral for ECMO of infants with severe hypoxemia and PPHN.

Implications for practice

PPHN results from right to left shunting at the foramen ovale and/or the ductus arteriosus and needs expert neonatal medical and nursing care. In order to minimise the shunt:
- The systemic blood pressure should be optimised with fluids and inotropes and carefully monitored.
- The oxygenation should be maximised to help reduce the pulmonary pressures
- Minimal handling is crucial to prevent stress and pulmonary vasoconstriction that increases pulmonary pressures.

Oxygen therapy and ventilatory support

Oxygen

Oxygen is a medication and it is essential in the management of preterm infants. However, oxygen also has risks, the most obvious of which is retinopathy of prematurity, and the optimal oxygen saturations for preterm infants remain unknown. Similarly, there have been no definitive studies to determine which oxygen tensions are ideal.

Oxygen saturation

The NeOProM (neonatal oxygen prospective analysis) collaboration is investigating the outcome of preterm infants in whom saturations are maintained in the range of 85–89% in comparison to those infants in whom saturations are maintained in the range of 91–95%.

Table 8.5 A comparison of nasal cannula oxygen with oxygen concentration of gas delivered to the hypopharynx.

Nasal cannulae oxygen flows (l/min)	Hypopharyngeal oxygen concentration
0.25	0.30–0.40 (30–40%)
0.5	0.35–0.55 (35–55%)
0.75	0.50–0.65 (50–65%)
1.00	0.55–0.75 (55–75%)

The relationship between oxygen saturation and partial pressure is shown below:

SpO_2 range 85–95% the 95% confidence intervals of PaO_2 were 3.8–8.9 kPa[35].

Oxygen administration

Infants with mild to moderate RDS can be managed in warmed and humidified ambient oxygen and many modern incubators now provide blended humidified oxygen without the need for a headbox. If the baby needs more than 50–60% oxygen, not only is it difficult to keep the concentration steady but it also suggests that the disease is severe and that alternative forms of therapy are indicated.

Oxygen can be administered by nasal cannulae for infants in long-term oxygen, typically those with CLD. These allow the baby to bottle or breast-feed, play, sit up and receive care while still receiving oxygen. An estimate of the oxygen concentration received is shown in Table 8.5.

Continuous positive airways pressure (CPAP)

The purpose of CPAP is to splint the alveoli open with applied pressures of between 6 and 10 cm H_2O and maintain lung volume. This is a similar mechanism to the grunting that infants employ themselves. The use of CPAP in an infant with mild to moderate respiratory distress will decrease the work of breathing and as well as preventing alveolar collapse this allows the infant to conserve energy.

Methods of CPAP administration

CPAP is usually administered with short prongs or a close fitting mask but nasopharyngeal CPAP can be provided in the short term via the ET tube. CPAP via ET tube should be avoided as it leads to increased work of breathing needed to overcome the resistive forces from the ET tube and ventilator tubing. There are three main ways in which the CPAP can be delivered:

- Most neonatal ventilators now have a CPAP mode, and can be used to administer the CPAP since this makes it easier to warm and humidify the inspired gas. The ventilator is instantly available should IPPV be necessary.
- Infant flow CPAP (Electro Medical Equipment Infant Flow Driver). This device gives continuous pressure with a 'fluidic flip' mechanism via double nasal prongs. The fluidic flip is designed to prevent the infant blowing against the CPAP pressure during expiration.
- Bubble CPAP: the expiratory limb is submerged in water to the depth of the desired nasal CPAP with flow set for constant bubbling. Evidence of its efficacy and safety is lacking, although one unit experienced decreased incidence of CLD in babies < 1500 g to < 5% by early initiation of bubble CPAP[36].

All CPAP machines have a gas flow meter for the air/oxygen pressure, a humidifier and a set of tubing which may include soft plastic nasal prongs or mask with Velcro® attachments for securing to the baby's hat. A CPAP of 5–6 cm H_2O is easily achieved by adequate seal of the prongs or mask with nose. It is very difficult to get CPAP pressures higher than 8 cm H_2O using nasal prongs.

Indications for using CPAP
The two main indications for CPAP are post-extubation of extreme preterm infants or in providing support for infants with mild respiratory distress. Many neonatal units in the Scandinavian countries and some in the UK are now using CPAP as the first mode of intervention in premature infants at risk of

RDS from the delivery suite due to decrease in chronic lung disease and ventilation days[37]. This is an alternative to intubation, early surfactant and early extubation onto CPAP.

CPAP is not an appropriate intervention in infants that have significant apnoeic episodes or who have become acutely unwell. Intubation and stabilisation should be considered in these infants.

Newer methods of CPAP delivery (SiPAP) (also refer to ventilator section)
Infant Flow® SiPAP™ provides bi-level (air delivered can be set at one pressure for inhaling and another for exhaling) nasal CPAP for the spontaneously breathing neonate through delivery of sighs above a baseline NCPAP pressure. These sighs may be timed, at a rate specified by the clinician, or triggered by the patient's own inspiratory efforts.

Complications of using prong CPAP
As with any neonatal intervention CPAP has well recognised complications:

- Nasal trauma leading to nasal deformity
- Gastric distension and perforations
- Feeding problems due to gastric distension
- Pneumothorax

Management of infants on CPAP
Infants on CPAP require all the biochemical and physiological monitoring described in RDS. Nursing care should ensure adequate seal of the prongs or mask to the nose and prevention of pressure leak from open mouth. Orogastric tube feeding is usually tolerated if the stomach is adequately deflated at regular intervals (nasogastric tubes will partially obstruct nasal passage) and many of the other complications can be avoided by careful nursing[38]. Nasal trauma can be reduced or prevented by frequent examination of the nasal area for signs of reddening, snubbing or flaring of nostrils[39]. Releasing nasal prongs or masks for a few minutes during care may also help prevent nasal trauma. Regular suctioning of the nose and nasopharynx will prevent obstructive apnoeas and failure of CPAP.

Weaning of infants on CPAP

There is no clear evidence of the best way in which CPAP should be weaned. A common strategy is to wean the CPAP by having periods where it is removed that are increased as tolerated. An alternative strategy is one where as the baby's condition improves the CPAP pressure is reduced by 1–2 cm at a time to 5–6 cm H_2O. The blood gases should be checked after each change. The CPAP can be discontinued once the blood gas has been satisfactory at 2 cm H_2O for 4–6 hours. If there is clinical deterioration with significant increase in respiratory distress or the gases deteriorate within 1–2 hours of discontinuing CPAP, it should be restarted.

Mechanical ventilation

The indications for starting intermittent positive pressure ventilation (IPPV) are as follows:

- Term infants that have required resuscitation at birth and do not quickly develop regular respiration
- Preterm low birthweight infants who fail to establish satisfactory respiration after resuscitation in labour ward
- Prophylactically in the extreme preterm low birthweight infants (< 1000 g)
- Sudden deterioration with apnoea or irregular respirations
- Preterm infants on CPAP with deteriorating blood gases
- Hypercarbia ($PCO_2 > 7.5$ kPa) associated with a pH of less than 7.2

The IFDAS (infant flow driver) trial compared infants that had the following management at delivery:

- Intubation and prophylactic surfactant and ventilation
- Intubation and prophylactic surfactant with early extubation to CPAP
- No intubation and CPAP from birth
- Clinical management at discretion of clinical team

There were no significant differences in the numbers of infants that developed chronic lung disease. The COIN Trial (CPAP or intubation at birth of 25–28 week preterm infants) did not show a reduction in mortality in those infants managed with initial CPAP but fewer infants needed oxygen at 28 days[40]. Other prospective randomised trials, the Vermont Oxford Network trial, and the SUPPORT trial may provide additional evidence for the potential benefit of CPAP compared with early surfactant in such infants.

Implication for practice

Nurses caring for infants receiving ventilatory support must have:
- Knowledge of how the equipment works and the ability to set it up and troubleshoot in the event of failure.
- Knowledge/understanding of the actions of the equipment modes.
- Knowledge/understanding of the complications of use.
- Be able to initiate resuscitation in the event of complications arising.

Intubation

An endotracheal tube can be passed orally or nasally to achieve access to the airways for ventilation and suction. Nasal intubation is more difficult but gives easy access to the mouth for suctioning, orogastric tube feeding and use of a pacifying dummy. Pressure necrosis to the anterior nares sometimes causes severe deformity requiring plastic surgery[41].

Oral intubation is a simpler technique but poses difficulty with securing, maintaining ET tube position and access to the mouth for suctioning. Oral tubes used for long-term ventilation may be responsible for distortion of the roof of the mouth in the form of a groove along the track of the tube, which may cause feeding and speech problems later[42].

Performing intubation

As with any clinical skill, preparation of the equipment, infant and team performing the intubation is essential. In an emergency intubation the procedure should be performed by an experienced member of staff. The following description refers mainly to an elective procedure and the main equipment required is listed below:

- The correct size ET tube and method of fixation
- An introducer, if required
- A laryngoscope with bright bulb and a suitable size blade (longer blade preferable)
- Bag and mask/Neopuff ™ set at appropriate inflation pressure
- Scissors to cut the tube to the correct size
- Hat to secure the ET tube holder
- Suction tube, wide bore (Yankuer) suction tube if available

The infants should be prepared by paying attention to the following factors:

- Aspiration of milk and air from the stomach prior to beginning the procedure
- Administration of premedication
- Thermoregulation
- Monitoring, particularly oxygen saturation and heart rate
- Ease of access for staff performing intubation
- Head position

Once the equipment has been prepared the infant should be placed supine with the neck in a neutral position and pre-oxygenated. This may be done using IPPV with a bag and mask or Neopuff ™, or if the infant is breathing spontaneously the ambient oxygen concentration can be increased. The aim of pre-oxygenation is to clear the lungs of nitrogen and carbon dioxide and fill them with oxygen so that there is an oxygen 'reserve' during the procedure. The premedication is then given (see Table 8.7) and allowed to work (this may take some minutes) and IPPV will then be necessary as the infant will be apnoeic. Awake intubation is painful and associated with a stress response

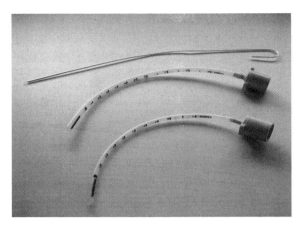

Figure 8.5 Examples of ET tubes with the black line visible to guide depth of insertion. An introducer is also shown which can be used with care by inserting through the ET (it must not protrude through the end).

which is detrimental to the baby. Therefore pre-medication should be used for all intubations except those on the labour ward or in an emergency. The ET is then inserted by a paediatrician or neonatal nurse with extended skills and this should take no longer than 20 seconds. Physiological stability in oxygen saturation and heart rate should be maintained throughout the procedure. The ET tube used in infants is non-cuffed and should extend to below the cords and just above the carina. The shouldered tube should rest its shoulders just above the cords and other tubes are usually marked with a black area to guide placement (see Figure 8.5). The size of the ET can be predicted using gestation (25 weeks = 2.5, 30 weeks = 3.0 etc.) and Table 8.6 shows a similar guide using birthweight.

A guide to depth of insertion of an oral ET tube is 6 + birthweight as a measurement of lip

Table 8.6 Endotracheal tube (ETT) sizes based on birthweight.

Baby's weight	ETT size
< 1000 g	2.5 mm
1000–2000 g	3.0 mm
2000–3000 g	3.0–3.5 mm
> 3000 g	3.5 mm

Figure 8.6 A disposable CO2 PEDICAP that *has not* been exposed to exhaled CO2 will appear purple. A disposable CO2-PEDICAP that *has* been exposed to exhaled CO2 will appear yellow.

to tip but bilateral symmetrical air entry and chest movement should always be confirmed following intubation. An additional method of confirming that the ET is in the trachea is the use of a CO_2-PEDICAP (see Figure 8.6), which changes colour when exposed to carbon dioxide. The tube is secured according to the local protocol.

A chest X-ray should be taken to ascertain the length and position of the tube. The ideal position for ET tube tip is 1–2 cm above the carina (bifurcation of the trachea into right and left main bronchus) which is at T3–T4. If the ET tube is too short, it is in danger of slipping out of the lungs into the oesophagus. If the ETT is too long, this will cause over inflation of the lung on that side (usually right lung). The ET tube should be withdrawn and the position confirmed once again. The correct length of placement of ET tube should be noted down for future intubations.

The need for intubation or not is one of the challenges of neonatology. It is vital to recognise when reintubation is required but equally ET tubes should not be changed unnecessarily as it can be associated with complications. Reintubation is only warranted if the tube is dislodged or blocked.

While intubated and ventilated the infant's head should be kept in a position of slight extension on the trunk. Flexing and extending the neck causes vast differences in ET tube position and can traumatise the laryngeal mucosa. There should also be only a small dead space between the ventilator circuit and the baby so the ET tube must be shortened appropriately.

Complications of a prolonged indwelling ET include:

- Laryngeal stenosis
- Tracheal stenosis
- Laryngomalacia/tracheomalacia
- Vocal cord palsy

Table 8.7 An example of pre-intubation medication.

Preintubation medications in elective and, if possible, in emergency intubations
• Morphine 50 mcg/kg (sedative, analgesic)
• Atropine 10–130 mcg/kg (inhibits vagal stimulation and bradycardia)
• Suxamethomium 1 mg/kg (paralysing agent)

Implication for practice

All neonatal nurses need the skills to assist with intubation, which include:
- Knowledge of the equipment required: including the ability to choose the appropriate size ET tube and assess the length for insertion.
- An understanding of the actions of drugs used when intubating.
- Skill in providing IPPV with a bag/valve mask or Neopuff ™.

Ventilatory strategies

There are an increasing number of ways in which infants can be ventilated and an increasing number of types of ventilators. It is important to be familiar with the types of ventilator and ventilatory strategies used locally[43]. The commonly used terminology is briefly defined below:

Classification of ventilators

Mechanical ventilators may be classified as described below.

Power supply

- Electrical requiring mains or battery
- Gas driven, requiring no external power but consuming a driving gas (pneupac)
- Gas driven, but electricity required to power display (Drager Babylog 8000)

Pressure limited or volume regulated

- Pressure generators deliver gas until a preset pressure is reached:
  - This protects lungs from high peak inspiratory pressures (PIP) and compensates for air leaks, but the tidal volume varies with lung compliance (as lung compliance decreases tidal volume increases with the same amount of pressure)
  - Risk of volutrauma
- Flow generators deliver a preset volume of gas:
  - This protects the lungs from excessive volume, but the pressure required will vary depending on lung compliance (if lung compliance increases, the pressure required to deliver the same volume will increase)
  - Risk of barotrauma
  - Small volumes may be absorbed by the compliance of the circuits resulting in hypoventilation.

The newer ventilators use both of these strategies and are known as pressure limited volume regulated but further studies are required to determine if they are superior to current methods[44–46].

Fundamental principles and terminology used in most ventilators

Cycling

- The term cycling refers to the stopping of inspiration and opening of the ventilator expiration valve
- The ending of the inspiration can be preset by volume-cycling, pressure-cycling or time-cycling

Limiting

- This term refers to the limit that causes the ventilator to cycle into expiration
- Limiting regulates the gas flow into the lungs; the limit may be volume or pressure or both

Trigger

This term refers to the signal that initiates the opening of the inspiratory valve allowing the pressurised gas to enter the infant's lungs. It is the capability of the ventilator to respond to the spontaneous breath of the infant and support spontaneous breathing.

Trigger sensitivity

Trigger should be sensitive enough for every breath to trigger ventilation without autocycling.

Tidal volume

- Tidal volume is the volume of gas inspired during one breath
- This is adjusted directly in volume limited mode but controlled indirectly in pressure limited mode

Minute volume

- Minute volume is the volume of gas inspired during one minute of ventilation
- Arterial pCO_2 is inversely proportional to minute volume

Rate

- Rate is the number of times inspiration occurs in one minute
- Arterial pCO_2 is inversely proportional to rate

I:E (inspiratory time: expiratory time) ratio

- This refers to the ratio of inspiratory time to expiratory time
- The expiratory time is normally longer than the inspiratory time to allow full clearance of carbon dioxide to occur

• Increasing the I:E ratio increases mean airway pressure (MAP) and improves oxygenation

Airway pressure
This can be categorised as:

• Mean airway pressure (MAP) is the area under the curve of time versus pressure throughout the respiratory cycle
• Peak inspiratory pressure (PIP) is recorded at end inspiration and results from increased pressure, volume, airway resistance, or pulmonary disease
• Plateau pressure is the pressure equilibration between the airways and alveoli

Peak inspiratory pressure (PIP)

• This refers to the highest pressure generated by the ventilator and is normally measured in the ventilator tubing upstream of the patient
• With normal lungs and low inspiratory gas flow rates alveolar pressure = PIP
• With high resistance in the circuit, ET tube or airways the alveolar pressure will be lower than the measured PIP
• If airway resistance is unevenly distributed the alveolar pressure (and hence the lung damage) will be greater in areas supplied by normal airways than those supplied by narrowed areas

PEEP (positive end expiratory pressure)

• This refers to the minimum pressure that is maintained by the ventilator during expiration phase (CPAP provides minimum pressure throughout respiratory cycle) and is measured in the ventilator tubing upstream of the patient
• It is usually 5–10 cm H_2O
• Splints the small airways preventing collapse in expiration
• Recruits alveoli, reducing intrapulmonary shunting
• Improves lung compliance

Modes of ventilation
The following modes of ventilation will be described:

• CMV (control mode ventilation)
• PS (pressure support) or ASB (assisted breath)
• VS (volume support)
• SIMV (synchronised intermittent mandatory ventilation)
• SIPPV (synchronised intermittent positive pressure ventilation) or PTV (patient triggered ventilation)
• BiPAP (bilevel positive airway pressure)
• HFOV (high frequency oscillatory ventilation)

CMV (control mode ventilation)
During CMV the ventilator delivers breaths *independently* of the patient's respiratory effort. This mode does not allow the patient to self-generate a tidal volume breath.

PS (pressure support) or ASB (assisted breath)
In this type of ventilation the infant is intubated and every spontaneous breath triggers the ventilator to provide pressure support to the infant's own ventilatory attempts.

VS (volume support)
In VS ventilation every spontaneous breath triggers the ventilator to provide volume support to the infant's own ventilatory attempts.

SIMV (synchronised IMV)

• This refers to a mode of ventilation in which there is a combination of mandatory breaths delivered by the ventilator and the possibility of some of these breaths being synchronised if the infant triggers a breath within a specific time window.
• Spontaneous ventilation (SV) earlier in the expiratory phase does not trigger as this would prevent adequate expiration and the spontaneous breath will not delay the ventilator breath which is *mandatory*.

- The rate will be set as will the time window (e.g. 50 msecs). If the infant breathes within this window the ventilator breath will be brought forward to coincide, i.e. *synchronised*.

SIMV (synchronised IMV) + PS (pressure support)/ASB (assisted breath)

The spontaneous breaths can also be boosted by assisting with a preset pressure, i.e. pressure support or assisted spontaneous breath. This method of ventilation is often used as a weaning strategy.

SIPPV (synchronised IPPV) or PTV (patient triggered ventilation)

In this mode of ventilation *every* spontaneous breath is supported by the ventilator, in contrast to SIMV. It can be considered as ASB with a back up rate, as the ventilator will deliver mandatory breaths if the respiratory rate falls below that set, but if all the back up ventilatory breaths are necessary the infant is receiving CMV.

BiPAP (bilevel positive airway pressure ventilation)

In BiPAP mode air delivered can be set at one pressure for inhaling and another for exhaling. A constant pressure is delivered as with CPAP but each breath that the infant makes is supported by a flow of gas at a higher pressure. As this is pressure limited ventilation the tidal volume will depend on lung compliance.

SiPAP (synchronised inspiratory positive airway pressure)

It is a form of non-invasive ventilation device designed to deliver extra 'sighs' to the babies with a set rate which synchronises with the infants' breathing movements, detected by an abdominal capsule. BiPAP can be delivered by SiPAP device.

HFOV (high frequency oscillatory ventilation)

- High frequency oscillators are essentially airways vibrators (a piston pump or vibrating diaphragm) that operate at frequencies at around 10 Hz (1 Hz = 1 cycle/sec).
- A continuous flow of fresh gas rushes past the vibrating source that generates the oscillation and a controlled leak or low-pass filter allows gas to exit the system. Pressure oscillations within the airway produce a tidal volume of 2–3 ml/kg around a constant mean airway pressure, which maintains lung volume in a manner equivalent to using very high levels of CPAP. The volume of gas moved in the tidal volume is determined by the amplitude of the airway pressure oscillation (ΔP).
- The strategy of HFOV is to inflate the lungs and recruit 'lung units' by applying a continuous distending pressure which keeps the lung at the optimal place of expansion.
- Oxygenation and carbon dioxide removal occurs via an oscillating pressure waveform superimposed on the MAP.
- During HFOV, inspiration and expiration are both active.

Indications for HFOV

- HFOV is generally used as a rescue therapy if conventional modalities of ventilation fail to achieve desired goals. There are some units which use prophylactic HFOV in preterm infants although there is no evidence of benefit.
- It is most useful for infants with homogeneous lung disease and has been used in severe RDS, meconium aspiration syndrome and severe bilateral uniform pulmonary interstitial emphysema (PIE) with hypercarbia.

Relative contraindication

It is relatively contraindicated in inhomogeneous lung disease as it can result in over ventilation of the relatively normal areas of the lung.

Complications

The major complications of HFOV if the infant is not closely monitored especially in the first 12–24 hours are hyperinflation and decreased venous return and pneumothorax. This is due to the fact that the MAP is continuous throughout the ventilatory cycle and it is possible to overinflate the lungs and reduce consequently venous return. Unlike in conventional ventilation, chest radiography is a useful measure to assess lung inflation and recruitment on HFOV especially if high MAPs are used.

Making changes in HFOV

- Improving oxygenation: in a similar way to CMV oxygenation it is dependent on MAP and FiO_2.
- Carbon dioxide elimination: this is mainly dependent on the amplitude and frequency. The frequency is not usually altered. If the $PaCO_2$ increases the amplitude should be increased to achieve a decrease in PaCo2. Frequency should be altered only as a last resort and a *reduction* in frequency will have the same effect as an *increase* in amplitude.

Implications for practice

- An understanding of the specific action of ventilator modes is vital.
- Recognition of changes in a ventilated infant's status may be subtle (gradual reduction in air entry with a coated ET tube) or dramatic (blocked ET tube or pneumothorax).

Interpretation of blood gases

One of the aims of neonatal care is to maintain physiological stability and this includes maintaining arterial blood gases within the optimal limits as shown in Table 8.8.

It is very important that the $PaCO_2$ is not allowed to drop below 4.5 kPa (33 mm Hg) as this increases the risk of brain damage and it is also very important that the PaO_2 does not rise above 11 kPa (82.5 mm Hg) as this may increase the risk of retinopathy of prematurity[47], and possibly bronchopulmonary dysplasia.

Steps to interpretation of an arterial blood gas

The arterial blood gas is used to evaluate both acid-base balance and oxygenation, each representing separate conditions. Acid-base evaluation requires a focus on three of the components: pH, $PaCO_2$ and HCO_3. This process involves three steps.

Step one

The pH is assessed to determine if the blood is within the normal range, alkalotic or acidotic. If the pH is above 7.45, the blood is alkalotic. If the pH is below 7.35, the blood is acidotic.

Step two

Once the primary problem has been identified as alkalosis or acidosis the next stage is to determine if it is caused primarily by a respiratory or metabolic problem. This involves assessment of the $PaCO_2$ level. In a respiratory problem, as the pH decreases below 7.35, the $PaCO_2$ should rise. If the pH rises above 7.45, the $PaCO_2$ should fall. Compare the pH and the PaCO2 values. If pH and $PaCO_2$ are indeed moving in *opposite directions*, then the problem is primarily respiratory in nature.

Step three

The final stage is to assess the HCO_3 value. In a metabolic problem, as the pH increases, the HCO_3

Table 8.8 Target arterial blood gases.

pH	7.27 to 7.35
PCO_2	4.5 to 6.0 kPa (33–45 mm Hg) (higher PCO_2 acceptable in CLD)
PO_2	6–10 kPa (45–75 mm Hg)
SaO_2	91–95%
HCO_3	The normal range is 22 to 26 mEq/litre
BE: the normal range is −2 to +2 mEq/litre.	The base excess indicates the amount of excess alkali such as bicarbonate. (A negative base excess indicates an excess of acid or a base deficit in the blood.)

Table 8.9 A summary of the common abnormalities seen in blood gases.

	pH	PaCO2	HCO3
Respiratory acidosis	↓	↑	normal
Respiratory alkalosis	↑	↓	normal
Metabolic acidosis	↓	normal	↓
Metabolic alkalosis	↑	normal	↑

should also increase. As the pH decreases, so should the HCO_3. Compare the two values. If they are moving *in the same direction*, then the problem is primarily metabolic in nature.

Table 8.9 summarises the relationships between pH, $PaCO_2$ and HCO_3.

Implication for practice

A basic understanding of the interpretation of blood gases is important for a neonatal nurse to fulfil his/her role with a ventilated infant:

- In respiratory acidosis the CO_2 will move in the opposite direction to the pH.
- In metabolic acidosis the CO_2 will move in the same direction to the pH.
- Infants who have been compromised at the time of delivery will have reverted to anaerobic metabolism and a mixed acidosis will develop.

Nursing an infant on conventional ventilation

It is important to be aware that a parent's perception of their infant being placed on a ventilator is that he/she is seriously ill, but this may not always be the case. They will often feel helpless and isolated and a detailed explanation may help to alleviate some of this pain and anxiety. It is always possible to involve parents with the care of their infant, such as helping with feeds, changing of nappies, cleaning, etc. Consideration should also always be given to kangaroo care if the infant is stable on a ventilator.

Setting up CMV

The ventilator should be plugged into the main power source and the wall oxygen and air inlets.

Table 8.10 Typical settings for conventional ventilation for preterm.

Oxygen	30–50%
IT	0.3–0.5 seconds
ET	0.7–0.5 seconds
I:E ratio	1:1–1:2
Rate	40–60/min
PIP	18–20 cm H_2O
PEEP	4–6 cm H_2O
Gas flow	6–8 l/minutes

The ventilatory circuits should be attached and the humidification set up. The sequence of setting up the mode of ventilation depends on the type of ventilator and the exact ventilator settings will vary depending on the specific clinical situation. A guide to initial ventilator settings for preterm and term infants is provided in Tables 8.10 and 8.11. This is only a guide as these settings should be influenced not only by the gestation of the infant but by other factors, which in the preterm include whether surfactant was given on the labour ward. Surfactant will improve lung compliance, which has the result of increasing the tidal volume for identical pressure settings. If this is not noted then the CO_2 may fall below 4.0 kPa, which may have effects on cerebral perfusion. It is extremely important to clinically assess chest movement and oxygen saturation on initial ventilation, and blood gases should be checked soon after ventilation has been established. On ventilators that also show tidal volume changes and compliance this will be indicated by an increase in tidal volume for the same pressure settings and some ventilators can be set to wean the pressures automatically to maintain a preset tidal volume. The underlying type of lung disease or reason for ventilation should also guide initial pressure settings.

Making changes in the ventilator settings

Changes in the ventilator settings are shown in Table 8.12.

Table 8.11 Typical settings for conventional ventilation for term.

Oxygen	40–50%
IT	0.5–0.6 seconds
ET	0.5–0.4 seconds
I:E ratio	1:1
Rate	50–60/min
PIP	22–24 cm H_2O
PEEP	4–6 cm H_2O
Gas flow	6–8 l/minutes

Table 8.12 Summary of effects of ventilation variables.

Increase in	Effect on PaO_2	effect on $PaCO_2$
Tidal volume	Increase (up to a point)	Decrease (up to a point)
FiO_2	Increase	No change
PIP	Increase	Decrease
Vt	Increase	Decrease
Rate	No change	Decrease
IT	Increase	No change
PEEP	Increase	Might rise if PEEP > 6

Troubleshooting basics

- If decrease in PaO_2: PaO_2 is dependent on FiO_2 and MAP (PIP × IT + PEEP). Therefore consider increasing FiO_2, PIP, IT, PEEP. Rate does not come into this equation.
- If increase in $PaCO_2$: $PaCO_2$ depends on minute ventilation. Therefore increase tidal volume by increasing the PIP or rate.
- If decrease in PaO2 and increase in PaCO2: use combination of the above
- Decrease in pH and increase in base: if respiratory, in most instances pH will improve with adjustment in ventilation. If pH does not improve, alkali may be used.

Care of the endotracheal tube

Maintaining the patency of the airway is paramount in preventing hypoxia and enabling efficient ventilation to take place. Strict aseptic precautions should be undertaken during routine care such as suctioning.

Endotracheal tube suction

The purpose of suctioning the ET tube is to remove airway secretions in order to prevent obstruction, lung damage and decreased lung compliance. This should improve oxygenation and ventilation. Suction is an important part of the care of the baby on the ventilator. However, suction has the potential to cause hypoxia, lung damage, periventricular haemorrhage and infection so should be done with care and knowledge.

Suctioning the ET tube should not be carried out routinely as it is a traumatic event for the baby, causing bradycardia (due to vagal stimulation), drop in oxygen levels and often a long recovery time afterwards. The need for suction should be assessed on increasing oxygen needs, alterations in heart or respiratory rate, the presence of visible secretions in ET tube, or if the blood gases show rising $PaCO_2$ levels, which could mean that the tube is blocked.

Ideally, each baby should have a tape measure cut to the length of the ET tube as a guide for measuring the depth of suction; allowance will be made for the holder of the tube. The suction catheter is gently but swiftly passed to the measured depth. If the catheter meets any obstruction it should be withdrawn by 0.5 cm, to prevent mucosal damage, before suction is applied. If the non-paralysed baby coughs on passage of the tube, it has been passed too far down the ET tube and may stimulate the vagal nerve to produce bradycardia.

Size and type of catheter
Suggested sizes of suction catheter are:

ET tube size	Catheter size
2.5–3.5 mm	6 Fr
4–5 mm	8 Fr

The suction catheters should be attached to negative pressure suction, ideally with a Y connection. This will ensure that the end is not occluded until the catheter is being withdrawn from the suction area. The recommended pressure is no more than 50–100 mmHg to prevent mucosal damage[48]. The length of time for which the baby is removed from the ventilator during suctioning should be as short as possible, preferably no more than 15 seconds[49].

It is common clinical practice to instil small amounts of normal saline into the endotracheal tube prior to suctioning procedures in the belief that this provides moisture and loosens tenacious secretions. A randomised controlled trial showed a lower ET tube resistance and less haemorrhagic secretions when periodic bolus instillations of normal saline solution were employed prior to suctioning in adults on mechanical ventilation[50]. It has been shown, however, that more than 80% of the instillate may remain inside the airway after suctioning and will probably later be absorbed or removed by the mucociliary system[51]. Suggested amounts of fluid to be used in infants vary widely from 0.1 to 0.5 ml/kg. However, saline may be detrimental to the innate immune system of the upper airway mucosa, rapidly unfolding and inactivating antimicrobial peptides such as LL-37[52].

Clinical deterioration on the ventilator

A sudden deterioration on the ventilator with an acute fall in PaO_2 and rise in $PaCO_2$ (blood gas or non-invasive transcutaneous monitoring) may be caused by DOPE:

- D   Displacement of ET tube
- O   Obstruction of ET tube
- P   Pneumothorax/pulmonary haemorrhage
- E   Equipment failure

There may be mechanical problems such as a leak around the ET tube or ventilator failure. Check all machinery for leaks, try hand-ventilating with a bag and mask/Neopuff ™ and insert a larger ET tube.

When the airway is blocked or the ET tube is displaced out of the trachea, there will be a sudden drop in oxygen saturations, possibly accompanied by bradycardia; there may be no movement of the chest wall. If ET tube block is due to secretions, suction should be performed using suction catheters that will pass easily into the ET tube with the help of normal saline irrigation. If the ET tube is thought to be displaced into the oesophagus, it should be removed immediately and the baby reintubated.

A slower deterioration accompanied by a slow fall in PaO_2 and rise in $PaCO_2$ may also be caused by the above factors or by the baby failing to synchronise its breathing with the ventilator. Other possible causes include:

- Intraventricular haemorrhage
- Patent ductus arteriosus
- Partial blockage of ET tube
- Hypotension
- Infection
- Anaemia
- Metabolic imbalance

Weaning off ventilation

Once a baby is stable on minimum ventilator settings (rate 10–15/minute, PIP 16, PEEP 4, IT 0.3–0.5, FiO2 < 35%) off paralysis, and blood gases have been satisfactory for 12 hours or so, the weaning process can begin. The baby may be extubated to nasal CPAP[53], or incubator oxygen.

Extubation of the baby

Most VLBW infants do not tolerate ET tube CPAP at all well when being weaned as it dramatically increases the work of breathing and should not be attempted[54]. The following precautions make successful extubation more likely:

- Check latest X-ray for pneumothorax, collapse consolidation, lung parenchyma and heart shadow
- Check work of breathing, blood gases, temperature, blood glucose, electrolytes and urine output
- Ensure the baby has received caffeine at least 2–4 hours prior, and morphine has been stopped or decreased to a minimum
- Stop oral feeds

- Carefully aspirate the baby's mouth and oropharynx
- Physiotherapy and suction may be useful in a baby who has been paralysed
- If planned to extubate onto CPAP or SiPAP ensure the baby is extubated straight onto nasal prongs with a minimum CPAP of 5–6 cm H_2O
- Ensure adequate humidification of the inspired gases
- Remember minimal handling

Implication for practice

The neonatal nurse should know:
- What size suction catheter to use.
- How far to insert the suction catheter to prevent inserting to below the end of the ET tube.
- The adverse complications of ET tube suctioning.

Monitoring

Arterial lines to monitor blood pressure

A central (umbilical) arterial line is easily accessed, secured and maintained in the newborn. However, peripheral arterial lines (radial, ulnar, brachial, posterior tibial and dorsal artery) could also be cannulated if needed. Brachial and dorsal arteries should be avoided if possible in neonates due to high risks of complications such as thrombosis and consequent necrosis of whole or distal parts. If the radial artery has been previously used or thrombosed due to prolonged use, the ulnar artery on the same side should be avoided. Arterial line patency should be maintained by running heparinised saline continuously at a concentration of (1 unit/ml).

Continuous blood pressure monitoring is possible but should be regularly recalibrated to get accurate readings, and the transducer must be placed level with the infant's heart.

If there is blanching distal to a peripheral arterial line or, in the case of an umbilical arterial line, the lower limbs or buttocks, the line should be removed immediately. Additional complications of an umbilical arterial line can include haematuria, which is also an indication for removal.

The removal of arterial lines also warrants care. An umbilical arterial line should ideally have the heparin infusion switched off for at least an hour to encourage clotting in the artery. A saline soaked gauge covering the dried umbilical stump will also aid easy removal of the catheter, especially if the cord has dried around the catheter. A ligature is tied around the umbilical stump and when the catheter has been removed the ligature can be tightened. If the umbilical stump bleeds heavily, firm pressure using index finger or thumb directly over the umbilical stump will immediately achieve haemostasis. Removal of peripheral arterial lines will require direct pressure on the site for up to five minutes.

Medication

Mechanical ventilation is a stressful experience, but not necessarily a painful one, for neonates. This may alter their neuroendocrine and physiological responses. Reasons to routinely sedate ventilated neonates include improved ventilator synchrony. Reasons not to routinely sedate include the well-known adverse side effects of pain medication, especially the opiates, including hypotension from morphine, chest wall rigidity from fentanyl, and tolerance, dependence and withdrawal from both opiates and benzodiazepines.

If patients are sedated, opiates are the most common class of drugs, with morphine the most well studied. Fentanyl may be advantageous in hypotensive, younger neonates because it has fewer cardiovascular effects. The benzodiazepines, midazolam and lorazepam, have been used in ventilated neonates, but midazolam has been associated with adverse effects in one small study, so concern remains regarding its use.

Continuous morphine infusion is a commonly used analgesia. However, evidence suggests that as well as affecting blood pressure morphine delays the attainment of full enteral feeds, partly by delaying the start of feeding[55]. Additionally, pre-emptive morphine infusions did not reduce the frequency of severe IVH, PVL, or death in ventilated preterm neonates, but intermittent boluses of open-label morphine were associated with an increased rate of the composite outcome[56]. Weaning after seven days' use of continuous morphine infusion should be slow. There is no need to wean morphine in babies requiring less than seven days as the morphine has a long half-life, especially in preterm infants.

Pancuronium and atracurium are paralysing agents and if paralysis is necessary analgesics should always be routinely commenced for pain relief. Pancuronium has a long half-life and therefore atracurium is preferred for its short half-life, but needs to be given as a continuous infusion to maintain paralysis. Caffeine is given to prevent apnoea of prematurity to infants who are being weaned off ventilation. It is given as a loading dose either orally or intravenously, followed by daily dose.

Implications for practice

The neonatal nurse needs to have knowledge of the actions and effects of drugs used to facilitate ventilation.

It is important that infants at risk of apnoea of prematurity are loaded with caffeine prior to extubation.

Additional nursing care of ventilated infant

All infants on a ventilator should be handled or disturbed as little as possible. The aim should be to do routine hygiene needs, suction and position changes when the baby is awake so that the baby gets uninterrupted sleep needed to gain weight, keep oxygen requirement to the minimum and have normal behavioural patterns. These interventions need only take place at 6–8 hourly intervals to prevent pressure sores and improve flexion and tension movements. Prone positioning improves oxygenation and behaviour in sick infants needing mechanical ventilation[57].

A paralysed infant cannot make any voluntary effort to breathe and will need hand bagging immediately if the endotracheal tube becomes displaced or blocked. Secretions from ET tube and nasopharynx tend to be copius and thick when using paralysis, so frequent suction is needed. The infant's position will need to be changed 4–6 hourly and attention given to pressure areas. Limbs should be put gently through a series of movements, flexion and tension, to ensure joints are correctly aligned. The baby cannot blink, so the eyes must be protected with drops of artificial tears such as hypomellose, to keep the corneas moist. Paraffin gauge can be used to prevent dust entering the eyes.

Nursing a baby on HFOV

The physical assessment of a baby on HFOV presents different challenges. New skills and an alteration of those learnt from using conventional ventilation are necessary. The baby will have the same type of endotracheal tube and connectors as for conventional ventilation but different assessments will be made about chest wall movement, behaviour state and colour. During this ventilation, vibrations of the chest wall must be even to give good gas exchange. The Sensormedics oscillator has a centring light that can be checked and adjusted after turning or moving the baby for X-ray. Small changes in symmetry and rates of vibrations are critical and can result in significant alteration in ventilation if left unchecked.

Chest auscultation is difficult because of the chest vibrations and noise. This should not be done frequently as the alveoli may collapse when the ventilator is off. When necessary it can be done by putting the ventilator alarm on standby for 5–10 seconds and switching off briefly to listen.

Suctioning can be done by using an ETT indwelling catheter so that the ventilator does not have to be discontinued. This suction has to be carried out with care. If the catheter is not fully retracted after suction, it can block the airway[58].

It should be remembered that babies on the Sensormedics oscillator will not alarm and will continue to demonstrate oscillations even if there is complete ET tube block.

Positioning and comfort

Infants can continue to breathe spontaneously while being oscillated and many of them settle easily. Some infants will be nursed on the Sensormedics HFOV, which has a long rigid arm from the ventilator to the ET tube so more attention needs to be paid to positioning. The rigid arm must be kept straight and slightly tilted downwards to the ventilator so that circuit condensation can flow way from the baby. Moving the baby for X-ray and position changes on this ventilator needs assistance of two or three people to prevent accidental ET tube dislodgement.

Weaning off HFOV

The aim during weaning is to maintain optimum lung volume:

- Reduce FiO$_2$ before MAP
- Once the FiO$_2$ is down to 30% then reduce MAP by ½–1 cm steps monitoring the blood gases regularly
- If PaO$_2$ decreases during weaning it is possible that one is reducing MAP too slowly; check for lung over inflation by chest X-ray
- Once the MAP is down to 10–12 cmH$_2$O change to IPPV
- The alternative is to wean directly from HFOV by reducing the MAP

Other treatments for respiratory problems

Nitric oxide

Nitric oxide is a highly diffusible gas and a potent pulmonary vasodilator that regulates vascular muscle tone at the cellular level. Inhaled nitric oxide (iNO) was originally described as having a role in the management of neonates with pulmonary hypertension in 1992[59]. It acts as a localised pulmonary vasodilator when introduced into the alveoli, diffusing directly across the cell walls, acting on and reducing pulmonary vascular resistance. It is also quickly inactivated, which minimises systemic side effects.

Nitric oxide can be given with CMV or HFOV and is an alternative to ECMO for term infants or infants > 33 weeks and < 28 days old with pulmonary hypertension[60,61]. This has not been confirmed in preterm infants < 34 weeks gestation[62,63]. Further research is ongoing in preterm infants to investigate if prophylactic nitric oxide from day one in preterm infants less than 1.5 kg can help prevent CLD.

Nitric oxide combines with oxygen to form toxic nitrogen dioxide, exposure to which can suppress platelet adhesion and aggregation and cause increase in bleeding time. Expired gas from the ventilator circuit is chemically scavenged to prevent occupational exposure to nitrogen dioxide. Monitoring of methaemoglobin at least twice a day is recommended to prevent toxicity.

Implication for practice

- Nitric oxide has a short half-life so must be supplied to bag/mask circuits too.
- Nitric oxide requires very careful weaning due to the risk of rebound effects.

Conclusion

Improved antenatal care, antenatal steroids, resuscitation in labour ward, post-natal surfactant and post-natal care have contributed to significant improvement in mortality especially in < 28 weeks and < 1000 g infants. However, the challenge for the future is to decrease morbidities such as chronic lung disease, retinopathy of prematurity and adverse neurodevelopment. Awaiting further answers, a comprehensive package of care involving prevention of antenatal infections and chorioamnionitis, respiratory therapies instituted in labour ward, gentle ventilation techniques, targeted oxygen saturations, prevention and prompt treatment of post-natal infections and patent ductus arteriosus and improved nutrition may improve outcomes.

References

1. Langston C, Kida K, Reed M, Thurlbeck WM (1984) Human lung growth in late gestation and in the neonate. *Am Rev Respir Dis*, **129** (4), 607–613.

2. Zeltner, TB, Burri PH (1987) The postnatal development and growth of the human lung. II. Morphology. *Respir Physiol*, **67** (3), 269–282.

3. Crowley P, Chalmers I, Keirse MJ (1990) The effects of corticosteroid administration before preterm delivery: an overview of the evidence from controlled trials. *Br J Obstet Gynaecol*, **97** (1), 11–25.

4. Jobe AH, Mitchell BR, Gunkel JH (1993) Beneficial effects of the combined use of prenatal corticosteroids and postnatal surfactant on preterm infants. Am *J Obstet Gynecol*, **168** (2), 508–513.

5. Sen S, Reghu A, Ferguson SD (2002) Efficacy of a single dose of antenatal steroid in surfactant-treated babies under 31 weeks' gestation. *J Matern Foetal Neonatal Med*, **12** (5), 298–303.

6. Peaceman AM, Bajaj K, Kumar P, Grobman WA (2005) The interval between a single course of antenatal steroids and delivery and its association with neonatal outcomes. *Am J Obstet Gynecol*, **193** (3 Pt 2), 1165–1169.

7. Ring AM, Garland J, Stafeil B, Carr M, Peckman G, Pircon R (2007) The effect of a prolonged time interval between antenatal corticosteroid administration and delivery on outcomes in preterm neonates: a cohort study. *Am J Obstet Gynecol*, **196** (5), 457.e1-457.e6.

8. Guinn DA, Atkinson MW, Sullivan L, *et al.* (2001) Single vs weekly courses of antenatal corticosteroids for women at risk of preterm delivery: a randomized controlled trial. *JAMA*, **286** (13), 1581–1587.

9. Jobe AH, Mitchell BR, Gunkel JH (1993) Beneficial effects of the combined use of prenatal corticosteroids and postnatal surfactant on preterm infants. Am *J Obstet Gynecol*, **168** (2), 508–513.

10. Morley CJ (1997) Systematic review of prophylactic vs rescue surfactant. *Arch Dis Child Foetal Neonatal Ed*, **77** (1), F70–F74.

11. Geary C, Caskey M, Fonseca R, Malloy M (2008) Decreased incidence of bronchopulmonary dysplasia after early management changes, including surfactant and nasal continuous positive airway pressure treatment at delivery, lowered oxygen saturation goals, and early amino acid administration: a historical cohort study. *Pediatrics*, 121 (1), 89–96.

12. Hansen TN, TN Mckintosh N (eds) (2000) Resuscitation of extremely preterm infants: the influence of positive pressure, surfactant replacement and supplemental oxygen on outcome. In: Hansen TN, TN Mckintosh N (eds), *Current Topics in Neonatalogy*, 4th edn. WB Saunders, London.

13. Raju TN, Langenberg P (1993) Pulmonary hemorrhage and exogenous surfactant therapy: a metaanalysis. *J Pediatr*, **123** (4), 603–610.

14. Horbar JD, Carpenter JH, Buzas J, *et al.* (2004) Timing of initial surfactant treatment for infants 23 to 29 weeks' gestation: is routine practice evidence based? *Pediatrics*, 113 (6), 1593–1602.

15. Halliday HL (2008) Surfactants: past, present and future. *J Perinatol*, **28** (Suppl. 1), S47–S56.

16. Horbar JD, Carpenter JH, Buzas J, *et al.* (2004) Timing of initial surfactant treatment for infants 23 to 29 weeks' gestation: is routine practice evidence based? *Pediatrics*, 113 (6), 1593–1602.

17. Finer NN, Carlo WA, Duara S, *et al.* (2004) Delivery room continuous positive airway pressure/positive end-expiratory pressure in extremely low birthweight infants: a feasibility trial. *Pediatrics*, 114 (3), 651–657.

18. Vanpée M, Walfridsson-Schultz U, Katz-Salamon M, Zupancic JA, Pursley D, Jónsson B (2007) Resuscitation and ventilation strategies for extremely preterm infants: a comparison study between two neonatal centers in Boston and Stockholm. *Acta Paediatr*, 96 (1), 10–6; discussion 8–9.

19. Lindner W, Pohlandt F (2007) Oxygenation and ventilation in spontaneously breathing very preterm infants with nasopharyngeal CPAP in the delivery room. *Acta Paediatr*, 96 (1), 17–22.

20. Northway WH Jr, Rosan RC, Porter DY (1967) Pulmonary disease following respirator therapy of hyaline-membrane disease. Bronchopulmonary dysplasia. *N Engl J Med*, **276** (7), 357–68.

21. Jobe AH, Bancalari E (2001) Bronchopulmonary dysplasia. *Am J Respir Crit Care Med*, **163** (7), 1723–1729.

22. Charafeddine L, D'Angio CT, Phelps DL (1999) Atypical chronic lung disease patterns in neonates. *Pediatrics*, **103** (4 Pt 1), 759–765.

23. Panickar J, Scholefield H, Kumar Y, Pilling DW, Subhedar NV (2004) Atypical chronic lung disease in preterm infants. *J Perinat Med*, **32** (2), 162–167.

24. Charafeddine L, D'Angio CT, Phelps DL (1999) Atypical chronic lung disease patterns in neonates. *Pediatrics*, **103** (4 Pt 1), 759–765.
25. Halliday HL, Ehrenkranz RA, Doyle LW (2003) Early postnatal (< 96 hours) corticosteroids for preventing chronic lung disease in preterm infants. *Cochrane Database Syst Rev* (1), CD001146.
26. Halliday HL, Ehrenkranz RA, Doyle LW (2003) Delayed (> 3 weeks) postnatal corticosteroids for chronic lung disease in preterm infants. *Cochrane Database Syst Rev* (1), CD001145.
27. Halliday HL, Ehrenkranz RA, Doyle LW (2003) Moderately early (7–14 days) postnatal corticosteroids for preventing chronic lung disease in preterm infants. *Cochrane Database Syst Rev* (1), CD001144.
28. Hodgman JE (2003) Relationship between Wilson-Mikity syndrome and the new bronchopulmonary dysplasia. *Pediatrics*, **112** (6 Pt 1), 1414–1415.
29. Morrison JJ, Rennie JM, Milton PJ (1995) Neonatal respiratory morbidity and mode of delivery at term: influence of timing of elective caesarean section. *Br J Obstet Gynaecol*, **102** (2), 101–106.
30. Alderdice F, McCall E, Bailie C, *et al.*(2005) Admission to neonatal intensive care with respiratory morbidity following 'term' elective caesarean section. *Ir Med J*, **98** (6), 170–172.
31. Kinsella JP (1999) Clinical trials of inhaled nitric oxide therapy in the newborn. *Pediatr Rev*, **20** (11), e110–e113.
32. Yoder BA, Kirsch EA, Barth WH, Gordon MC (2002) Changing obstetric practices associated with decreasing incidence of meconium aspiration syndrome. *Obstet Gynecol*, **99** (5 Pt 1), 731–739.
33. Wiswell TE, Gannon CM, Jacob J, *et al.* (2000) Delivery room management of the apparently vigorous meconium-stained neonate: results of the multicenter, international collaborative trial. *Pediatrics*, **105** (1 Pt 1), 1–7.
34. Vain NE, Szyld EG, Prudent LM, Wiswell TE, Aguilar AM, Vivas NI (2004) Oropharyngeal and nasopharyngeal suctioning of meconium-stained neonates before delivery of their shoulders: multicentre, randomised controlled trial. *Lancet*, **364** (9434), 597–602.
35. Quine D, Stenson BJ (2009) PaO$_2$ values in infants < 29 weeks of gestation at currently targeted saturations. *Arch Dis Child Foetal Neonatal Ed*, **94** (1, Jan.), F51–F53. Epub 19 Feb 2008.
36. Polin RA, Sahni R (2002) Newer experience with CPAP. *Semin Neonatol*, **7** (5), 379–389.
37. Morley CJ, Davis PG, Doyle LW, Brion LP, Hascoet JM, Carlin JB (2008) Nasal CPAP or intubation at birth for very preterm infants. *N Engl J Med*, **358** (7), 700–708.
38. McCoskey L (2008) Nursing Care Guidelines for prevention of nasal breakdown in neonates receiving nasal CPAP. *Adv Neonatal Care*, **8** (2), 116–124.
39. Robertson NJ, McCarthy LS, Hamilton PA, Moss AL (1996) Nasal deformities resulting from flow driver continuous positive airway pressure. *Arch Dis Child Foetal Neonatal Ed*, **75** (3), F209–F212.
40. Morley CJ, Davis PG, Doyle LW, Brion LP, Hascoet JM, Carlin JB (2008) Nasal CPAP or intubation at birth for very preterm infants. *N Engl J Med*, **358** (7), 700–708.
41. Crawford D, Dixon M (eds) (2004) *Neonatal Nursing*. Chapman and Hall, London.
42. Crawford D, Dixon M (eds) (2004) *Neonatal Nursing*. Chapman and Hall, London.
43. Snow TM, Brandon DH (2007) A nurse's guide to common mechanical ventilation techniques and modes used in infants. Nursing implications. *Adv Neonatal Care*, **7** (1), 8–21.
44. D'Angio CT, Chess PR, Kovacs SJ *et al.* (2005) Pressure-regulated volume control ventilation vs synchronized intermittent mandatory ventilation for very low-birth-weight infants: a randomized controlled trial. *Arch Pediatr Adolesc Med*, **159** (9), 868–875.
45. Grover A, Field D (2008) Volume-targeted ventilation in the neonate: time to change? *Arch Dis Child Foetal Neonatal Ed*, **93** (1), F7–F13.
46. McCallion N, Lau R, Morley CJ, Dargaville PA (2008) Neonatal volume guarantee ventilation: effects of spontaneous breathing, triggered and untriggered inflations. *Arch Dis Child Foetal Neonatal Ed*, **93** (1), F36–F39.
47. Flynn JT, Bancalari E, Snyder ES, *et al.* (1992) A cohort study of transcutaneous oxygen tension and the incidence and severity of retinopathy of prematurity. *N Engl J Med*, **326** (16), 1050–1054.
48. Hodge D (1991) Endotracheal suctioning and the infant: a nursing care protocol to decrease complications. *Neonatal Netw*, **9** (5), 7–15.
49. Runton N (1992) Suctioning artificial airways in children: appropriate technique. *Pediatr Nurs*, **18** (2), 115–118.
50. Tenaillon A, Boiteau R, Perrin-Gachadoat D, Burdin M (1990) Humidification and aspiration of the respiratory tract in patients with mechanical ventilation. *Rev Prat*, **40** (25), 2315–2319.

51. Hanley MV, Rudd T, Butler J (1978) What happens to intratracheal saline instillations? *Am Rev Respir Dis*, **177** (Suppl.), 1245.

52. Christensen RD, Rigby G, Schmutz N, *et al.* (2007) ETCare: a randomized, controlled, masked trial comparing two solutions for upper airway care in the NICU. *J Perinatol*, **27** (8), 479–484.

53. Davis PG, Henderson-Smart DJ (2003) Nasal continuous positive airways pressure immediately after extubation for preventing morbidity in preterm infants. *Cochrane Database Syst Rev* (2), CD000143.

54. Davis PG, Henderson-Smart DJ (2001) Extubation from low-rate intermittent positive airways pressure versus extubation after a trial of endotracheal continuous positive airways pressure in intubated preterm infants. *Cochrane Database Syst Rev* (4), CD001078.

55. Menon, G, Boyle EM, Bergqvist LL, McIntosh N, Barton BA, Anand KJ (2008) Morphine analgesia and gastrointestinal morbidity in preterm infants: Secondary results from the NEOPAIN Trial. *Arch Dis Child Foetal Neonatal Ed*, **93** (5, Sept.), F362–F367. Epub 18 Dec. 2007.

56. Anand K, Hall RW, Desai N, *et al.* (2004) Effects of morphine analgesia in ventilated preterm neonates: primary outcomes from the NEOPAIN randomised trial. *Lancet*, **363** (9422), 1673–1682.

57. Chang YJ, Anderson G, Dowling D, Lin C (2002) Decreased activity and oxygen desaturation in prone ventilated preterm infants during the first postnatal week. *Heart Lung*, **31** (1), 34–42.

58. Avila K, Mazza L, Morgan-Trujillo L (1994) High-frequency oscillatory ventilation: a nursing approach to bedside care. *Neonatal Netw*, **13** (5), 23–30.

59. Roberts JD, Polaner DM, Lang P, Zapol WM (1992) Inhaled nitric oxide in persistent pulmonary hypertension of the newborn. *Lancet*, **340** (8823), 818–819.

60. Field D, Elbourne D, Hardy P, *et al.* (2007) Neonatal ventilation with inhaled nitric oxide vs. ventilatory support without inhaled nitric oxide for infants with severe respiratory failure born at or near term: the INNOVO multicentre randomised controlled trial. *Neonatology*, **91** (2), 73–82.

61. Finer NN, Barrington KJ (2006) Nitric oxide for respiratory failure in infants born at or near term. *Cochrane Database Syst Rev* (4), CD000399.

62. Field D, Elbourne D, Truesdale A, *et al.* (2005) Neonatal ventilation with inhaled nitric oxide versus ventilatory support without inhaled nitric oxide for preterm infants with severe respiratory failure: the INNOVO multicentre randomised controlled trial (ISRCTN 17821339). *Pediatrics*, **115** (4), 926–936.

63. Barrington KJ, Finer NN (2006) Inhaled nitric oxide for respiratory failure in preterm infants. *Cochrane Database Syst Rev* (1), CD000509.

Chapter 9

NEONATAL SURGERY

Shawqui Nour and Maggie Hallsworth

Learning outcomes

After reading this chapter the reader will be expected to be able to:

- Discuss the antenatal management of a foetus who has been diagnosed with a congenital surgical anomaly
- Discuss the clinical history, diagnosis and management of an infant with a surgical condition
- Explain the general principles of pre and post-operative care of an infant with a surgical condition
- Discuss the long-term implications of surgical conditions and their prognoses

---

Introduction

Neonatal surgical conditions include congenital abnormalities and those that arise as a complication of prematurity. Prior to 1930 very few infants with congenital surgical conditions survived either their condition or the surgical procedure. With a multidisciplinary team approach in the management of these patients, survival of those infants in whom parents have decided to continue the pregnancy has improved[1,2]. Other factors which have contributed to greater survival are advances in surgical techniques, understanding of the congenital abnormality and its physiological impact and the introduction of antibiotics.

Surgical conditions that are due to the complications of prematurity include:

- Necrotising enterocolitis (NEC)
- Persistence of the ductus arteriosus (pDA)
- Retinopathy of prematurity (ROP)

Persistence of the ductus arteriosus will be discussed in Chapter 11, retinopathy of prematurity in Chapter 5 and necrotising enterocolitis will be discussed in this chapter.

The greatest improvement in survival of neonates with a surgical diagnosis was seen from the 1970s onwards and it coincided with the introduction of intravenous feeding and advances in neonatal intensive care and anaesthesia. At the present time the vast majority of newborns with a congenital surgical anomaly will survive and the leading cause of death will be associated lethal anomalies, e.g. severe lung hypoplasia, major cardiac defects or lethal syndromes.

This chapter will begin with antenatal care and the general principles of post-natal surgical management, before discussing specific surgical diagnoses.

Antenatal diagnosis and counselling

Over the last 20 years there has been a tremendous advance in the field of foetal medicine. It has been helped by the great sophistication in ultrasound machine technology which provides clear images and views of the foetus, therefore allowing an early diagnosis of many surgical conditions. The following are a few examples:

- Congenital lung malformation
- Oesophageal atresia
- Congenital diaphragmatic hernia
- Duodenal atresia
- Abdominal wall defects (gastroschisis and exomphalos)
- Renal abnormality
- Spina bifida
- Hydrocephalus

Although antenatal scanning will not provide a 100% accurate diagnosis, in most common conditions it provides a highly accurate diagnosis which will allow antenatal counselling.

The major advantages of antenatal diagnoses are:

- Counselling of future parents: it allows the parents to meet the paediatric surgeon, neonatologist, geneticist and obstetrician and discuss the antenatal management plan, the delivery plan and the post-natal care. Such dialogue with the parents aims to offer them a clearer picture and improve their understanding of the diagnosis and planned neonatal care. It also takes away the element of shock and surprise of an unexpected major congenital anomaly discovered at birth.
- Planning of the delivery in a tertiary centre close to paediatric surgeons: this will aim to minimise separation of the family, which can occur when an infant is transferred to a tertiary surgical centre having been born in a peripheral unit. It will also prevent a delay in surgery while transfer is awaited.
- Planned induction of labour: this will enable detailed post-natal planning and will prevent the spontaneous onset of labour resulting in the mother being admitted to a more local hospital without the surgical expertise.

It is also important to explain to the future parents that the antenatal diagnosis, although it is highly accurate, will require further evaluation following delivery and may rarely be incorrect.

The antenatal counselling session should also include a visit to the labour ward and the neonatal unit, which allows future parents to meet the teams who will be looking after their infant. The neonatal team should meet with them again prior to delivery in order to answer any questions that they may have.

Implications for practice

- Antenatal diagnosis will facilitate delivery of the infant at the optimal place for ongoing care.
- A proposed plan of care may be developed following discussion with the prospective parents.

Post-natal management

General principles

Most infants born with a surgical condition require a standardised approach that includes a detailed clinical assessment, certain routine and diagnosis specific investigations and a clear management plan. This standardised approach should be discussed with the surgical team.

It will always include:

- A detailed birth history: weight, gestation and any antenatal abnormalities should be recorded
- A detailed post-natal clinical examination: to detect any associated anomalies, e.g. heart defects
- Nursing in an incubator to facilitate a thermoneutral environment, monitoring:
  - Skin colour, temperature
  - Abdominal care, bowel action and type of stool
  - Respiration, oxygen saturation
  - Ventilatory requirements, blood gases
  - ECG, blood pressure
  - Intravenous cannulation
  - Antibiotics
  - Intravenous fluid administration
- Vitamin K_1: this should be administered routinely intramuscularly for infants with surgical conditions

- Investigations: the general investigations include full blood count, urea and electrolytes, clotting screen, group, and save and cross match if blood required
- Breast milk: the provision of expressed milk should also be discussed with the parents as infants with a surgical diagnosis often find expressed milk easier to absorb than formula.

The following management will be needed in a large number of specific surgical conditions:

- The passage of a nasogastric tube of adequate size according to the size of the infant:
  - Placed on free drainage and aspirated four hourly
  - Replacement of losses with normal saline (0.9% sodium chloride) and added potassium chloride.
- Radiology: X-ray investigations are often required in such infants, e.g. abdominal and chest X-rays as well as an upper or lower gastrointestinal water soluble contrast studies.
- Ventilation: this may be required pre-operatively in an unwell infant or post-operatively as routine and will help with the administration of appropriate analgesia in the form of morphine, which will require close monitoring.
- Central venous access: a central venous catheter is often needed for intravenous feeding in these neonatal surgical infants as they may not be able to feed enterally for a few days.
- Pain relief: infants with a surgical diagnosis are often in pain pre-operatively and will almost certainly require pain relief post-operatively. This often takes the form of a morphine infusion, which may have complications such as respiratory depression and hypotension. Paracetamol is also used.
- Chromosomal analysis: this is often needed in this group of newborn infants and certainly if a chromosomal abnormality is suspected then a blood sample must be obtained prior to any blood transfusion.
- Genetic investigations: Delta 508 blood investigation is needed in certain conditions if the possibility of cystic fibrosis exists.

It is essential to have excellent communication between the neonatal intensive care team and the paediatric surgical team in order to provide a plan of management which is clear to the parents. The parents need to be fully informed of the management plan for the infant by explaining the abnormality to them, its effect on their infant, the management options, details of the surgical procedure, especially if a stoma is going to be constructed, the immediate post-operative care, the short and long-term outcome. The last thing these anxious parents need is differences of opinion and it is helpful if the nurse looking after the infant can be present during these discussions[3].

A consent form will be required by the surgeon who is going to operate on the infant and it is the responsibility of the surgeon to gain informed consent by explaining the procedure to the parents in detail. The consent form needs to be signed either by the mother, or by the father if they are married, or if his name will appear on the birth certificate.

Implications for practice

- A detailed assessment to facilitate accurate diagnosis and close communication with the parents is vital.
- Consent for surgery should be taken by a member of the surgical team.

Preoperative assessment

The infant should be resuscitated and stabilised prior to theatre unless it is an absolute surgical emergency (e.g. volvulus). There is good evidence in adults, paediatric and neonatal practice that the outcome from surgery is improved when patients have been stabilised prior to theatre.

Resuscitation and stabilisation can be considered under the areas of:

- Thermoregulation
- Ventilation
- Fluid balance and glucose status
- Cardiovascular
- Haematological

Most neonatal units and theatres have a detailed checklist to work through prior to leaving the neonatal unit and entering the theatre for surgery. An example of this is shown in Figure 9.1.

Post-operative care

Post-operative care should begin with a full clinical assessment of the infant on return from theatre. This should involve a clinical examination of the infant, recalculation of all of the infusions, examination of cannulae and central venous access sites and in many cases a repeat CXR and AXR. The surgical notes should be consulted and the operation discussed with the surgeon so that accurate advice will be given to parents. Further care can also be considered under the headings:

- Thermoregulation
- Ventilation
- Fluid balance and glucose status
- Cardiovascular
- Haematological

Necrotising enterocolitis

Necrotising enterocolitis (NEC) is a common acute inflammatory condition with high morbidity and mortality, which affects mainly preterm infants[4,5]. As the title suggests it consists of ischaemia and necrosis of the gastrointestinal tract, which may lead to perforation.

The exact aetiology is unknown but it is almost certainly multifactorial. The combination of intestinal immaturity, the presence of inflammation or infection, hypoxia and enteral feeding will all contribute to the risk of development of necrotising enterocolitis in the preterm infant[6]. A patent ductus arteriosus and treatment with indomethacin are also added risk factors[7,8]. Breast milk has a protective effect and it has also been demonstrated that the use of a standardised feeding regime may be protective[9-11]. The exact way in which feeds should be introduced and increased until an infant is on full feeds continues

to be studied but evidence is accumulating that a rapid increase in feed volume may be an added risk factor[12]. There is also some concern about the widespread use of ranitidine as this prevents gastric acid formation and may be an additional risk factor for the development of NEC[13].

Clinical features

NEC most commonly presents between the third and tenth day of life but it can occur as early as within 24 hours of birth and the extreme preterm infant often presents later than the moderately preterm infant[14].

A strong index of suspicion combined with early recognition and treatment will improve the mortality and morbidity of the disease as it does progress through well defined stages, although in some infants this progression is rapid and devastating. Modified Bells criteria for diagnosis are shown in Table 9.1[15].

Clinically, the symptoms and signs can be divided into systemic or specific to the gastrointestinal tract and some of these are listed below:

- Systemic
  - Temperature instability
  - Tachycardia
  - Thrombocytopenia
  - Apnoea and bradycardic episodes
- Specific to the gastrointestinal tract:
  - Feed intolerance increasing aspirates, bile stained aspirates and vomiting
  - Abdominal distension
  - Abdominal tenderness
  - Bleeding per rectum

If the pre-term infant is ventilated the ventilation requirements may increase. Abdominal examination will reveal a distended and tender abdomen and in the late stages of the disease erythema of the abdominal wall and a mass will be palpable.

Investigations include FBC, U & E, clotting, group and save, and abdominal X-ray. The latter is often diagnostic. It may show gas in the

University Hospitals of Leicester **NHS**

NHS Trust

Theatre Checklist

Consultant	
Ward	
Intended Procedure	
Date of Procedure	☐☐ ☐☐ **20** ☐☐

Name _____

Address _____

_____

_____

DOB _____

Patient label

Check 1 (Surgeon on ward)	**Action** • Check patient's identity (ID) • Check reliable documentation and/or images to ascertain intended surgical site • Mark the intended site according to UHL policy	**Confirm Check Complete** Signature _____ Print name _____
Check 2 (Registered Nurse / Midwife on ward)	**Check** • Identification band x 2 • Consent form signed • Consent form checked with reliable documentation, e.g. case notes, operating list etc • Operation Mark (if appropriate)	**Confirm Check Complete** Signature _____ Print name _____

RECORD ALL OBSERVATIONS OVERLEAF

My last feed was at:	My nappy was last changed at:	I am allergic to:	My Mum and Dad are coming to theatre with me: Yes / No

Documents to Theatre

Prescription chart ☐   Obschart ☐   Fluid chart ☐   Notes ☐   X-rays ☐

Latest Blood Results

Sodimu	Potassium	Urea	Hb	Platelets	Clotting

Has blood been ordered? Yes / No   Where stored: Blood Bank / LW fridge / Theatre Fridge

Check 3 Theatre Staff in Theatre Reception	In the theatre suite and prior to anaesthesia parent or accompanying nurse to state name, DOB, intended procedure and anatomical site of procedure. Theatre staff to check this information against:	**Check**	**Sign**	**Print name**
		ID Band		
		Consent Form		
		Operating List		
		Operation Mark (if appropriate)		
		Confirm details in CHECK 2		
Check 4 Operating Staff in Theatre	In the operating theatre and prior to commencement of surgery, the operating surgeon or a senior member of the clinical team must carry out the following:	**Check** • Check the surgical mark against the supporting documentation • Re-check imaging studies are available in operating theatre • The availability of the correct implant / central line (if applicable)	**Confirm check complete** **Signature** Print name	
		• Verbal check with: Name of Operating Surgeon (Print Name)		

Figure 9.1   Theatre checklist. Reproduced by kind permission of University Hospitals of Leicester NHS Trust.

Return to Ward

Ventilated / O_2 / Self- ventilating in air _____

Drains in situ:_____

Returned:　**X-rays** [　]　　**Notes** [　]　　**Unused central lines** [　]

Pain Control:

Post-operative instructions: _____
_____
_____
_____
_____
_____

Mum and Dad contacted?

OBSERVATIONS

	WORKING WEIGHT (KG)					
On leaving NNU	Temp	Pulse	Resps	BP	O₂Sats	Blood Glucose
On arrival in Theatre	Temp	Pulse	Resps	BP	O₂Sats	Blood Glucose
On collection from Theatre	Temp	Pulse	Resps	BP	O₂Sats	Blood Glucose
On arrival in NNU	Temp	Pulse	Resps	BP	O₂Sats	Blood Glucose

National Patient Safety Agency Information on Correct Site Surgery

Circumstances where marking may not be appropriate

1. Emergency surgery should not be delayed due to lack of pre-operative marking.
2. Teeth and mucous membranes.
3. Cases of bilateral simultaneous organ surgery such as bilateral tonsillectomy, squint surgery.
4. Situations where the laterality of surgery needs to be confirmed following examination under anaesthesia or exploration in theatre such as revision of squint corrections.

Pre-operative marking recommendations

The National Patient Safety Agency (NPSA) and the Royal College of Surgeons of England (RCS) strongly recommend preoperative marking to indicate clearly the intended site for elective surgical procedures.

1. How to mark

An indelible marker pen should be used. The mark should be an arrow that extends to, or near to, the incision site and remain visible after the application of skin preparation. It is desirable that the mark should also remain visible after the application of theatre drapes.

2. Where to mark

Surgical operations involving side (laterality) should be marked at, or near, the intended incision. For digits on the hand and foot the mark should extend to the correct specific digit. Ascertain intended surgical site from reliable documentation and images.

3. Who marks

Marking should be undertaken by the operating surgeon, or nominated deputy, who will be present in the operating theatre at the time of the patient's procedure.

4. With whom

The process of pre-operative marking of the intended site should involve the patient and/or family members/significant others wherever possible.

5. Time and place

The surgical site should, ideally, be marked on the ward or day care area prior to patient transfer to the operating theatre. Marking should take place before pre-medication.

6. Verify

The surgical site mark should subsequently be checked against reliable documentation to confirm it is (a) correctly located, and (b) still legible. This checking should occur at each transfer of the patient's care and end with a final verification prior to commencement of surgery. All team members should be involved in checking the mark.

Ref: NPSA, Patient Safety Alert 06, 2005, Correct site surgery (CSS)

Figure 9.1　(Continued)

Table 9.1   Modified Bells criteria for diagnosis.

Stage	Systemic signs	Intestinal signs	Radiologic signs	Treatment
(1) Suspected				
(a)	Temperature instability, apnoea, bradycardia	Elevated pregavage residuals, mild abdominal distension, occult blood in stool	Normal or mild ileus	NPO, antibiotics × 3 days
(b)	Same as (1)(a)	Same as (1)(a), plus gross blood in stool	Same as (1)(a)	Same as (1)(a)
(2) Definite				
(a) Mildly ill	Same as (1)(a)	Same as (1), plus absent bowel sounds, abdominal tenderness	Ileus, pneumatosis intestinalis	NPO, antibiotics × 7 to 10 days
(b) Moderately ill	Same as (1), plus mild metabolic acidosis, mild thrombocytopenia	Same as (1), plus absent bowel sounds, definite abdominal tenderness, abdominal cellulitis, right lower quadrant mass	Same as (2)(a), plus portal vein gas, with or without ascites	NPO, antibiotics × 14 days
(3) Advanced				
(a) Severely ill, bowel intact	Same as (2)(b), plus hypotension, bradycardia, respiratory acidosis, metabolic acidosis, disseminated intravascular coagulation, neutropenia	Same as (1) and (2), plus signs of generalised peritonitis, marked tenderness and distension of abdomen	Same as (2)(b), plus definite ascites	NPO, antibiotics × 14 days, fluid resuscitation, inotropic support, ventilator therapy, paracentesis
(b) Severely ill: bowel perforated	Same as (3)(a)	Same as (3)(a)	Same as (2)(b), plus pneumoperitoneum	Same as (3)(a), plus surgery

bowel wall (pneumointestinalis), and dilated bowel loops and free gas in the abdominal cavity in advanced NEC with bowel perforation. A normal X-ray does not exclude NEC.

Medical care

The infant with NEC should obviously be resuscitated as the clinical condition dictates. A wide bore nasogastric tube should be sited and the stomach regularly aspirated before placing the nasogastric tube on free drainage. This may facilitate decompression of the intestine and limit mucosal damage. Feeds should be stopped and intravenous broad spectrum antibiotics

commenced. The mainstay of medical conservative treatment consists of intravenous antibiotics, nil by mouth and intravenous feeding, with repeated abdominal X-rays when indicated.

As well as the specific management of NEC as documented above, the infant will require neonatal intensive care, including:

- Assisted ventilation:
  - The infant will require close monitoring of respiratory status and many of these infants will need ventilation in view of apnoeas and bradycardias and to improve oxygen delivery to the damaged tissues as well as facilitate adequate and appropriate pain management.

○ In infants that are ventilated a high PEEP will help to prevent the overdistended abdomen from compressing the lungs.

○ In some infants pulmonary hypertension may develop which will require aggressive management.

- Nutrition:

  ○ The infant with NEC will initially be in a highly catabolic state, using all of its energy to survive. Following the acute episode it will need to be supplied with adequate nutrition to enable it to enter an anabolic state and repair the damaged tissues as well as grow.

  ○ The placing of a long line will provide access for the administration of intravenous feeding (TPN) which will be essential to maintain adequate nutrition since the infant will not be fed orally during the course of the treatment.

- Fluid balance:

  ○ It is not uncommon for an infant with NEC to become hypoalbuminaemic and oedematous.

  ○ Obsessive attention to fluid input and output is necessary to maintain optimal fluid balance.

- Coagulopathy: thrombocytopenia or deranged clotting may accompany severe NEC and will need monitoring and management such as platelet transfusion and fresh frozen plasma.

Surgery

Surgical intervention will be required in up to 30% of the patients and the indications include:

- Free air in the abdominal cavity, indicating bowel perforation and peritonitis
- Failure of improvement with medical treatment

The main surgical interventions are:

- Bowel resection with end-to-end anastomosis
- Bowel resection with defunctioning ileostomy/colostomy

Post-operative

The post-operative care and management of the infant with NEC must be carefully managed. The sick infant who has had surgery may become even sicker in the immediate post-operative period. Optimising oxygen delivery to the damaged tissues will promote healing and careful ventilation management will facilitate this. In addition, the infants will require adequate pain relief.

Surgery may have resulted in the formation of a stoma or an end-to-end anastomosis, following resection of necrotic bowel, and observation of both wound and stoma for leakage, colour and tension are essential observations. Third space fluid losses into the abdominal cavity can result in a distended abdomen becoming increasingly hard and shiny. This can put additional tension upon the wound and cause increased pain and distress to the infant. These third space losses must be considered in the management of the overall fluid balance. A urinary catheter, monitoring of the infant's toe/core temperature deficit, capillary refill time, blood pressure and regular infant weights will all facilitate careful fluid management.

Care of the parents is crucial; they will be anxious to speak to the surgeon at the earliest opportunity to discuss the operation findings and long-term implications and prognosis, with regular further updates as needed. If a stoma has been performed the parents will be shown how to care for this. Depending on the amount of bowel loss and the site of the stoma it can have implications for the long-term nutrition of the infant. It may be that he/she will require long-term nutritional support with TPN to promote growth and development. Most infants will have reversal of the stoma prior to discharge home, or soon after.

Prognosis

Infants that have had NEC are at risk of developing strictures and so further investigation with contrast investigations and surgery may be indicated if they show signs of abdominal distension and vomiting. The parents are likely to be especially disappointed and distressed when their infant once again develops vomiting and abdominal distension; it is vital, therefore, that they are informed of these risks before the symptoms show.

Gastroschisis

Gastroschisis is a congenital abdominal wall defect that may be diagnosed antenatally as early as 12 weeks gestation. It is an abdominal wall defect to the right of the umbilicus in the majority of cases, and as a result of this defect the small and large bowel, the stomach, Fallopian tubes and ovaries may protrude through this opening. There is no membrane or sack covering these structures, in contrast to infants with an exomphalos or omphalocele[16]. The incidence of gastroschisis has been rising over recent years and the exact reason for this is unknown, but it does seem to be a condition that occurs most frequently in infants of young mothers[17,18].

Clinical features

Gastroschisis is usually an isolated abnormality which is easily noted at birth (see Figure 9.2). In most cases of antenatal diagnosis the labour is induced so that surgery can be planned and these

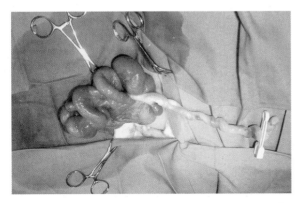

Figure 9.2 Gastroschisis seen at surgery. The bowel is pink and healthy but is lying exposed without a peritoneal covering.

infants may be born vaginally or by caesarean section if there are obstetric indications.

Medical care

Once the infant is born it should be placed in a special plastic bag with a purse string ribbon up to the nipples. The main objective of this bag is to keep the infant warm and to decrease insensible losses from the exposed intestine. These losses can be significant. In addition, the use of a plastic bag facilitates observation of the exposed bowel for colour and circulation. It is vital that this exposed bowel does not become kinked and its blood supply compromised. The use of cling-film to wrap around the infant and the defect will achieve similar aims.

A wide bore nasogastric tube should be passed whilst still in the delivery room, as the stomach often contains a large volume of bile stained fluid which needs draining to reduce the risk of vomiting and associated complications. Intravenous access should be established in order to ensure hydration with maintenance fluids as well as with bolus fluids of 10 ml/kg if required. Regular assessment of the clinical signs of hydration as well as monitoring of fluid input and output are essential to ensure adequate hydration prior to surgery. Antibiotics that are active against both aerobic and anaerobic bacteria should be administered and routine blood investigations as detailed above should be performed.

Surgery

Once the infant is haemodynamically stable, he/she is taken to the operating theatre and under general anaesthesia the bowel is cleaned, the abdominal wall is gently stretched and the bowel contents returned to the abdominal cavity (primary closure). If the bowel is severely matted together or the abdominal cavity is too small then part of the bowel is reduced and the rest is put in a special silo sac sutured to the abdominal wall. During this period the silo will be gently suspended from the incubator roof and the effects of gravity, reduction in bowel swelling and increase in abdominal space will facilitate a later return of the bowel to the abdomen. The nursing staff will play an active role in maintaining the integrity of the bag during this period. Leakage of fluid into the bag will make assessment of fluid losses difficult. It is critical that there is attention to detail in the observation of blood pressure, toe/core temperature gap, capillary refill time and other fluid losses/gains. Seven to ten days after initial surgery the infant will return to theatre to have the bag removed and the rest of the bowel inserted into the abdominal cavity (secondary closure).

Post-operative care and long-term prognosis

Intravenous feeding (parental nutrition) is essential in these infants as the bowel may be non-functioning for up to three or four weeks. This will delay the commencement and advancement of enteral feeding. Initially, the infants will produce copious amounts of gastric aspirate which will be markedly bile stained. Replacement of these losses with normal saline and added potassium will prevent metabolic alkalosis and electrolyte imbalance. Once the aspirates have reduced and bowel sounds are heard the gradual introduction of feeds may be commenced, which will be a very slow process initially. In the majority of infants with gastroschisis the bowel will begin to work after the second or third week, although some infants take longer. This post-operative course may be complicated by NEC or bowel strictures and some of these infants will develop a conjugated hyperbilirubinaemia as a complication of prolonged TPN. Most infants, however, will be home within four or five weeks after delivery.

The long-term outcome in gastroschisis infants is generally good and apart from gastrointestinal abnormalities (initial paralytic ileus, the occasional bowel atresia); these infants do not usually have associated congenital anomalies[19]

Implications for practice

Fluid balance is one of the keys to managing these infants well:

- Prior to surgery: placing the infant in a plastic bag up to the armpits at the time of delivery, will reduce heat and fluid loss from the defect.
- Post-surgery: these infants will initially lose copious amounts of fluid from their nasogastric or orogastric tubes. These losses are usually replaced by saline with added potassium.

Exomphalos

Exomphalos is another congenital abdominal wall defect that may be diagnosed antenatally. The defect is based at the umbilicus where the abdominal muscles and the skin remain wide apart with abdominal viscera protruding. Exomphalos are classified as:

- Exomphalos minor: the small bowel protruding
- Exomphalos major: the diameter is more than 8 cm in diameter and the liver is also included in this defect

There are two main differences between exomphalos and gastroschisis:

- In an exomphalos the viscera are protected by their peritoneal covering. In a gastroschisis there is no peritoneal covering present; the viscera are therefore more easily damaged.
- Exomphalos is often associated with congenital anomalies such as congenital heart defects, chromosomal abnormalities (trisomy 13, 18 or 21) and Beckwith-Wiedemann syndrome. Gastroschisis is usually not associated with other anomalies.

Clinical features

A full clinical examination should be conducted for signs of associated cardiac or chromosomal abnormalities and echocardiography and karyotype are important investigations to perform prior to surgery.

Medical care

The initial management is similar to the management of an infant with gastroschisis: a wide bore nasogastric tube should be passed, an intravenous cannula inserted and intravenous antibiotics commenced. After birth the exomphalos is wrapped in a clean sheet of cling-film, or the infant is placed in a drawstring plastic bag.

These infants do not usually require aggressive fluid management because the bowel is protected by the peritoneal covering. However, they should be carefully examined for features of chromosomal abnormalities or Beckwith-Wiedemann syndrome and appropriate genetic investigations should be sent. It is also usual to perform a cardiac echo prior to surgery.

Surgery

Depending on the size of the exomphalos, primary closure is attempted and the object is to repair the abdominal wall and to obtain skin cover. In a large exomphalos major this might not be possible and in these cases conservative management consists of keeping the membrane clean and dry and applying an antiseptic solution in order to thicken the wall of the sac and perform a secondary repair months later.

Post-operative care

Intravenous feeding will be necessary until the newborn is ready to feed enterally. Infants with an exomphalos should be able to commence and tolerate enteral feeds much more quickly than infants with gastroschisis as their bowel was not bathed in amniotic fluid and was protected by the peritoneum. In a similar way to infants with gastroschisis, feeds should not be commenced until bile stained aspirates have cleared and bowel sounds are heard.

Prognosis

The prognosis of infant's with exomphalos is dependent upon the associated anomalies and the size of the exomphalos.

Implications for practice

The long-term outlook for infants with exomphalos is dependent on the presence of and severity of other abnormalities and screening for these should have been commenced in the pre-operative period.

Hirschsprung's disease

Hirschsprung's disease (HD) is a congenital anomaly due to a deficiency of enteric ganglion cells within the bowel (aganglionosis). These cells normally have a role in maintaining smooth muscle tone and coordinating peristalsis. The clinical result of aganglionosis is functional obstruction of the bowel and dilatation of the normal bowel proximal (prior) to the defect. The amount of bowel affected by the disease varies between individual infants. In most infants the disease extends upwards from the rectum to the rectosigmoid junction and in a minority of cases the infant may have a total colonic aganglionosis. Most patients with Hirschsprung's disease present in the first month of life.

Clinical features

Clinically, the infants present with poor feeding, bile stained vomiting, abdominal distension and delay in the passage of meconium. A delay in passage of meconium of over 24-hour duration in a term infant should alert the clinician as to the possibility of Hirschsprung's disease as most infants pass meconium within 24 hours, although some may be delayed until 48 hours[20–22]. Examination reveals a distended abdomen which is tender. Rectal examination will show a tight grip on the examining finger and a gush of faecal matter on withdrawal of the finger.

Infants with trisomy 21 have an increased risk of Hirschsprung's disease and it can also be associated with other related congenital anomalies which include cardiac defects and Ondine's curse (cerebral apnoea). It is important to make the diagnosis of Hirschsprung's disease as an early diagnosis will mean that appropriate medical or surgical care is instituted and that parents are made aware of the complications of Hirschsprung's and the clinical features of these complications. These include enterocolitis which can lead to perforation and faecal peritonitis, which has a significant mortality and morbidity.

Medical care

The main features of acute resuscitation are:

- Airway and breathing support as required: this is not usually necessary unless the infant has developed enterocolitis
- Fluid rehydration
- Insertion of a wide bore naso/orogastric tube
- Antibiotics that are effective against pathogens found within the gastrointestinal tract

Insertion of a wide bore nasogastric tube is essential to decompress the distended gut. Blood investigations as detailed above should be requested. An abdominal X-ray will show a dilated bowel and a contrast enema can be diagnostic in showing collapsed distal bowel with dilatation above. The diagnosis can be confirmed by performing a rectal biopsy and this will establish the diagnosis in the vast majority of these patients.

Once the diagnosis is made a full discussion and explanation is given to the parents. The current management of Hirschsprung's disease in infants includes twice daily rectal washouts by the parents for 4–6 weeks, followed by a primary one stage surgical procedure. In many neonatal units, parents of infants with Hirschsprung's disease who are awaiting surgery will be taught how to perform the rectal washouts. As long as these are effective in promoting defaecation the

infant may be discharged home, whilst awaiting surgery. Ongoing support may be given by the community neonatal team during this time.

Surgery

The primary elective surgical procedure is performed either by an open technique or laparoscopically, and involves removal of the affected bowel and primary anastomosis. On occasions these infants are too ill or present late and conservative management with washouts will not be effective, and on these occasions a colostomy or ileostomy will be performed with a pull-through end-to-end anastomosis performed a few weeks later.

Post-operative care and long-term prognosis

Although most of these patients will have a good long-term outcome some of the.
patients will suffer from chronic constipation, soiling and faecal incontinence but generally these children improve as they grow older.

Implications for practice

- Healthy newborns should generally pass meconium within 24 hours of delivery.
- Once the diagnosis has been made, screening for associated anomalies should be undertaken

Oesophageal atresia and tracheo-oesophageal fistula

Congenital atresia of the oesophagus and tracheo-oesophageal fistula are common anomalies, with a combined incidence of 1:4500 births. The primary defect results from failure of separation of the trachea from the oesophagus. The common types of oesophageal atresia are shown in the Figure 9.3.

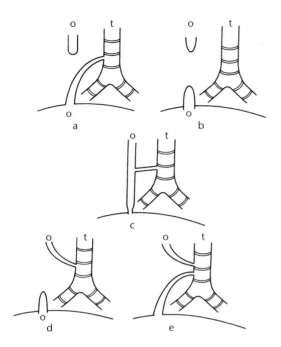

Figure 9.3 Types of tracheo-oesophageal atresia.

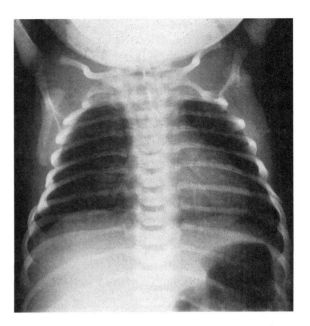

Figure 9.4 A CXR of an infant with oesophageal atresia. The gastric tube will not advance further than T4. The presence of a stomach bubble indicates that there is also a tracheo-osophageal fistula.

Newborns with this congenital anomaly often have associated anomalies such as congenital heart defects, renal abnormalities and vertebral anomalies. VATER or VACTERL are acronyms describing these abnormalities (Vertebral, Anal, Cardiac, Tracheo Oesophageal, Renal and Limb abnormalities).

Clinical features

The demonstration of a small or absent stomach in the foetus on an antenatal ultrasound scan with the presence of maternal polyhydramnios should alert the clinician to the possibility of oesophageal atresia.

These infants can present with frothy secretions in the mouth, requiring frequent suction. Often they present with respiratory distress and cyanosis if a feed is attempted. Occasionally the newborn will present with a chest infection secondary to aspiration. If at all possible CPAP or artificial ventilation should be avoided in these infants as it may increase the risk of stomach perforation.

Once the diagnosis is suspected an attempt to pass a large bore nasogastric or Replogle tube should be made and in oesophageal atresia it will not pass beyond 10–12 cm from the lips. The Replogle tube is a wide bore tube which has the facility to attach to low vacuum suction and drain continuously; it is valuable in draining the upper pouch whilst awaiting surgery and preventing aspiration of secretions. A chest X-ray taken with the tube in situ will demonstrate the tube located in the upper chest (see Figure 9.4). An abdominal radiograph is also required and if there are gas shadows in the abdomen it implies that there is a fistula between the lower oesophagus and the trachea. A gasless abdomen on the X-ray means that there is oesophageal atresia without a fistula.

Medical care

The infant is nursed with the head elevated to prevent aspiration of stomach contents through a fistula, and kept nil by mouth. A Replogle tube is inserted into the upper pouch and connected to gentle suction. Antibiotics are commenced as well as intravenous fluids.

A thorough clinical examination is performed in order to rule out associated congenital abnormalities. Echocardiography is essential to establish the presence of heart defects and also the site of aortic arch prior to surgery. Renal ultrasound scan and spinal X-rays need to be performed at some stage.

Surgery

Once the infant is stable, repair of the oesophageal atresia and tracheo-oesophageal fistula is performed through a right thoracotomy. In oesophageal atresia without fistula the gap between the two ends of the oesophagus may be too wide to anastomose immediately and therefore a gastrostomy is inserted for feeding, with a delayed anastomosis performed 8–10 weeks later. During this period the infant remains in the neonatal unit and assessment with X-rays is performed periodically. During the period the infant remains on the neonatal unit, the Replogle tube is vital in preventing aspiration of oral secretions while the infant is growing. The neonatal nurse will be required to ensure this tube remains in situ and patent with regular flushes with normal saline. These infants are not given the opportunity to suck feeds and the association of sucking and swallowing with the introduction of food to the stomach will be compromised. The use of a dummy during gastric feeds is therefore important. If the gap remains too wide then the infant will need an oesophageal replacement a few months later.

Post-operative care

Post-operatively the infant remains nil by mouth with intravenous fluids and antibiotics. Often these infants are ventilated for a few days postoperatively, depending on the degree of tension at the anastomosis. Adequate pain relief and the use of paralysing drugs during the period of ventilation are vital in ensuring the infant does not become distressed and agitated, which may put undue tension on the healing anastomosis. It is important to keep the neck in a flexed position to prevent excessive pressure on the surgical anastomosis. Trans-anastomotic tube feeding (a nasogastric tube which is passed at the time of the surgery down the oesophagus and into the stomach) commences 3–5 days post-operatively and some surgeons obtain a contrast study to check the anastomosis at day six. If this is normal, showing no leak, oral feeding will commence and be built up gradually.

It is important to keep the trans-anastomotic nasogastric tube in situ in these infants as it is the only access to the stomach and if it does come out it would be very difficult to reinsert it due to the danger of perforating the anastomosis. The tube should be clearly marked TAT and the infants will have mittens on their hands to prevent them pulling the tube out.

Prognosis

The long-term prognosis of these infants is usually good if there are not other serious congenital abnormalities, although gastro-oesophageal reflux is common and some of them will need surgical intervention such as oesophageal dilatation. Some infants will also have problems with disordered oesophageal peristalsis which can make feeding particularly challenging.

Implications for practice

- Pre-op: infants with oesophageal atresia should be nursed head up, with a Replogle tube on low suction.
- Post-op: the infant should initially be nursed with the neck slightly flexed and measures should be in place to prevent accidental removal of the trans-anastomotic tube by the infant or staff

Congenital diaphragmatic hernia

Congenital diaphragmatic hernia is the term used to describe herniation of the abdominal contents into the chest and it has the major complication of restricting lung growth on that side. During embryological development the thoracic and abdominal cavities are one cavity until the development of the diaphragm and closure of the pleuro-peritoneal membrane at eight weeks gestation. The defect is much more likely to occur on the left side through a posterior lateral defect (known as the foramen of Bochladek). Less commonly the defect can be central (Morgagni hernia) or bilateral. Lung hypoplasia and pulmonary hypertension are the common factors which determine the prognosis of these infants.

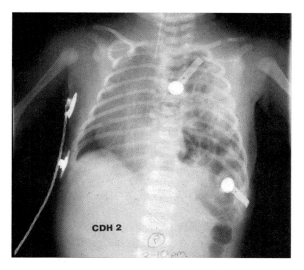

Figure 9.5 A CXR showing a left-sided congenital diaphragmatic hernia with gas filled bowel.

Clinical features

CDH is often diagnosed antenatally as early as 12–16 weeks gestation. If not diagnosed antenatally some infants will present with profound respiratory distress (gasping, tachypnoea and cyanosis) post-natally that causes a rapid clinical deterioration. The presence of a scaphoid abdomen, displaced heart sounds and reduced breath sounds on the left may alert the resuscitation team to the potential diagnosis. The presence of the bowel and the stomach in the chest cavity, which will expand with air, as a result of the infant gasping to breathe, or, because of bag and mask ventilation, will compromise the position of the mediastinum and the function of the contralateral lung. With prolonged resuscitation using bag and mask the chest may take on a barrelled appearance as the stomach and bowel within the chest are distended with air. Chest X-ray will confirm the presence of a gas filled stomach and bowel loops in the chest cavity.

Eighty five percent are left diaphragmatic hernias and almost 15% are right diaphragmatic. In less than 1% it is bilateral (see Figure 9.5).

Medical care

If the diagnosis has been made antenatally the delivery should be planned to occur in a tertiary level neonatal unit with access to neonatal surgery. The neonatal team should be available in the delivery suite. Following delivery, which may be vaginal unless obstetric issues have occurred, the infant should be immediately sedated and paralysed, and intubated and ventilated. The sedation and paralysis which may be administered by the intramuscular route for speed of administration, is to prevent the infant from dilating the stomach during spontaneous breathing or by swallowing air. The intubation and ventilation is to ensure that the lungs are expanded without inflating the stomach which would happen if IPPV with a bag and mask were to be performed. Minimising the air flow into the gastrointestinal tract in these ways will prevent dilatation of the gastrointestinal tract occupying the chest and maximise the available lung expansion. A large bore nasogastric tube should also be passed at the time of delivery to further decompress the stomach. An IV cannula should be sited to commence fluid infusions and antibiotics.

It is important to appreciate that CDH is a major physiological challenge to the infant. Ventilation requirements may include standard ventilation, high frequency oscillation, surfactant therapy and nitric oxide inhalation. Extracorporeal membrane oxygenation (ECMO) is only very rarely indicated as the pulmonary hypertension in CDH is usually secondary to pulmonary hypoplasia, which is *not* reversible (one of the criteria for starting ECMO). Following delivery, infants with CDH may show signs of persistent pulmonary hypertension of the newborn (PPHN) and the pre-operative stabilisation aims are to facilitate a reduction in the right to left shunting of blood at both ductal and atrial levels, thus improving oxygenation to the tissues. The infants will require continuation of the paralysis and sedation given at the time of delivery and should be nursed in a quiet environment to reduce stress and distress.

It is important to search for associated congenital abnormalities such as neural tube defects, chromosomal and cardiac defects (e.g. trisomy 18).

Surgery

Once the infant is stable, repair of the diaphragmatic hernia is performed through an abdominal approach. The viscera and solid organs are returned to the abdominal cavity and the defect in the diaphragm is closed with sutures if it is small or a patch if large.

Post-operative care and long-term prognosis

The PPHN may persist in the post-operative period since the infants will always have a degree of pulmonary hypoplasia. They will often be ventilated for a period until their pulmonary hypertension settles down and they are able to gas exchange adequately. Frequently they may have an initial period of relative stability (honeymoon period) followed by an exacerbation of the PPHN. Fluid losses into the chest cavity to occupy the space previously occupied by the bowel may further increase the mediastinal shift. Allowing time for reabsorption of this fluid rather than removing it by insertion of chest drains is recommended. In spite of all the new advances in management the mortality remains up to 50% and the outcome generally depends on the degree of pulmonary hypoplasia, the pulmonary hypertension and the associated abnormalities. The prognosis is also known to be worse when the CDH is on the right side and when the liver has herniated into the chest.

The general long-term prognosis of the surviving infants is good although there is an increase in respiratory and gastrointestinal morbidity[23].

Implications for practice

The extent of the pulmonary hypoplasia in CDH is what determines prognosis.

Current theories of acute management suggest that bag and mask ventilation should be avoided at the time of delivery and immediate intubation, sedation and paralysis and the insertion of a wide-bore nasogastric tube are a priority

Malrotation and volvulus

Malrotation is a congenital abnormality where there is abnormal fixation of the small and large bowel and the presence of bands (Ladd's bands) crossing over and obstructing the duodenum. During foetal life the gut initially develops as a straight tube and it moves out of the embryo and into the base of the cord at about six weeks. It then undergoes a 270° counterclockwise rotation before returning to the embryo and fixing in its anatomical position at about 12 weeks. If there is any problem with this important embryological stage the infant's gastrointestinal tract will be malrotated and not rigidly fixed in position by peritoneum. As a result it is susceptible to constriction by Ladd's bands and volvulus and if the blood supply becomes compromised during this process part of the bowel will become ischaemic.

Clinical features

The infant may be clinically well but if part of the bowel is obstructed by Ladd's bands there will be symptoms of poor feeding and bilious vomiting. If a volvulus has occurred the infant will be shocked, with anaemia, hypotension and metabolic acidosis. Abdominal examination will reveal a tender abdomen, which may also be distended, and the infant may pass bloody stools.

Diagnosis is established with an upper gastrointestinal contrast study, which will show the abnormal position of the bowel. In some centres abdominal ultrasound scan can be used to diagnose the condition.

Medical care

A diagnosis of volvulus is one of the indications for immediate surgery and there is no role for medical management aside from acute ventilatory and fluid resuscitation.

Surgery

Once the diagnosis of a malrotation is established laparotomy is performed urgently in view of the possible risk of volvulus and loss of bowel. At laparotomy the Ladd's bands will be divided and the bowel dissected in order to widen the small bowel mesentery and reduce the risk of future volvulus. Evaluation for the presence of necrotic bowel may result in resection at the time of the initial surgery, or further surgery 24–48 hours later to re-evaluate for recovery once the blood supply has been restored.

Post-operative care

Post-operatively the infant is kept nil by mouth with free drainage of the nasogastric tube. The NG losses are replaced and intravenous feeding is commenced until the infant is ready to feed enterally.

Prognosis

Long-term prognosis is good unless there has been a major loss of bowel due to volvulus and gangrene.

Implications for practice

Bile stained vomiting is an abnormal occurrence in the newborn infant, which always requires investigation and management.

Anorectal malformation

This is a common congenital abnormality whereby the anal opening is either absent or located in an anterior position, in females close to the vagina. It is therefore important to thoroughly examine the perineum of all infants after delivery. See Figure 9.6. There is a wide spectrum of abnormalities as shown in Table 9.2.

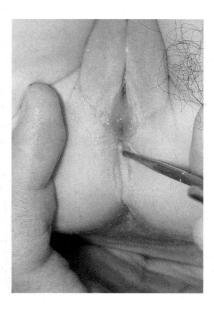

Figure 9.6 An anterior anus in a female infant.

Table 9.2 Spectrum of anorectal malformation.

Males	Females
Anal stenosis	Anal stenosis
Covered anus	Covered anus
Anterior anus	Anterior anus
Recto-urethral bulbar fistula	Vestibular anus
Recto-urethral prostatic fistula	Recto-vaginal fistula
Recto-bladder neck fistula	Cloacal malformation
Anal atresia	Anal atresia

Clinical features

It is important to conduct a full clinical examination in infants with anorectal malformation, due to the presence of other anomalies, e.g. the VACTERL associations. In particular renal abnormalities are common in these infants, e.g. vesicoureteric reflux, renal dysplasia, absent kidney and horseshoe kidney.

Medical care

These infants are generally well at the time of presentation and the initial stabilisation will involve ensuring all pre-operative investigations are performed, and IV cannulation for administration of fluids. This condition is often a postnatal diagnosis and pre-operative counselling of the parents is therefore crucial.

Surgery

Management depends on the type of abnormality. The low anorectal malformation (anal stenosis, covered anus and anterior anus) requires a simple repair which is performed in the neonatal period without colostomy. In intermediate and high anorectal malformation a staged repair is performed with a colostomy in the first instance followed by definitive repair and closure of colostomy in the future. The parents of an infant with a colostomy will need support and guidance to care for their infant, which may initially be provided by the neonatal nurses and later by the stoma care and neonatal community teams.

Post-operative care and long-term prognosis

The prognosis depends upon the level of abnormality associated with the presence of other congenital malformations.

Implications for practice

Renal and other conditions are commonly associated with anorectal anomalies; screening for these should be commenced in the pre-operative period.

Conclusion

The general principles of care for the infant who requires surgery for whatever condition are as for the care of any sick infant. Newborn infants may not tolerate changes in their physiological condition due to the surgical condition and can very quickly become compromised by these changes. Meticulous attention to stabilisation of the infant's condition prior to surgery will facilitate their tolerance of the procedures performed. Neonatal surgery requires a coordinated approach from all personnel involved in the procedure – surgeons, anaesthetists, neonatal staff and parents. Consideration of temperature control to, from and in theatre, and consideration of pain relief prior to leaving theatre are just two of the essential considerations to be made. By working as a coordinating team the tolerance of the procedure, together with the surgical outcome, for the infant may be enhanced.

References

1. Roberton RS, Rennie JM (eds) (1999) *Textbook of Neonatology*. Churchill Livingstone, New York.
2. Fisher R, Attah A, Partington A, Dykes E (1996) Impact of antenatal diagnosis on incidence and prognosis in abdominal wall defects. *J Pediatr Surg*, **31** (4), 538–541.

3. Farrell MF, Frost C (1992) The most important needs of parents of critically ill children: parents' perceptions. *Intensive Crit Care Nurs*, 8 (3), 130–139.

4. Parker LA (1995) Necrotizing enterocolitis. *Neonatal Netw*, 14 (6), 17–26.

5. Holman RC, Stoll BJ, Curns AT, Yorita KL (2006) Necrotising enterocolitis hospitalisations among neonates in the United States. *Paediatr Perinat Epidemiol*, 20 (6), 498–506.

6. Caplan MS, Jilling T (2001) New concepts in necrotizing enterocolitis. *Curr Opin Pediatr*, 13 (2), 111–115.

7. van de Bor M, Verloove-Vanhorick SP, Brand R (1988) Patent ductus arteriosus in a cohort of 1338 preterm infants: a collaborative study. *Paediatr Perinat Epidemiol*, 2 (4), 328–336.

8. Fujii AM , Brown E, Mirochnick M, O'Brien G (2002) Neonatal necrotizing enterocolitis with intestinal perforation in extremely premature infants receiving early indomethacin treatment for patent ductus arteriosus. *J Perinatol*, 22 (7), 535–540.

9. Fasoli L, Turi RA, Spitz L, Kiely EM, Drake D (1999) Necrotizing enterocolitis: extent of disease and surgical treatment. *J Pediatr Surg*, 34 (7), 1096–1099.

10. Patole SK, de Klerk N (2005) Impact of standardised feeding regimens on incidence of neonatal necrotising enterocolitis: a systematic review and meta-analysis of observational studies. *Arch Dis Child Foetal Neonatal Ed*, 90 (2), F147–151.

11. Premji SS (2005) Standardised feeding regimens: hope for reducing the risk of necrotising enterocolitis. *Arch Dis Child Foetal Neonatal Ed*, 90 (3), F192–F193.

12. Henderson G, Craig S, Brocklehurst P, McGuire W (2007) Enteral feeding regimens and necrotising enterocolitis in preterm infants: multicentre case-control study. *Arch Dis Child Foetal Neonatal Ed*, 92, F236–F238.

13. Basaran UN, Celayir S, Eray N, Ozturk R, Senyuz OF (1998) The effect of an H2-receptor antagonist on small-bowel colonization and bacterial translocation in newborn rats. *Pediatr Surg Int*, 13 (2–3), 118–120.

14. Wilson R, Del Portillo M, Schmidt E, Feldman RA (1982) Age at onset of necrotizing enterocolitis. Risk factors in small infants. *Am J Dis Child*, 136 (9), 814–816.

15. Walsh MC, Kliegman RM (1986) Necrotizing enterocolitis: treatment based on staging criteria. *Pediatr Clin North Am*, 33 (1), 179–201.

16. Grosfeld JL, Weber TR (1982) Congenital abdominal wall defects: gastroschisis and omphalocele. *Curr Probl Surg*, 19 (4), 157–213.

17. Alvarez SM, Burd RS (2007) Increasing prevalence of gastroschisis repairs in the United States: 1996–2003. *J Pediatr Surg*, 42 (6), 943–946.

18. Keys C, Drewett M, Burge DM (2008) Gastroschisis: the cost of an epidemic. *J Pediatr Surg*, 43 (4), 654–657.

19. Grosfeld JL, Weber TR (1982) Congenital abdominal wall defects: gastroschisis and omphalocele. *Curr Probl Surg*, 19 (4), 157–213.

20. Clark DA (1977) Times of first void and first stool in 500 newborns. *Pediatrics*, 60 (4), 457–459.

21. Ogala WN, Amiebenomo CS (1986) The time of passage of the first urine and stool by Nigerian neonates. *Trop Geogr Med*, 38 (4), 415–417.

22. Chih TW, Teng RJ, Wang CS, Kit Y(1991) Time of the first urine and the first stool in Chinese newborns. *Zhonghua Min Guo Xiao Er Ke Yi Xue Hui Za Zhi*, 32 (1), 17–23.

23. Adzick NS, Filly RA, Stringer MD, Harrison MR (1985) Diaphragmatic hernia in the foetus: prenatal diagnosis and outcome in 94 cases. *J Pediatr Surg*, 20 (4), 357–361.

Chapter 10
CONGENITAL CONDITIONS

Mandy Barry

Learning outcomes

After reading this chapter the reader will be expected to be able to:

- Recognise that basic genetic knowledge is essential for all health professionals and especially those involved in the care of neonates[1,2]

- Discuss the difference between congenital and genetic conditions

- Explain basic genetic terminology

- Describe some of the more common chromosome aneuploidies

- Distinguish different patterns of Mendelian inheritance

- Discuss the role of the genetic service and the aims of genetic counselling

---

Introduction

This chapter will give an overview of genetic principles in relation to conditions which may be encountered in neonatal nursing practice. Case studies of common genetic conditions will be used to illustrate the implications for practice from both the clinical genetic and neonatal nursing perspective. The role of the clinical genetic service in the management of the neonate, parental counselling and prenatal diagnosis will also be discussed. Finally, the limitations of current genetic testing methods will be considered in relation to both diagnostic and screening tests.

Congenital and/or genetic conditions

A congenital condition is one that is present at birth. In some cases the condition, whilst congenital in origin, is not recognised until the individual is older (e.g. some renal conditions, heart conditions and deafness). Congenital conditions can result from single gene mutation (alteration, like a misprint), chromosome anomalies (alterations in number or structure), the intra or extra-uterine environment or as a result of multiple different factors. They can be inherited or acquired at the point of gametogenesis, fertilisation or during foetal development. The cause of a considerable number of congenital disorders remains unknown and their effects can be relatively minor through to very severe, in some cases being incompatible with life. Some congenital conditions occur spontaneously, that is purely by chance. The challenge is to determine if the condition is one that having occurred spontaneously can be inherited in future generations or whether the condition is *sporadic* (occurs by chance) and thus the risk of recurrence is small.

A *genetic condition* is a disorder which can be passed from one generation to another. Many genetic conditions are inherited according to the mechanisms described by Gregor Mendel in 1866 (Mendelian inheritance). In some cases, however, the genetic alteration occurs for the first time in the individual who has the condition. This is known as a *de novo* (new) event; once the change has occurred in this way it can be passed on in future generations. Asking questions about family history in order to record the family tree (*pedigree*) can help to establish the way in which a condition is inherited.

Implications for practice

All genetic conditions are congenital but not all congenital conditions are genetic.

The dysmorphic infant

Dysmorphology is defined as 'the branch of clinical genetics that specialises in birth defects and combines knowledge of genetic principles, developmental mechanisms and the natural history of a wide variety of congenital abnormalities'[3].

When an infant is examined the clinician looks for and notes any physical features which are unusual for the child's age, sex or ethnic background. However, dysmorphology relates to internal as well as external structural features. Consideration of all such features can inform diagnosis of the condition as a result of recognition of the association of features (*syndromes, sequences and associations*). For instance, if an infant has a cardiac defect such as atrial septal or ventriculo septal defect, and also has a cleft palate and hypocalcaemia, this is suggestive of a chromosome abnormality (22q11 deletion syndrome).

Consideration of family history is also important. For instance, an infant may present with severe respiratory problems and hypotonia. When talking to the parents the clinician notices

that the mother has a paucity of facial movements. This might be as a result of undiagnosed myotonic dystrophy (MD) in the mother, which has been inherited by the child in severe congenital form (see case study 5).

The family pedigree

Drawing a pedigree of at least three generations is an invaluable tool to aid understanding of the family situation. It will help to determine whether a condition is inherited or not and if so will help with determining the mode of inheritance. This information can then be used to provide more accurate evaluation of risk to the nuclear family and other blood relatives (see Figure 10.1).

Basic principles of genetics

Our bodies are made up of billions of cells. Within the nucleus of our cells are found the rod like structures known as *chromosomes*. Human beings usually have 46 chromosomes (23 pairs) in each cell. We inherit one of each chromosome pair from our mother and the other from our father. We have 22 pairs of *autosomes* which are the chromosomes which are alike in both males and females and one pair of *sex* chromosomes. A female (XX) has two X chromosomes one inherited from her mother and one from her father. A male (XY) has an X chromosome inherited from his mother and a Y chromosome inherited from his father which makes him male. The full set of chromosomes which an individual has is known as their *karyotype* (see later section for further discussion of karyotype).

Located on the chromosomes are the 25,000 or so *genes*, which are the units of genetic information that make us what we are. This is how we inherit characteristics from our parents. In general, our genes also come in pairs and we inherit one copy from our father and one from our mother. These gene copies are known as *alleles* and the *genotype* refers to the full set

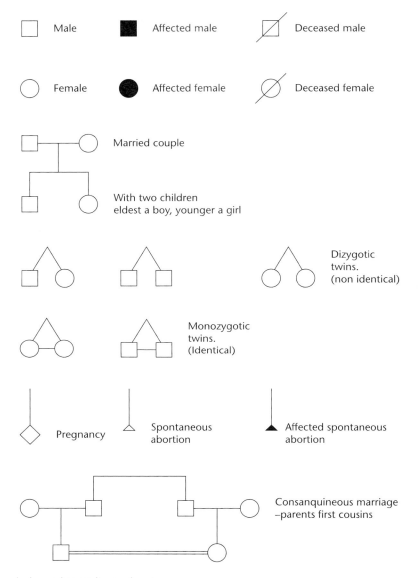

Figure 10.1 Symbols used in pedigree drawing.

of alleles which a person has – their genetic blueprint. Another important concept is that of *phenotype* which refers to the identifiable features which relate to a specific genotype. For instance a child with Down syndrome has an extra copy of chromosome 21 and thus an extra copy of all the genes packed onto that chromosome. The phenotype which results is recognisable by observable *dysmorphic* features such as upslanting palprebral fissures, protruding tongue, single palmar crease, etc. Other phenotypic features are less obvious at birth, for instance developmental delay and the increased risk of childhood leukaemia.

Genetic conditions may occur as a result of:

- Chromosomal anomalies
- Mutations in the DNA of single genes

We can think of all our genetic material as being the information contained in a large book. The chromosomes are the various chapters within the book. Some chapters are large and others small; however, each contains essential information for the book to be fully understood and interpreted. Within the chapters are the paragraphs which can be likened to our genes. Each paragraph may be short or long but will contain specific information in each of the sentences (the different sections of the gene). Any alterations to the book, for instance the loss of a chapter, a paragraph, a sentence or indeed the loss of or change of a single letter can result in the information being misinterpreted. Genetic conditions ar the result of such alterations.

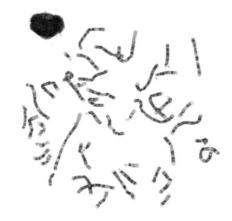

Figure 10.2   Metaphase spread.

- Multifactorial conditions – changes in multiple genes +/− environment
- Mitochondrial gene mutations
- Mosaicism

Chromosome abnormalities and karyotyping

The human chromosome set (karyotype) contained in a cell can be visualised using a microscope after appropriate preparation. The chromosome spread seen at the period of cell division (mitosis) known as *metaphase* can then be analysed by the cytogeneticist (see Figure 10.2). The chromosomes can be sorted and numbered according to size. In this way the cytogeneticist is able to determine that the correct number of chromosomes is present. Each chromosome has a short arm known as the 'p' arm and a long arm known as the 'q' arm. Between the p and q arms is the centromere which is the constricted area of the chromosome. Identification of any additional, missing or altered chromosomes is facilitated by the 'banding' pattern which is apparent as a result of the staining method used in cell preparation (see, for example, Figure 10.3). Any loss or gain of chromosome material will be expected to have a phenotypic effect.

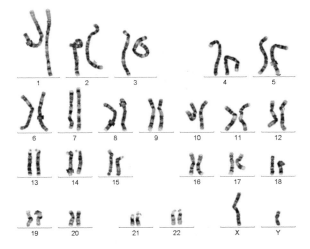

Figure 10.3   G banded karyotype.

The cytogeneticist will use an internationally agreed standard form of nomenclature to report the karyotype. For instance a normal female karyotype will be reported as 46, XX (the number of chromosomes counted and the type of sex chromosomes identified).

Aneuploidy

Aneuploidy refers to an alteration in the number of whole chromosomes which can occur as a result of errors of cell division. Any alteration in the number of whole chromosomes will have a phenotypic effect. In most cases this will be incompatible with life and result in spontaneous abortion. However, the following aneuploidies are viable:

- Down syndrome – trisomy 21 (47, XX, +21 or 47, XY +21)
- Edwards' syndrome – trisomy 18 (47, XX, +18 or 47, XY +18)
- Patau syndrome – trisomy 13 (47, XX, +13 or 47, XY +13)
- Sex chromosome aneuploidies such as Turner's syndrome (45,XO), Klinefelter's syndrome (47, XXY), Triple X syndrome (47, XXX) and XYY male (47, XYY)

Trisomy 21 (Down syndrome)

This is the most common viable chromosome aneuploidy, occurring in about 1 in 650 live births[4]. Advancing maternal age is known to increase the risk of trisomy 21 although many such pregnancies abort spontaneously. The majority of Down syndrome babies have an extra copy of chromosome 21, which occurs as a result of an error of cell division.

Affected babies have a characteristic phenotype which includes hypotonia, upslanting palpebral fissures, epicanthic folds, protruding tongue, flat nasal bridge, low set ears, short neck with loose neck skin, single transverse palmar crease and a sandal gap between the first and second toes. There is also an increased incidence of other abnormalities such as congenital heart disease (30%), tracheo-oesophageal fistula and duodenal atresia. The diagnosis may therefore be made prior to confirmation by karyotyping. However, it is also possible for Down syndrome to result from a chromosome translocation (discussed in the section on chromosome alterations). It is therefore important that the child's chromosomes are analysed as the risk of recurrence is high if the condition has occurred as a result of an inherited translocation.

Case study 1

Jennifer was born following a normal vaginal delivery at 38 weeks gestation with good Apgar scores. The midwife who examined Jennifer immediately following delivery noted that she appeared rather hypotonic, had a protruding tongue and other characteristics which suggested Down syndrome. The paediatrician who examined Jennifer also noted a cardiac murmur which required further investigation. Jennifer was therefore transferred to the neonatal unit.

Clinical genetic implications

It is important to establish the type of Down syndrome. A blood sample was therefore taken for urgent karyotyping, the result of which showed that Jennifer had trisomy 21. She therefore had 47 chromosomes with an extra copy of chromosome 21. This is written scientifically as 47, XX, +21. Having established this result the geneticist would know that the parents' risk of having another child with Down syndrome was in the region of 1%, although the actual risk would be further informed by the age of the mother. If Jennifer's Down syndrome had been a result of a chromosome translocation the recurrence risk would have been much higher and would be determined by the type of translocation and be dependent on which parent was the carrier of the translocation.

Implications for practice

A senior paediatrician should meet with the parents to discuss the implications of a diagnosis of trisomy 21. This verbal communication should be backed up by written information.

The karyotype should be sent marked urgent and this usually means that a provisional result will be available in 48 hours.

These infants do not require routine admission to the neonatal unit but they often require feeding support in view of the hypotonia and require assessment for congenital heart disease (clinical assessment with ECG, oxygen saturations and echocardiogram (urgent if ECG shows a superior axis)).

Additional acute problems are polycythaemia and jaundice, which should be evaluated.

Trisomy 18 (Edwards' syndrome)

Trisomy 18 occurs in about 1 in 7500 live births[5], although the incidence at conception is much higher as over 90% of trisomy 18 conceptions are aborted spontaneously. Maternal age (over 35) is known to be a factor.

Affected babies have a characteristic phenotype which includes intrauterine growth retardation, failure to thrive, hypotonia, receding jaw, low set ears, short sternum, clenched fists with the second and fifth fingers overlapping the third and fourth and rocker bottom feet. Prognosis is poor, with 90% of affected babies dying within a few months of birth.

Case study 2

David was born at 37 weeks gestation after labour was induced because of the obstetrician's concerns relating to intrauterine growth retardation. His birthweight was 2200 g. On examination he was noted to have many of the features outlined above and a clinical diagnosis of Edwards' syndrome was made. This was later confirmed as David was shown to have an abnormal male karyotype with an extra copy of chromosome 18 (written scientifically as 47, XY, +18)

Clinical genetic implications

The parents will wish to understand the cause of David's condition and the chance of recurrence in a future pregnancy. However, the most important aspect of their care immediately following David's diagnosis will be his prognosis and care. Whilst input from the genetic service may be required, at this point David's management will be the responsibility of the neonatal team.

Implications for practice

A lead consultant and neonatal nurse should meet with the parents to discuss the future plan of care for David. It is important that a detailed clinical assessment is done to identify the associated medical conditions that will guide his prognosis. This can raise some ethical dilemmas regarding treatment but it is important that his parents have quality time with him and that all management decisions are taken with his interests at heart. It may be possible for him to be discharged home with supportive (palliative) care to be provided at home.
Clear plan of care
Quality time for David and his parents
Facilitating home care if parents wish

Trisomy 13 (Patau syndrome)

This only occurs in about 1 in 20,000 live births, as most trisomy 13 conceptions result in spontaneous abortion. Like the other trisomies maternal age is a risk factor but in general the recurrence risk is low provided karyotyping confirms it is due to trisomy 13 and not as a result of a chromosome translocation.

Affected babies have characteristic features which include intrauterine growth retardation, failure to thrive, microcephaly, microphthalmia, malformed ears and cleft lip/palate. Most affected babies will die within the first month of life.

Case study 3

Pam and her husband, Adam, knew that their baby daughter had trisomy 13 after an amniocentesis was performed, at their request, because of Pam's age (41). Once the result was known they were offered a termination of pregnancy but decided that this was not an option for them. Gemma was born normally at 37 weeks gestation. A sample of cord blood was taken which confirmed that she had an abnormal female karyotype with an extra copy of chromosome 13 (written scientifically as 47, XX, +13).

Clinical genetic implications

Following the amniocentesis result Pam and Adam had had a long discussion with the geneticist so that they understood the cause of Gemma's condition and the chance of recurrence in a future pregnancy. They were also fully aware of her prognosis and had had the opportunity to discuss their wishes in relation to her post-natal care with the paediatric team.

Implications for practice

This situation is similar to that of David (above) but the parents have had time to prepare for Gemma's birth. Parents sometimes find it difficult to accept results such as these until they see the infant at birth. Clinical staff should be sensitive to this but consistent in the information that they tell parents.

Other chromosome anomalies (rearrangements)

These anomalies include chromosome translocations, inversions, duplications, deletions, as well as mosaicism.

Translocations

There are two types of translocation (*Robertsonian* and *Reciprocal*) both of which can occur in a *balanced* form where there is no resultant loss or gain of chromosome material. Conversely, the rearrangement can result in loss or gain of chromosome material, in which case it is known as an *unbalanced* translocation. It is important to understand that loss or gain of chromosome material will usually have an adverse phenotypic effect.

Robertsonian translocations (see Figure 10.4)
This type of translocation is found in about 1 in 500 of the population. The rearrangement involves two of the *acrocentric* chromosomes (chromosomes 13, 14, 15, 21 and 22) which have their *centromere* very close to one end of the chromosome. Two acrocentric chromosomes join together with the loss of their very small p arms but since they do not carry unique genes there is no deleterious effect[6]. Chromosome analysis would therefore reveal a balanced karyotype with only 45 chromosomes since two had joined together. There is, however, a risk that in a pregnancy the balanced translocation in the parent can be inherited in an unbalanced form by the offspring. One example of this would be a Down syndrome baby who inherited a third copy of chromosome 21 as a result of a Robertsonian translocation between

chromosome 21 and another acrocentric chromosome, commonly chromosome 14.

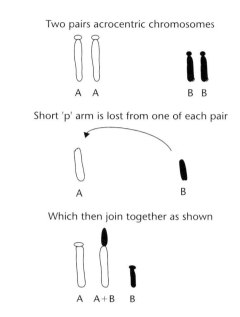

Figure 10.4 Robertsonian translocation.

Reciprocal translocations (see Figure 10.5)
This type of rearrangement occurs when two non-homologous chromosomes (different chromosomes, e.g. chromosome 1 and 6) break and exchange chromosome material. For instance an individual could have one normal copy of both chromosome 1 and 6, but the other copies have broken and become rearranged so that chromosome no.1 has lost some material which has become attached to chromosome no. 6. Conversely, chromosome no. 6 has lost some material (which has become attached to chromosome no. 1) and has gained some material from chromosome no. 1. Provided no chromosome material has been lost or gained this would be a balanced translocation. However, as with Robertsonian translocations there is a possibility that the rearrangement could be inherited in an unbalanced form, which could result in spontaneous abortion or a child with physical handicap and/or learning difficulties.

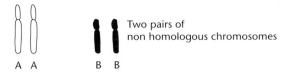

Two pairs of
non homologous chromosomes

A A   B B

The chromosomes break a exchange material

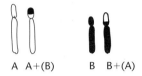

A A+(B)   B B+(A)

Figure 10.5 Reciprocal translocation.

Chromosome inversions

This occurs when a single chromosome breaks in two places and the broken piece rotates 180° before joining back up. There are two types: *pericentric* (where the chromosomes break with the centromere within the broken segment – see Figure 10.7) or *paracentric* (where the breaks occur in either the short or long arm of the chromosome and do not include the centromere – see Figure 10.6).

Chromosome deletions

This occurs when part of a chromosome is lost, with resultant phenotypic effect. Examples include 22q11 deletion, also known as Velocardiofacial and DiGeorge syndromes. In general, deletion of chromosome material is more deleterious than chromosome duplication.

Case Study 4

Penny and her husband, Tom, are very concerned when their baby daughter, Julie, is found to have a cleft palate and a heart murmur. Further investigations are initiated to determine the severity of her heart condition. The staff ask also for the parents' permission to take blood for calcium levels and also to look at Julie's chromosomes.

Clinical genetic implications

A geneticist may be asked to assess Julie, especially if she has other dysmorphic features which might suggest a syndrome. One possible diagnosis is 22q11 deletion (DiGeorge syndrome) which results from a deletion of a small part of one copy of chromosome 22. Phenotypic findings in babies with this deletion

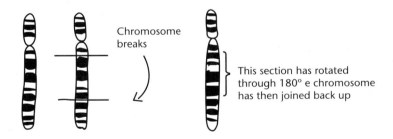

Chromosome breaks

This section has rotated through 180° e chromosome has then joined back up

Figure 10.6 Paracentric inversion.

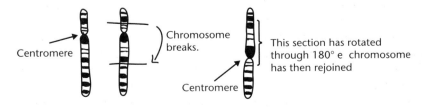

Centromere

Chromosome breaks.

Centromere

This section has rotated through 180° e chromosome has then rejoined

Figure 10.7 Pericentric inversion.

include significant heart problems such as tetral-ogy of Fallot, cleft palate (although this may not be immediately apparent as submucosal) and hypocalcaemia.

There are also implications for the baby's future health as the immune system can be affected in the early years. As the child grows, recognisable but subtle facial features are present. Growth retardation, delayed speech and learning difficul-ties are also common.

The genetic service will also offer to screen the parents to see if the deletion is a de novo event or if it has been inherited. If it is inher-ited, cascade screening for at risk relatives will be offered.

Implications for practice

The diagnosis of any congenital condition is obviously distressing and investigating for genetic conditions can stimulate feelings of guilt in the parents, which need to be handled sensi-tively by the clinical staff. It is obviously helpful if the neonatal staff understand the genetic tests that have been performed and their implica-tions so that they can support the work of the genetic team.

Chromosome duplications

This occurs when part of a chromosome is dupli-cated. For instance this may occur as a result of a chromosome translocation being inherited in an unbalanced form

Chromosome rings

This occurs when a chromosome breaks at both ends (the telomeres) and some chromosome material is lost, the 'sticky' ends of the remain-ing p and the q arms then fuse to form a ring. The ring chromosome so formed can disrupt mitosis (cell division).

Marker chromosomes

These are small additional pieces of chromosome material. Whilst the presence of a marker may be found during karyotyping, actually identifying

the origin of the marker is more problematic. Predicting the phenotypic effect is also difficult as some markers are familial and thus a nor-mal phenotype in a parent who also has the marker is reassuring. If the marker is de novo, special cytogenetic techniques such as FISH (Fluorescent In Situ Hybridisation – a chromo-some painting technique which uses fluorescent probes) may be required to identify the origin of the marker.

Mosaicism

Most chromosome rearrangements are appar-ent in all the cells of an affected individual. In mosaicism an individual has two or more differ-ent chromosome complements (cell lines). For instance some of the cells may have a normal karyotype whilst others only have one sex chro-mosome (Mosaic Turner's syndrome). Another example is Mosaic Down syndrome, where some cells have a normal karyotype and others have an extra chromosome 21. As with any ane-uploidy prenatal diagnosis should be offered in a future pregnancy.

There can also be evidence of mosaicism in other tissues, for instance in association with abnormal skin pigmentation. The blood karyo-type may be normal, and confirmed as such even when additional cells are analysed, because of the skin pigmentation. However, if a skin biopsy is performed a mosaic karyotype may be found in the skin cells. Such findings are relatively rare but require considerable input from experienced paediatricians, geneticists and laboratory staff to ensure realistic information is given to parents.

Implications for practice

The hardest concept for parents to understand when told of unbalanced chromosome rear-rangements as a result of any of the causes dis-cussed above is that it can be very difficult or even impossible to predict what the outcome will be for the child.

Single gene disorders

There are over 9000 known single gene conditions and more are being identified as knowledge increases as a result of the Human Genome Project and other research[7]. The conditions are individually rare but within an affected family the chance of recurrence is high. The risk can be predicted, as single gene disorders are inherited according to Mendelian mechanisms, which include the following:

- Autosomal dominant inheritance
- Autosomal recessive inheritance
- X-linked recessive inheritance
- Other modes of inheritance (de novo, mitochondrial, mosaicism)

Autosomal dominant inheritance

An affected individual has one normal copy of the gene responsible for the condition and one altered copy. The altered copy is different, as a mutation (like a misprint) has occurred when the DNA sequence of the gene was copied. This mutation results in the 'instructions' conveyed being faulty and consequent disruption of gene function and protein synthesis. Male and female children of an affected individual all have a 1 in 2 (50%) chance of inheriting the condition.

In Figure 10.8 it should be noted that:

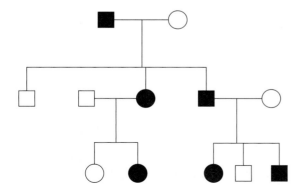

Figure 10.8   Consider the above pedigree.

- There are affected individuals in each generation
- The condition is passed by affected males or affected females to children of either sex
- On average males and females are affected in equal proportions
- On average one in two children of affected individuals inherit the condition (see Figure 10.9)

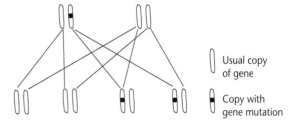

Usual copy of gene

Copy with gene mutation

1 in 2 (50%) chance in every pregnancy of affected offspring

Figure 10.9   Autosomal dominant inheritance.

Case Study 5

Danielle was born by normal delivery at 39 weeks. At birth the delivery staff were very surprised that whilst she had good Apgar scores she was very floppy. As she was experiencing considerable difficulty with respiration the paediatrician was called urgently. Danielle required significant ventilatory support before adequate oxygenation could be achieved.

Once Danielle had been stabilised, the consultant paediatrician spoke with her shocked parents Rebecca and Stephen. During the conversation he noted that Rebecca had a paucity of facial expression. When questioned about her family history Rebecca stated that her mother was alive and well and that her father had died shortly after her birth. The only other history of note was that she was aware of an uncle who had a muscle problem which required him to use a wheelchair.

Clinical genetic implications

A geneticist was asked to see Danielle and was also concerned about Rebecca's paucity of facial expression, especially when further examination revealed other evidence of muscle weakness. After full discussion with Rebecca and Stephen molecular analysis was requested and confirmed that both Rebecca and Danielle had myotonic dystrophy (MD).

MD is due to an expansion in the MD gene, resulting in a recognisable but variable clinical presentation. As the condition is dominant, any child of an affected individual will have a 1 in 2 (50%) chance of inheriting MD. If passed from mother to child the expansion is unstable and can enlarge further, resulting in the baby inheriting the severe congenital form of MD (CMD). This was the explanation for Danielle's floppiness and respiratory problems. If, like Rebecca, a mother has neuromuscular involvement the chance of a baby with CMD is 10–30%[8].

Follow-up genetic counselling will be offered to discuss the diagnosis, possible long-term complications, monitoring and prognosis in more detail. Risk of recurrence and possibility of prenatal diagnosis in a future pregnancy and implications for relatives will also be discussed.

Implications for practice
The parents will want to know why a genetic opinion might be helpful and the mother will require psychological support when she becomes aware of her own diagnosis and the fact that her daughter has inherited the condition from her. The parents will be trying to come to terms with Danielle's uncertain prognosis as well as the implications for future pregnancies.

Conditions which are inherited in this way include osteogenesis imperfecta, neurofibromatosis, tuberous sclerosis, achondroplasia, congenital myotonic dystrophy, as well as adult onset conditions such as Huntington's disease, myotonic dystrophy, familial cancer syndromes, adult polycystic kidney disease.

Autosomal recessive inheritance

An affected individual has two non-functioning copies of the gene responsible for the condition. Often there is no history of the condition in the family as it has been inherited from parents who are healthy carriers. Carriers are individuals who have one normal copy of the gene which is functional and one copy of the gene with a mutation which is non-functioning. They are healthy, as the functioning copy of the gene is producing enough of the gene product to maintain their health.

In Figure 10.10 it should be noted that:

- Affected individuals occur in a single generation only
- On average males and females are affected in equal proportions
- Siblings have a 1 in 4 risk of being affected (see Figure 10.11)
- Risk of recurrence in the extended family is low unless there is consanguinity, when the chance of parents carrying the same mutated gene is increased

Conditions which are inherited in this way include cystic fibrosis, sickle cell anaemia, beta thalassaemia major, spinal muscular atrophy, Tay Sachs disease, phenylketonuria, MCAD (medium chain acyl-CoA dehydrogenase deficiency) and many other metabolic conditions

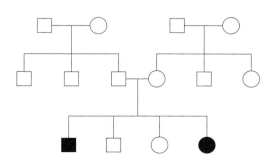

Figure 10.10 Consider the above pedigree.

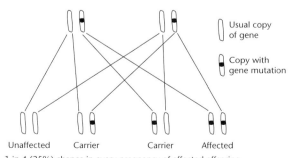

Unaffected   Carrier   Carrier   Affected
1 in 4 (25%) chance in every pregnancy of affected offspring

Usual copy of gene

Copy with gene mutation

Figure 10.11 Autosomal recessive inheritance.

Case Study 6

Fleur and Pierre were concerned when their baby was found to have an echogenic bowel during a routine antenatal scan. Soon after birth their daughter, Josie, was admitted to the neonatal unit in preparation for surgery after meconium ileus was diagnosed. Echogenic bowel is a common finding in antenatal scans; however, it is known that 3% of babies with hyperechogenic bowel will have cystic fibrosis (CF)[9]. Of those neonates who develop meconium ileus 10–20% will have CF [10].

Clinical genetic implications

Clinical genetic input will be most important once Josie has recovered from her surgery and there is confirmation of cause of meconium ileus. This will include risk of recurrence, possibility of prenatal diagnosis and the implications for the extended family.

Implications for practice

The parents will need to discuss the implications of Josie's diagnosis and possible causes with the clinician and senior neonatal nurse. They will need information regarding the procedure and completion of a sweat test to confirm or refute possible clinical diagnosis of CF. To appreciate why a sweat test is performed they will need to have an appreciation of the limitations of molecular analysis for CF.

Josie's parents would also benefit from the opportunity to contact other parents with a child with CF, ongoing support after discharge and help with coming to terms with ongoing treatment and the uncertain prognosis.

X-linked recessive inheritance

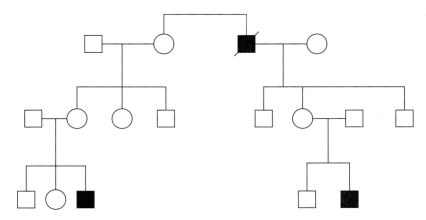

Figure 10.12 Consider the above pedigree.

In Figures 10.12 and 10.13 it should be noted that:

- Affected individuals are male
- All male children of affected males are unaffected
- All female children of affected males will be obligate carriers of the condition
- In some X-linked conditions the female carriers of the condition can be affected by the condition but their *phenotype* is generally milder

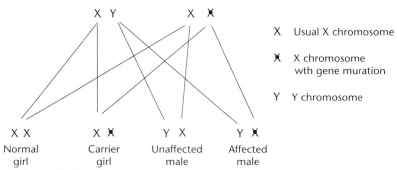

Figure 10.13   X-linked recessive inheritance.

Conditions which are inherited in this way include haemophilia, Duchenne muscular dystrophy, adrenoleucodystrophy, Alport syndrome, X-linked microcephaly, Menkes syndrome

Multifactorial conditions

Conditions such as those discussed in the previous two sections are the result of single gene mutations (*monogenic*) or chromosomal abnormalities and thus the risk of recurrence can be determined by consideration of the known modes of inheritance.

However, many other conditions are the result of the interaction of many genes (*polygenic*), the interaction of genes and environment, or environmentally based, so estimation of risk is more difficult. Examples of conditions resulting from the interaction of genes and environment include congenital heart disease, clefting, congenital dislocation of the hip and spina bifida (see Chapter 13) all of which can cluster in families but are also affected by the environment. Conditions which result from environmental factors include foetal alcohol syndrome, rubella and talipes. Other sporadic conditions can result from associated malformations; examples include tracheo-oesophageal fistula (TOF), CHARGE and VATER syndromes which are discussed in Chapter 8.

In order to give the parents an estimation of risk of recurrence the geneticist will base his/her answer on *empiric* data (that is data derived from observation and experience of comparable populations).

Mitochondrial gene alterations

Single gene disorders occur as a result of mutations in nuclear DNA. The cell cytoplasm also contains numerous organelles. One type of organelle, known as mitochondria, is concerned with energy transfer. There are numerous mitochondria in each cell, each of which contain mitochondrial DNA (mtDNA). It is possible that some mitochondria contain mutations in the mtDNA. Since the mitochondria are important in the body's energy systems, mutations can result in a severe phenotype. All organs with high demands for energy, such as skeletal and cardiac muscle, the central nervous system, liver and pancreas, are potentially affected.

Mitochondrial conditions are maternally inherited. Each ovum contains approximately 100,000 mitochondria[11]. Some of the mitochondria may have normal mtDNA whilst others have the mutant mtDNA. For this reason, prediction of the likely phenotype if the condition recurs is problematic, as the proportion of mutant mtDNA inherited can vary considerably.

Mosaicism

A new mutation for a single gene disorder can arise during gametogenesis (germline mosaicism). Neither parent has the disorder as their somatic cells are not involved and their karyotypes are normal. However, their off-spring can still be affected. This is why unaffected parents who have a child affected by a single gene disorder (autosomal dominant or X-linked) are offered prenatal diagnosis in a subsequent pregnancy as there may be a significant recurrence risk.

Genetic counselling

Genetic counselling is defined by the American Society of Human Genetics (1975) as:

'A communication process which deals with human problems associated with the occurrence, or the risk of occurrence, of a genetic disorder in a family. This process involves an attempt by one or more appropriately trained persons to help the individual or family to (1) Comprehend the medical facts, including the diagnosis, probable course of the disorder, and the available management; (2) appreciate the way heredity contributes to the disorder, and the risk of recurrence in specified relatives; (3) understand the alternatives for dealing with the risk of recurrence; (4) choose the course of action which seems to them appropriate in view of their risk, their family goals and their ethical and religious standards, and to act in accordance with that decision; and (5) make the best possible adjustment to the disorder in an affected family member and/or the risk of recurrence of that disorder[12]'.

Genetic professionals strive to ensure that the individuals with whom they come into contact are given full and up-to-date information in a non-directive and non-judgmental manner. Ethical dilemmas are regularly encountered during such interactions and resolution is considered by the whole genetic team on a case-by-case basis. The four biomedical principles: autonomy, non-maleficence, beneficence and justice are central to these discussions[13]. Ethical issues related to genetic counselling are outside the scope of this chapter but are considered in relation to neonatal nursing in Chapter 18.

Who provides genetic counselling?

Traditionally, genetic services are provided by specialist clinical and laboratory departments at tertiary level. Genetic counselling is provided by consultant geneticists, specialist registrars and genetic nurses/counsellors. Individuals or families affected by, or at risk of, genetic conditions are referred by other clinicians to discuss the implications of the condition and their options for the future. This might include discussion in relation to prenatal diagnosis, cascade screening or management of risk as a result of familial cancer.

Whilst there has always been a close working relationship with foetal medicine and neonatology, it is only in recent years that more joint clinics have evolved. Many centres have now also initiated joint clinics with foetal medicine, community paediatrics, ophthalmology, cardiology, neurology, renal services, etc.

Increasingly, health professionals from all disciplines are becoming aware of the relevance of genetics to their everyday practice. The Government White Paper, *Our Inheritance Our Future* (June 2003)[14] resulted in considerable investment in genetic services. Some of the investment was specifically aimed at developing models of care that would improve integration of genetics into everyday practice as well as promote a more multidisciplinary approach to patient care. Studies have identified the genetic competencies required by clinicians and nurses, midwives and health visitors in order to fulfil this extended role[15,16]. The establishment of the National Genetics Education Centre will further support these developments by addressing the training needs.

Why is genetic counselling important?

A basic understanding of genetics is essential for all those working in neonatal units. Parents with a sick child will want as much information as possible about their child's condition and prognosis. In particular, the information given could inform decisions relating to the management of the sick neonate. For instance, if a serious genetic condition is diagnosed and the child's prognosis is extremely poor the parents may value the opportunity to discuss with the clinical team involved if further active treatment would be appropriate. If it was agreed that active treatment should be withdrawn they could then spend precious time with their child without the hindrance of intravenous infusions, monitoring and ventilation equipment.

All readers will recognise the importance of working in partnership with parents, discussing their child's condition openly and honestly so that they have realistic expectations with regard to the outcome. This is often made more difficult because of the phenotypic variability found in some conditions or in those resulting from chromosomal anomalies.

Parents are also likely to want to know what the chances are of having another baby with the same condition and whether any tests can be offered in pregnancy. These tests may include detailed ultrasound scanning or specific prenatal diagnosis to facilitate karyotyping, single gene analysis or biochemical tests. Some couples may also like to investigate the possibility of *pre-implantation genetic diagnosis*. The risk of recurrence as a result of single gene conditions or inherited chromosome rearrangements is high. In other cases there is no clear pattern of inheritance and therefore the recurrence risk is calculated using *empiric* (experiential) data. Whatever the risk of recurrence couples are likely to need support as they consider their options and the seriousness of the condition before deciding to embark on another pregnancy.

Overview of embryological principles in relation to the genetic consultation

An overview of embryological principles is provided in Chapter 5 and this foundation is expanded on in subsequent chapters in relation to the specific subject matter. From a genetic perspective the nature of the congenital abnormality can provide insight into the timing, cause and recurrence risk of the condition.

Congenital abnormalities can result from many factors:

- Before conception: possible factors include environment, diet, exposure to teratogens or infection, pre-existing maternal conditions, sporadic events all of which could affect reproductive fitness and/or gametogenesis
- Single gene disorders either de novo or inherited
- Errors in cell division at, or immediately following, fertilisation can result in chromosome anomalies
- The intrauterine environment can be compromised by the formation of amniotic bands, exposure to teratogens, placental insufficiency, infection and oligohydramnios
- Foetal malpresentation during labour, hypoxia and infection can all result in the birth of an ill neonate

The clinician will consider the possible causes of an abnormality in relation to when the adverse event may have occurred and determine if it could be the result of:

- Malformation: this occurs when a normal embryological developmental process does not occur and thus an abnormality results, e.g. anencephaly
- Deformation: this occurs when a normal development process is distorted in some way, for instance as a result of restriction of foetal movement in relation to oligohydramnios
- Disruption: this occurs when a normal developmental process is interrupted, for instance amputation of part of a normally developing limb as a result of amniotic bands

Screening to predict or prevent congenital conditions

Screening can be undertaken as part of a general public health programme for instance screening for cervical cancer, or as part of the care offered to an individual as a result of a specific episode of care such as that related to pregnancy. This would include the mainstream antenatal screening discussed in Chapter 2.

In families where there is a known genetic condition it may be possible to screen the foetus for the condition. However, this is better described as prenatal diagnosis as the test is offered so that the parent can consider their options if the child they are expecting is predicted to be affected by the genetic condition. Genetic tests carried out after birth (other than those undertaken as part of the neonatal screening programme) are also often described as screening but again they would be better viewed as diagnostic tests.

Neonatal screening programme

In recent years the availability of screening tests in the neonatal period has increased and this trend is likely to continue. However, it remains essential to ensure that any screening test adopted fulfils the widely agreed essential criteria for such tests[17]. These are that the test should be for an important health problem which will benefit from early treatment, easy to perform and interpret, acceptable, accurate, reliable, sensitive, specific and cost effective.

The neonatal screening programme currently screens for phenylketonuria (PKU), hypothyroidism, haemoglobin disorders (sickle cell and thalassaemia), cystic fibrosis and in some areas MCAD (medium chain acyl-CoA dehydrogenase deficiency). Each of these conditions fulfils the criteria outlined above. For instance, normal development can be achieved with appropriate treatment for PKU or hypothyroidism and a child with CF benefits from early physiotherapy. Also, the parents of a child known to have MCAD are made aware of the importance of avoiding hypoglycaemia, thereby reducing the risk of sudden death. And finally, a child with a sickle cell disorder benefits from prophylactic antibiotics to help avoid infections which may precipitate sickle cell crisis.

Neonatal nurses need to be aware that there may be reasons why this screening needs to be repeated in the ill neonate. For example, the PKU test requires feeding to be established when it is taken. Blood transfusions can also negate the results obtained, e.g. when screening for the haemoglobin disorders.

Screening for these conditions may also identify some neonates who are carriers of the condition. This is true for sickle cell and cystic fibrosis. This has implications for their parents as it is possible that they are both carriers of these recessively inherited conditions and are therefore at risk of having an affected child in a future pregnancy.

Limitations of genetic testing

Testing for single gene disorders is only feasible after full clinical assessment of the individual and the identification of the possible differential diagnoses. Tests for specific conditions can then be requested. Whilst the number of genetic tests which can be offered is increasing, there remain many conditions for which testing is not yet possible or is technically difficult. Even if a test is available, it should be noted that current techniques do not generally allow us to rule out a diagnosis entirely.

For instance, in cystic fibrosis (CF) there are over 1000 known gene mutations, many of which may be unique within a family. It is not feasible to test for all such mutations. Consequently, when individuals are tested to see if they are carriers for the condition the most common 29–30 mutations are looked for as they actually account for 90% of the known mutations. In this way an individual's risk of being a CF carrier can be reduced but not ruled out entirely.

If a child is thought to have CF but only one mutation has been found the diagnosis can be confirmed clinically by means of a sweat test. Once the diagnosis is confirmed further mutation analysis will be requested in a specialist laboratory to try to identify the second mutation.

Identification of a rare CF mutation may take many months or years and in some instances, may be elusive, until new techniques are available.

In order for prenatal diagnosis for a single gene disorder to be offered the gene mutation must have been identified in a family. However, in some conditions it may still be difficult to interpret the result obtained because of the possibility of instability in the mutation or variation in phenotype (see Case study 5).

Implications for practice

A normal karyotype does not necessarily mean that the chromosomes are normal in structure – small deletions may be difficult to see on standard karyotype screening.

In some diseases such as cystic fibrosis (CF) large numbers of mutations have been identified. In any screening programme only the most common mutations can be tested for. It is therefore possible for a person to have CF despite no mutations for CF being identified by the genetic screening tests.

Management of a neonate with congenital abnormality

The information above has focused on specific conditions and modes of inheritance. But an accurate diagnosis can only be reached if the newborn with congenital abnormalities is fully assessed. This assessment should include consideration of all systems and a thorough head-to-toe examination. But when a neonate is extremely ill the plethora of tubes, treatment in progress, etc. can make it very difficult for any clinician to achieve this ideal. So often, very subtle clues to a genetic diagnosis can be missed due to the more pressing demands of maintaining ventilation, temperature, hydration and nutrition. Accurate observation by all members of staff, with discussion of concerns raised, can help minimise this difficulty.

If, sadly, the infant dies the neonatal unit staff will need to discuss the option of a post-mortem sensitively (see Chapter 14). Whilst not acceptable to some the PM can give considerable information for the management of future pregnancies. Blood samples for cytogenetic, metabolic and molecular analysis are also important but can only be utilised effectively if phenotypic features are noted to inform identification of appropriate tests. Clinical photography can also be invaluable when recording features that are hard to describe.

Some generic implications for practice

- Increased recognition of the importance of genetics in relation to health; therefore all nursing staff need to develop basic genetic competencies at the point of registration[18].
- As the nurse's experience grows so should his/her knowledge of genetics[19].
- A basic understanding of the way in which conditions are inherited is essential when discussing genetic conditions with parents.
- All health professionals need to be aware of the limitations of their own knowledge. For instance, it is easy to give parents false expectations in relation to genetic testing, in terms of test availability, time to result and interpretation of result in relation to prognosis or phenotype.
- Neonatal nurses should have a basic knowledge of the genetic service available in their area and the non-directive, non-judgemental philosophy that clinical genetic professionals strive for.
- See above case studies for more specific implications for practice.

Conclusion

This chapter has given a basic overview of congenital conditions and a basic knowledge of genetics, which can help neonatal staff in their discussions with parents. However, the most important aim of the chapter is to ensure that the reader also recognises the possible complexities of making and interpreting a genetic diagnosis, as well as the limitations of genetic testing. In this way it is hoped that parents will have realistic expectations of what a genetic opinion or referral can offer.

Glossary of genetic terms

Acrocentric – A chromosome with the centromere near one end as in chromosomes 13, 14, 15, 2 and 22 where the p arms are very small.

Allele – One copy of a gene pair. For instance, we inherit one cystic fibrosis (CF) allele from our mother and a second CF allele from our father.

Amniotic bands – Fibrous cords which arise from the amnion which may constrict part of the developing foetus, such as limb buds.

Associations – A recognisable collection of anomalies.

Aneuploidy – An alteration in the number of chromosomes, may be more or less, with a resultant phenotypic effect.

Autosomes – Chromosomes which are alike in both males and females.

Balanced translocation – This is one where the chromosome is rearranged but there is no loss or gain of chromosome material.

Centromere – The constricted area of a chromosome that is important in cell division.

Chromosomes – Rod-like structures found in the cell nucleus, made up of coiled DNA.

De novo – A new event, e.g. loss of part of a gene, which can then be inherited by the individual's offspring.

Deletion – When part of a chromosome or gene is lost.

Disruption – When a normal developmental process is interrupted.

DNA – Deoxyribonucleic acid: our genetic blueprint.

Duplication – When there is an additional copy of a part of a chromosome or gene.

Dysmorphology – Study of malformations which may be congenital or genetic in origin.

Empiric – Risk calculation based on observed data.

Gametogenesis – Formation of the gametes (ova or sperm), which involves production of cells with a half set of chromosomes (haploid set).

Genes – Genetic blueprint for a specific protein or protein component.

Genotype – The genetic makeup of an individual.

Inversion – A chromosome inversion is when a section of chromosome has broken in two places and turned through 180° prior to rejoining the chromosome.

Karyotype – The number and structure of the chromosomes as viewed under the microscope and after G banding to show the banding patterns.

Malformation – When a developmental process is abnormal.

Meiosis – The cell cycle which results in the formation of the gametes with a half set of chromosomes.

Metaphase – The phase in the cell cycle when the chromosomes can be visualised under the microscope.

Mitochondria – Found in the cytoplasm and concerned with energy production. Contains mitochondrial DNA (mtDNA).

Mitosis – Process of cell division resulting in cells with normal diploid (full set) of chromosomes.

Monogenic – Relating to a single gene.

Mosaicism – When there is more than one cell line in an individual or tissue.

Nonhomologous – Not the same, i.e. different.

Paracentric inversion – Where the breaks occur in either the short or long arm of the chromosome and do not include the centromere.

Pedigree – Pictorial representation of a family tree, which can facilitate determination of mode of inheritance and risk calculations.

Pericentric – Where the chromosome breaks occur in either the short or long arm of the chromosome and do not include the centromere.

Phenotype – Signs and symptoms observed as a result of a condition.

Polygenic – The result of the interaction of more than one pair of genes.

Reciprocal translocation – Where material from different chromosomes is exchanged.

Robertsonian translocation – Reduction in the number of chromosomes as a result of two acrocentric chromosomes joining together.

Sequences – A recognisable pattern of birth defects which result from a single primary defect.

Sporadic – A chance event.

Syndromes – A combination of abnormalities which form a recognisable pattern.

Translocation – A chromosome rearrangement

Unbalanced translocation – This is one where the chromosome is rearranged and there is loss or gain of chromosome material which will have a phenotypic effect.

Bibliography

Clarke A (1994) *Genetic Counselling; Practice & Principles*. Routledge, London.

Kingston H (2002) *ABC of Clinical Genetics*, 3rd edn. Blackwell Publishing Ltd, London.

Skirton H, Patch C (2002) *Genetics for Healthcare Professionals. A Lifestage Approach*. Bios Scientific Publishers, Oxford.

Support group information

Contact a Family: www.cafamily.org.uk
209–211 City Road, London EC1V
Tel: 020 7608 8700

This directory provides information about UK family support groups, specific conditions and rare disorders. Within the directory there is also a brief description of the condition and method of inheritance.

References

1. Kirk MM, K Longley, M Anstey S, *et al.* (2003) *Fit for Practice in the Genetics Era; Defining what Nurses, Midwives and Health Visitors Should Know and be Able to do in Relation to Genetics.* University of Glamorgan, Pontypridd.

2. Burton H (2003) *Addressing Genetics Delivery Health*, in *Public Health Genetics*. Public Health Genetics Unit, Cambridge.

3. Nussbaum RL, McInnes RR, Willard HF (2001) *Thompson and Thompson Genetics in Medicine*. Saunders, Philadelphia, USA.

4. Harper PS (2004) *Practical Genetic Counselling*. Arnold, London.

5. Nussbaum RL, McInnes RR, Willard H F (2001) *Thompson and Thompson Genetics in Medicine*. Saunders, Philadelphia, USA.

6. Rose P, Lucassen A (1999) *Practical Genetics for Primary Care*. Oxford University Press, Oxford.

7. Rose P, Lucassen A (1999) *Practical Genetics for Primary Care*. Oxford University Press, Oxford.

8. Firth HV, Hurst JA (2005) *Oxford Desk Reference – Clinical Genetics*. Oxford University Press, Oxford.

9. Firth HV, Hurst JA (2005) *Oxford Desk Reference – Clinical Genetics*. Oxford University Press, Oxford.

10. Nussbaum RL, McInnes RR, Willard HF (2001) *Thompson and Thompson Genetics in Medicine*. Saunders, Philadelphia, USA.

11. Firth HV, Hurst JA (2005) *Oxford Desk Reference – Clinical Genetics*. Oxford University Press, Oxford

12 American Society of Human Genetics, Ad Hoc Committee on Genetic Counselling (1975) Genetic Counselling. *Am J Hum Genetics*, 27, 240–2.

13. Beauchamp TL, Childress JF (1994) *Principles of Biomedical Ethics*. Oxford University Press, Oxford.

14 Department of Health (2003) *Our Inheritance, Our Future: realising the potential of genetics in the NHS*. The Stationery Office: London.

15. Kirk MM, K Longley, M Anstey S, *et al.* (2003) *Fit for Practice in the Genetics Era; Defining what Nurses, Midwives and Health Visitors Should Know and be Able to do in Relation to Genetics.* University of Glamorgan, Pontypridd.

16. Burton H (2003) *Addressing Genetics Delivery Health*, in *Public Health Genetics*. Public Health Genetics Unit, Cambridge.

17. Wilson JM, Jungner G (1968) *Principles and Practice of Screening for Disease*, in *Public Health Paper No. 34*. WHO, Geneva.

18. Kirk MM, K Longley, M Anstey S, *et al.* (2003) *Fit for Practice in the Genetics Era; Defining what Nurses, Midwives and Health Visitors Should Know and be Able to do in Relation to Genetics.* University of Glamorgan, Pontypridd.

19. Kirk MM, K Longley, M Anstey S, *et al.* (2003) *Fit for Practice in the Genetics Era; Defining what Nurses, Midwives and Health Visitors Should Know and be Able to do in Relation to Genetics.* University of Glamorgan, Pontypridd.

Chapter 11

NURSING NEWBORN BABIES WITH CONGENITAL HEART DISEASE

Frances Bu'Lock, Andrew Currie and Venkatesh Kairamkonda

Learning outcomes

After reading this chapter the reader will be expected to be able to:

- Describe an approach to the cardiovascular examination of a neonate

- Describe a management approach for hypotension in a neonate

- Identify the causes of neonatal congenital heart disease (CHD)

- Demonstrate a knowledge of neonatal heart failure and its treatment

- Explain why the term HSDA is more useful than always using the term pDA

- Compare the risks of medical or surgical management of a HSDA

Introduction

This chapter is divided into three main parts. It will begin with a brief overview of cardiac physiology and a structured approach to cardiovascular clinical assessment as well as the management of hypotension. The second section is devoted to congenital heart disease and the prevention of heart failure and the final section is devoted to the ductus arteriosus and its importance in the preterm infant.

In the term infant congenital cardiac abnormalities can present immediately after birth but their presentation may also be delayed secondary to closure of the arterial duct or changes in pulmonary pressures. Aside from these congenital abnormalities cardiac function is usually compromised secondarily to systemic illness or respiratory compromise. A structured approach

to cardiac examination and investigation is therefore necessary to differentiate cardiac conditions from systemic or respiratory conditions. In the preterm infant a ductus arteriosus that remains patent and haemodynamically significant will considerably increase the risk of morbidity. The final part of this chapter discusses the evaluation of a haemodynamically significant duct and the management strategies.

Cardiac physiology and clinical assessment of cardiac function

Embryology

The cardiovascular system is the first system to function in the embryo. Blood begins to circulate by the middle of the third week after conception to provide the rapidly growing embryo with nutrients and to dispose of waste products.

The critical period for developmental faults occurs at approximately the twenty-eighth day, when the major chambers are evolving. At this time blood is flowing through the heart and septation of the heart and great vessels occurs[1].

Foetal circulation and changes following birth

The heart of the foetus beats throughout pregnancy, but the placenta supplies oxygen and nutrition to the foetus and removes carbon dioxide through the umbilical vessels. The foetal circulation is reviewed in detail in Chapter 3 but the changes that occur following birth are summarised in Figure 11.1.

Post-natal circulation

The normal neonatal circulation is essentially similar to that of the adult circulation. The right ventricle pumps deoxygenated blood to

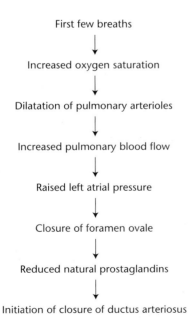

First few breaths
↓
Increased oxygen saturation
↓
Dilatation of pulmonary arterioles
↓
Increased pulmonary blood flow
↓
Raised left atrial pressure
↓
Closure of foramen ovale
↓
Reduced natural prostaglandins
↓
Initiation of closure of ductus arteriosus

Figure 11.1 Changing from foetal to adult circulation.

the lungs where it picks up oxygen, discharges carbon dioxide and recirculates to the left side again (see Figure 11.2). The left atrium receives oxygenated blood from the pulmonary circulation and this passes through the mitral valve into the left ventricle which then drives the blood forwards through the aortic valve to the systemic circulation. The pulmonary vascular resistance normally falls through the first six weeks or so of life, and the right ventricle, having been dominant in foetal life, involutes as the left ventricle takes over the majority of the responsibility for circulatory integrity.

Common cardiac physiological terms

Cardiac output

Cardiac output is defined as the volume of blood that is ejected from the heart each minute. It is the product of heart rate and stroke volume:

Cardiac output (ml/minute) = heart rate (number heart beats per minute) × stroke volume (ml/beat)

The heart rate falls from a neonatal rate of around 130–150 beats per minute throughout infancy and childhood. Heart rate is determined by the spontaneous rate generated at the cardiac pacemaker (sinoatrial node) which is under the influence of the autonomic nervous system and responds to changes in arousal state and exertion to respond to the body's energy demands. Stimulation of the parasympathetic nervous system (e.g. vagal nerve stimulation during suction or intubation) and hypothermia decrease heart rate; stimulation of the sympathetic nervous system (e.g. following adrenaline/epinephrine release) and factors that increase metabolic demand increase heart rate.

The stroke volume is influenced by three primary factors and these are described below.

Preload
- This term refers to the ventricular volume at the end of diastole (ventricular end-diastolic volume). It is influenced mainly by venous

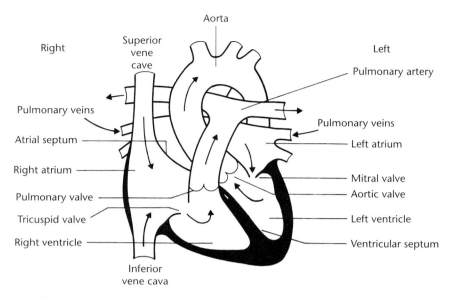

Figure 11.2   Blood flow through the heart of a healthy neonate.

return which itself is affected by blood volume and tone in the venous system.

• The relationship between ventricular end-diastolic volume and stroke volume is governed by Starling's law (see Figure 11.3) which states that the force of contraction of the heart muscle is proportional to the initial length of the muscle fibre. If the ventricular end-diastolic volume doubles then stroke volume will double until the point of over-stretching.

Afterload
This term refers to the ventricular pressure at the end of systole or the resistance to ventricular ejection. It is influenced mainly by systemic vascular resistance (determined by diameter of the arterioles) and blood viscosity.

Contractility
This is the intrinsic ability of a cardiac muscle to contract at a given fibre length. In other words it is the 'power' or inotropic ability of the heart.

A summary of factors controlling cardiac output is provided in Figure 11.4.

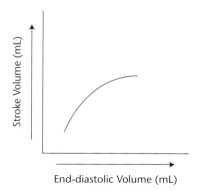

Figure 11.3   Starling's law of the heart; an increase in end-diastolic volume will lead to an increase in stroke volume until the maximum limit is reached.

Implications for practice

• Hypothermia induces bradycardia.
• The contractility of the heart is decreased during periods of hypoxia and acidosis.
• The contractility of the heart is increased by calcium and inotropic support.

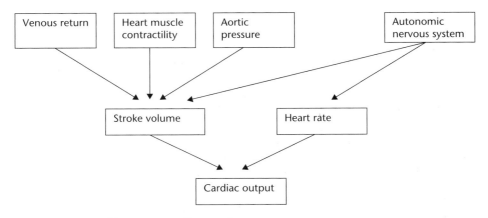

Figure 11.4 The summary of factors controlling cardiac output.

Blood pressure

Adequate blood pressure is essential to maintain tissue perfusion and is defined as the product of blood flow and resistance:

Blood pressure (mm Hg) = speed of blood flow × resistance

An understanding of these components is necessary to ensure that the aetiology of hypotension is accurately defined and the appropriate management instituted. The resistance in the blood vessels is affected by the length and radius of the individual blood vessels or the total surface area of vessels available for blood flow.

- *Systolic blood pressure* is the maximum pressure recorded by the contraction of the ventricles. Systolic blood pressure is a measure of left ventricular function and is directly influenced by contractility.
- *Diastolic blood pressure* is the minimum pressure recorded during the relaxation phase of the cardiac cycle. It is directly influenced by resistance to blood flow.

The systolic and diastolic blood pressures are both also influenced by blood volume and viscosity.

Pulse pressure is determined by subtracting diastolic blood pressure from systolic blood pressure. A wide pulse pressure is greater than 50% of the systolic blood pressure and may occur when resistance is low (e.g. in infants with a large PDA).

Mean arterial pressure (MAP) is the product of cardiac output and total peripheral resistance:

MAP = cardiac output × total peripheral resistance

MAP represents the best measure of organ perfusion as it is the difference between MAP and the venous pressure that drives blood through the capillaries of the organs. Because more time is spent in diastole than in systole, MAP is not simply the average of the systolic and diastolic pressures but is defined as:

MAP = diastolic pressure + 1/3 pulse pressure

Implications for practice

- Blood pressure is influenced by cardiac function and blood volume.
- Non-invasive blood pressure measurements are not reliable in sick neonates.
- An acute rise and fall in invasive blood pressure may be due to problems with the transducer and therefore should be checked before clinical interventions are made.

Cardiovascular assessment

Cardiovascular assessment should always begin with a general examination to identify features suggestive of congenital heart disease or cardiac dysfunction. These are summarised below.

General examination and inspection

- Dysmorphic features and evidence of syndromes known to be associated with congenital heart disease: e.g. trisomy 21 (Down's syndrome), trisomy 18 (Edwards' syndrome), trisomy 13 (Patau syndrome), Turner's syndrome (X0), DiGeorge syndrome (22q11-).
- Skin and mucous membranes:
  - Colour: look for pallor (anaemia), cyanosis (e.g. PPHN or cyanotic heart disease), mottling (e.g. hypoplastic left heart, sepsis) or flushing (warm sepsis). It is important to note that blue or dusky mucous membranes are consistent with cyanosis.
  - Temperature: cool (e.g. hypovolaemia, congestive cardiac failure due to significant PDA), cold (e.g. hypoplastic left heart, septic shock) or hot (sepsis, vasodilatation). A core-peripheral temperature difference suggests poor cardiac function or peripheral oedema
  - Hydration: capillary refill time (CRT): the skin is pressed for five seconds to occlude capillary blood flow and on release the time taken for the skin to become pink again is measured; 2/3 seconds is normal. Core CRT should be assessed on the sternum. Peripheral CRT can be influenced by the environmental temperature and is assessed on the forearm, and feet of the neonate.
  - Tissue turgor: this assesses interstitial fluid. Decreased turgor is when the skin appears less elastic and remains elevated.
- Palpation:
  - Pulses: palpate the radial, brachial, femoral pulses to assess rate and volume.
  - Generalised decreased pulses may indicate hypovolaemia, hypotension, severe vasoconstriction, hypoplastic left heart syndrome, aortic stenosis or cardiac failure.
  - Bounding pulses may indicate a patent ductus arteriosus.
  - Absent or decreased femoral pulses (and sometimes left brachial pulse) are a reliable indicator of coarctation of aorta[2].
- Auscultation:
  - During auscultation the quality of the first and second heart sounds should be assessed and additional heart sounds (third or fourth heart sounds producing a 'gallop' rhythm) or murmurs should be listened for.
  - A heart murmur is heard when there is turbulent blood flow.

Cardiovascular investigations and monitoring

If readily available, echocardiography is the investigation of choice to diagnose underlying cardiac abnormalities and to assess cardiac function.

Other useful parameters of cardiovascular stability are:

- Blood pressure
  - Cuff blood pressures are usually higher than arterial line readings, up to 15 mmHg[3], and may be falsely reassuring. Invasive blood pressure is more accurate and therefore recommended in the sick infant[4].
  - Non-invasive blood pressure measurement of four limbs may be useful for providing *supportive* evidence for a coarctation of the aorta (difference between upper limb and lower limb blood pressure > 20 mmHg). However, this is not a reliable test in isolation as it has an 8% false positive rate[5].
- Oxygen saturation: the comparison of a pre-ductal (right arm) and postductal oxygen saturation can be a very useful investigation. A higher preductal saturation suggests differential cyanosis that can be seen in PPHN and left ventricular outflow tract obstruction when deoxygenated blood from the pulmonary circulation enters into the descending aorta through the ductus arteriosus.

- Hyperoxia test: this is also known as the nitrogen washout test and can be performed in a neonate with cyanosis and circulatory collapse. The test involves measurement of pre-ductal arterial PaO_2 with the infant breathing room air ($FiO_2 = 0.21$) and then repeating the measurement after breathing in 100% oxygen ($FiO_2 = 1.00$) for ten minutes. A rise in PaO_2 above 20 kPa in 100% oxygen makes congenital cyanotic heart disease unlikely. The test should be avoided in an infant with a strong suspicion of a duct dependent heart condition, such as interrupted aortic arch and with better access to echocardiography it is not used as commonly.
- Electrocardiogram tracing: each cardiac cycle is represented by a series of waves, explained below in Figure 11.5.

The following approach to examination of the ECG trace may help identify underlying abnormalities.

- Rate: normal (90 to 160/ min), slow (< 90/ min in complete heart block), fast (> 200/min in tachyarrhythmias such as supraventricular tachycardia, atrial flutter).
- Rhythm: regular (apparently one P wave before each QRS complex), regularly irregular (atrial bigemini) and irregularly irregular (atrial fibrillation). In complete heart block,

the P wave has no fixed relationship with QRS complex).
- P, QRS and T wave morphology: inverted P wave in left atrial isomerism (no right atrium = no sinus node) or dextrocardia; peaked P wave in pulmonary hypertension, AVSD (atrioventricular septal defect), cardiomyopathy; Ebstein's anomaly; broad P waves (P mitrale) in left heart disease.
- Peaked T wave in hyperkalaemia and digoxin toxicity. Normally T waves are upright in V1 from 1 week to > 16 years.
- Intervals: PR interval shortened in babies with SVT due to ventricular pre-excitation (accessory pathway).
- QT interval (prolongation causes abnormal T wave and a slow heart rate (e.g. hypothermia, hypocalcaemia, hypokalaemia, prolonged QT syndromes). Associated with paroxysmal ventricular fibrillation.

Implications for practice

- Central capillary refill time (CRT) is prolonged when the peripheral circulation is poor due to hypovolaemia or a poor cardiac output.
- Absent or deceased femoral pulses are reliable indicators of coarctation of aorta.
- Oxygen is a potent pulmonary vasodilator and stimulates ductal closure.
- Supplemental oxygen should be used cautiously in a duct dependent congenital cyanotic heart disease.

Hypotension

The incidence of hypotension in the preterm-neonatal population has been estimated at 20–45% and is inversely proportional to gestational age[6,7]. One of the challenges has been to define normal values for mean arterial blood pressure in the well preterm infant, as a significantly low blood pressure has been shown to be associated with a worse outcome[8].

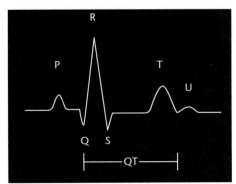

Figure 11.5 An ECG trace representing one cardiac cycle.

Table 11.1 Birthweight and tenth percentile for MAP.

Birthweight	Tenth percentile for mean BP
500–750 grams	26 mmHg
750–1000 grams	28 mmHg
1000–1250 grams	29 mmHg
1250–1500 grams	30 mmHg
1500–2000 grams	31 mmHg
2000–2999 grams	32 mmHg
3000–3999 grams	36 mmHg
4000 grams	42 mmHg

Table 11.2 Birthweight and average MAP with 95% upper confidence intervals.

Birth weight	Average MAP	95% upper CI
500–750 grams	35 mmHg	44 mmHg
750–1000 grams	38 mmHg	47 mmHg
1000–1250 grams	39 mmHg	48 mmHg
1250–1500 grams	40 mmHg	49 mmHg
2000–2999 grams	41 mmHg	50 mmHg
3000–3999 grams	47 mmHg	55 mmHg
4000 grams	52 mmHg	62 mmHg

Table 11.3 Indicators of clinically significant hypotension.

Appearance	Pale, cold, clammy
Toe – core temperature difference	> 2°C
Capillary refill time	Delayed (> 3 seconds)
Acid base balance	Metabolic acidosis with an elevated lactate
Urine output	<1 ml/kg/hr
Oxygenation/ventilation	High mean airway pressure (MAP) or oxygenation index (OI)*
Cardiac function	Echocardiographic evidence of poor cardiac contractility

*OI = FiO_2 X MAP X 100 / PaO_2 where measurement are in mmHg

Many neonatal units use the easily remembered gestation rule, i.e. A MAP above or equal to gestational age in completed weeks is acceptable[9]. Alternatively, Table 11.1 provides the tenth percentile for MAP plotted against birthweight[10].

In reality, a MAP that provides adequate blood perfusion to vital organs and therefore produces a well baby, i.e. one that is passing urine, has good perfusion, is easy to ventilate, is not acidotic, does not have a high lactate, or is not septic, is likely to be appropriate[11,12].

In critically sick infants with sepsis or PPHN the blood pressure should not be allowed to fall to the tenth percentile as this MAP is likely to be too low to maintain organ perfusion or to reverse the shunts in PPHN. Table 11.2 gives the average MAP measured invasively and the upper confidence interval for that mean. In critically sick infants one should aim for at least the average, and possibly for the 95% upper confidence limit of the average[13,14].

The causes of hypotension can be summarised as:

- Hypovolaemia, e.g.:
  - Blood loss prior to or at delivery, e.g. foetomaternal haemorrhage, maternal abruption
  - Large post-natal haemorrhage, e.g. intraventricular, sub-galeal
  - Blood loss secondary to frequent blood tests
- Abnormal distribution of blood, e.g.:
  - Large patent ductus arteriosus: wide pulse pressure
  - Infection: vasodilatation

- Cardiogenic, e.g.
  - Ductal closure in duct dependent cardiac lesions
  - Infection
  - Cardiomyopathy, myocarditis

In a baby with a low blood pressure, by either weight or gestational age criteria, any one of the indicators in Table 11.3 may indicate clinically significant hypotension.

Pharmacology of commonly used inotropes

Inotropes help to achieve delivery of oxygenated blood to the tissues by maintaining or improving blood pressure in infants with clinically significant hypotension. They do this by improving contractility of the heart and increasing vascular resistance but their specific effects vary depending on the receptors that they bind to. Adrenoreceptors include α1, β1, and β2. The α1 receptors are found in the coronary, pulmonary and skin vasculature and their activation causes vasoconstriction. The β1 receptors are located in the sinoatrial node and the myocardium. Their activation results in an increase in heart rate and contractility. The β2 receptors are found in the bronchi, gastrointestinal system and skeletal muscle and their activation results in vasodilatation.

The adverse effects of inotropes can be predicted from a knowledge of the receptors that they predominantly bind to, and include excessive chronotropy (increased heart rate),

tachyarrhythmias and an increase in afterload, which may cause tissue/end organ ischaemia.

The commonly used inotropes in neonatal medicine are summarised in the Table 11.4.

Treatment of clinically significant hypotension

One of the goals of intensive care management is the delivery of oxygenated blood to the tissues, which requires an effective blood pressure. The two most important aspects of management of clinically significant hypotension are:

- Treatment with fluid and inotropic support
- Identification of the cause in order to guide management

Table 11.4 Commonly used inotropes in the neonatal intensive care units.

Inotrope	Receptors	Predicted actions
Dopamine	2–5 microgram/kg/min Dopaminergic receptors	At low dose, dopamine acts on dopaminergic receptors – predominantly in the kidney, so increasing renal perfusion
	5–10 microgram/kg/min-Alpha and beta 1 Adrenoreceptors	At intermediate doses, dopamine has beta 1 effects and increases cardiac output
	> 10 microgram/kg/min-alpha effects predominate	At higher doses alpha effects predominate, and cause peripheral vasoconstriction
Dobutamine	Mainly beta 1 Adrenoreceptors	Dobutamine acts on beta 1 receptors, and has a predominantly cardiac effect, increasing heart rate and contractility and improves diastolic relaxation. It causes less extravasation injury than dopamine and is safer to use peripherally if no central access is available
Adrenaline/epinephrine	Potent agonist of α + β receptors	Low dose infusion predominantly β receptor activation (increased HR + contractility; decreased SVR (dilatation of vascular beds)) Higher doses stimulate α receptors (increased SVR + MAP; +/− increased myocardial oxygen demands)
Hydrocortisone	Dosing: range from 0.5 to 3 mg/kg/day. The most common regimen was 1 mg/kg (approximately 10 mg/m^2) every eight to twelve hours. Hydrocortisone was continued in most of the trials for three to five days [15–18].	Gastrointestinal perforation is one of the primary adverse effects associated with steroid administration in neonates.

Although there is no evidence based guideline, the following treatment strategy may be employed:

Volume and fluid type
- Volume: a dose of up to 20 mL/kg (usually given in separate boluses of 10 ml/kg) may be enough to bring up the blood pressure with no further intervention[19,20]. Further fluid volumes may be associated with worse outcome, e.g. chronic lung disease, symptomatic arterial ducts and death[21–23].
- Fluid type: normal saline (0.9% saline) is the first fluid of choice. It is effective, cheap and there is no evidence of any advantages to routinely using colloid in neonates[24–28]. However, 4.5% human albumin can be considered in severe sepsis, the post-operative period of certain surgical conditions and acute blood loss awaiting transfusion.

Inotropic support
- Dopamine and dobutamine: the Cochrane reviews of hypotension in neonates identified dopamine as the most effective agent at increasing blood pressure[29]. Dopamine may be used as the first line agent in babies with low systemic vascular resistance and high pulmonary vascular resistance when the arterial duct is still open. In other infants, where the pulmonary vascular resistance is low, the vasoconstrictive actions may increase shunting through the duct[30]. In these situations and those where there is no central access or there are concerns about poor myocardial function then dobutamine may be the first choice. Dobutamine mainly works through increasing myocardial contractility and heart rate. It also has mild vasodilating properties which is why it can be given as a peripheral infusion, although central access is preferred. Regardless of whether dopamine or dobutamine is started first, the other may be added if further inotropic support continues to be required and both are frequently used together.

- Hydrocortisone: recent evidence has supported the use of hydrocortisone to acutely raise blood pressure in premature neonates[31,32]. It is thought to work through improving the immature neonatal stress response and by increasing the number of receptor sites for inotropes. As steroids work by increasing gene expression, it may take several hours for a response to be seen. Hydrocortisone may be a useful adjunct to traditional therapies for the treatment of refractory hypotension in neonatal patients.
- Adrenaline: adrenaline should only really be administered through a central line. There is a Cochrane protocol to review the use of adrenaline and its publication is awaited[33]. A proposed treatment algorithm for hypotension in the neonatal unit is shown in Figure 11.6.

Implications for practice

- Skin temperature, capillary refill, pulse rate and volume and urine output are reliable markers of cardiac output.
- Lines to be used for infusions of inotropes should be primed with the specific inotropic first. These lines *must* not be flushed.
- Dopamine and adrenaline should be given via central lines.

Congenital heart defects

Congenital heart defects affect between 5 and 8 in every 1000 live born babies[34]. About one-third of these will develop life-threatening symptoms requiring treatment in the first few days of life[35]. There have been dramatic improvements in both the diagnosis and treatment of congenital heart disease over the last 10–15 years so that now more than 85% of people born with a heart defect are expected to survive to adulthood, although few are truly 'cured'[36]. Consequently, for most patients and their families, this is a lifelong disease and the risks of heart failure, cardiac arrhythmias, infective endocarditis,

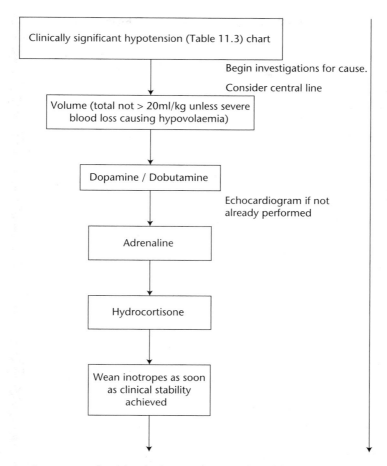

Figure 11.6 A proposed treatment algorithm for hypotension on the neonatal unit.

pulmonary vascular disease and sudden cardiac death mean that there is also a lifelong need for expert follow-up[37]. Mortality for congenital heart disease is highest in the first year of life but also rises again in the current population of > 45-year-olds[38]. Congenital heart defects have an overall statistical recurrence risk of between 2 and 4% for the next baby born to the same parents, whatever the cause, but for some families the risk may be much higher (or lower).

Although congenital heart problems are mainly structural defects, there are also babies born with abnormalities of the heart rhythm or muscle function (cardiomyopathies) which may require treatment in the first few days or even hours after birth.

Causes of congenital heart defects

The precise causes of congenital heart defects are not clearly known for all babies and are thought to be influenced by a number of factors.

Chromosomal/genetic abnormalities

Along with the well known major chromosome abnormalities like trisomies 13, 18 and 21, and Turner's syndrome (XO), many more abnormalities of chromosomes, and single gene defects (such as Holt-Oram syndrome) associated with congenital heart disease are now recognised. These are frequently 'new mutations' but it is increasingly clear that some (e.g. 22q deletion syndrome and Noonan's syndrome) may be present in a parent or siblings as well. Children of consanguinous parents are also at significantly increased risk of congenital heart disease. In such familes, recurrence risks are much higher than the 2–4% generally quoted overall.

Infections
Maternal infections can cause problems, especially rubella, cytomegalovirus and toxoplasmosis.

Drugs
Some drugs may affect the cardiac development of the foetus. These include anticonvulsants (such as phenytoin and sodium valproate), antidepressants (such as lithium), alcohol and cocaine.

Maternal ill health
A mother with diabetes mellitus carries a 4–5% risk of having a baby with congenital heart defects. The most common defects are transposition of the great vessels, ventricular septal defect, patent ductus arteriosis and cardiomyopathy, a disorder of the heart muscle. Phenylketonuria and systemic lupus erythematosus (SLE) in the mother are also known to be associated with congenital heart problems in the baby.

Exposure to teratogens
Teratogens are substances capable of disrupting foetal growth and producing malformations. Exposure to radiation, chemicals or any substance that has an adverse effect on foetal development can cause problems if exposure takes place very early in pregnancy.

Antenatal diagnosis of congenital heart disease

Ultrasound scanning
This was also discussed in Chapter 2.

Many heart defects are now diagnosed prenatally on ultrasound scan screening from as early as 13–14 weeks gestation, although significant defects can still be missed for a variety

of reasons. Detailed foetal ultrasound examination around 20 weeks gestation should include visualisation of all four main cardiac chambers and the walls between them. Sonographers are also encouraged to look at the great arterial connections as well. When a cardiac abnormality is suspected or when other major anomalies (e.g. exomphalos, tracheo-oesophageal fistula or diaphragmatic hernia) are detected, referral to a specialist foetal cardiologist is required for detailed cardiac scanning and careful counselling. More recently, foetuses with markedly increased nuchal translucency at dating scan (13–14 weeks) are also referred as there is a high incidence of congenital heart disease in these foetuses even when the karyotype is normal[39,40]. Foetal karyotyping and examination of the rest of the foetus by a foetal medicine specialist is generally recommended if this has not already been done.

Counselling of parents
The proportion of pregnancies terminated for congenital heart disease varies markedly, both with the severity of the cardiac condition, other associated problems and long-term prognosis and with the parents' social, cultural and religious background. This needs to be well understood by the counselling team and time for consultation with other family or community members is invaluable before a course of action is confirmed.

Implications for practice

- Congenital heart disease affects 5–8 /1000 live births.
- A concise maternal and family history is essential when evaluating an infant for possible CHD.
- Some CHD may be diagnosed prenatally from as early as 13–14 weeks gestation.

Antenatal care
Early diagnosis of CHD allows the opportunity to optimise plans for delivery and immediate post-natal care, which may have long-term

benefits for both the baby and the family. Indications for antenatal treatment include foetal arrythmias such as supraventricular tachycardia, which can lead to hydrops or death. Treatment of the mother with anti-arrhythmic drugs which cross the placenta may improve the chance of the baby's survival[41]. A small number of babies each year may benefit from *in utero* balloon dilatation of either the aortic or pulmonary valves, or even atrial septostomy, but this can only be offered to a few and performed in a very limited number of very specialist centres.

Some babies with severe heart disease (especially arryhthmias, cardiomyopathy and Ebstein's anomaly may develop hydrops (fluid retention causing oedema, ascites and pleural effusions) and these babies may well die *in utero*. Early delivery may be beneficial for these babies despite the increased risks from preterm delivery, as there are more treatment options available in this extreme situation. Caesarian delivery is required for babies with arrythmias, as reliable monitoring of the foetal heart rate is not possible, and is often performed for those with foetal hydrops.

If the pregnancy is to continue parents are advised to have the delivery in a hospital with high-level neonatal care facilities where the baby can be assessed and stabilised immediately after birth and then safely transported to their regional cardiac unit. Few paediatric cardiac units, at least in the UK, are in the same hospital, or even on the same site, as a maternity and neonatal unit and hence high quality transport expertise is mandatory. Babies with transposition of the great arteries should be delivered as close as possible to a cardiac unit in case atrial septostomy is required very soon after delivery, but the majority of babies with other conditions can be delivered reasonably close to home and transferred after delivery[42].

For most babies with heart disease, normal vaginal delivery as close to term as possible is preferred in order to optimise foetal somatic growth and lung maturity. Induction of labour close to term may be useful to facilitate transport or childcare arrangements, especially for multiparous women.

Post-natal care of a baby with congenital heart disease

Nursing a neonate with a congenital heart defect requires careful assessment and early recognition of the clinical signs that may affect the outcome of the infant. If the baby has a defect that obstructs normal circulation, life will depend on the foetal ductus arteriosus remaining open. When the duct starts to close (usually 24–48 hours) after birth, the baby will start to develop symptoms including dyspnoea, tachycardia or failure to complete feeds. If these signs go unnoticed and untreated the baby may deteriorate suddenly with either severe cyanosis or circulatory failure which will rapidly progress to shock and death without strenuous resuscitation.

In these days of early maternal discharge and the small but steady increase in home births, the diagnosis may not be made until the baby is examined for discharge or when at home. A murmur may be heard on auscultation of the chest during the CVS examination. A soft systolic murmur is common in newborn babies due to the changes from foetal circulation to adult circulation and this disappears later. A loud systolic murmur is a reason for immediate cardiac investigation and the baby should be fully assessed and is likely to be admitted to the neonatal unit for this assessment.

Many neonatal units now have a 'neonatologist with an interest in cardiology', who can perform echocardiography, make a provisional diagnosis, begin initial management and discuss transport arrangements with the cardiac referral centre. The baby will need at least a secure airway, good intravenous access for drugs and fluids, good thermal management and a stable blood sugar (see Chapter 13). This will ensure the baby will travel safely and arrive in the best condition possible at the receiving unit. Babies with known duct dependent heart disease will be started on intravenous prostaglandin treatment shortly after delivery to prevent ductal closure. This can be given at relatively low doses

(3–5 ng/kg/min) and apnoea is rare at these doses so the baby may well not need to be ventilated for transport[43]. However, it is important to check the blood gases prior to departure to ensure the baby is stable for the journey. Babies who are sick or with suspected/newly diagnosed duct dependent conditions may need higher doses of prostaglandin +/− other drugs and ventilation prior to transfer.

The neonatal team have a major role in providing crucial early support to the family as well as their baby. Parents of babies with prenatally diagnosed heart disease may have been to the unit before the birth, met the staff and seen the equipment. They will be prepared for problems and this will help them to understand what is happening, but does not mean they will find the course of their baby's illness and treatment any easier to bear. If the parents are not able to accompany their baby to the specialist cardiac centre they must be told of the possible need for emergency surgery and what the surgery will entail. A signed consent form should then be obtained. It may be impossible to tell the parents exactly what the operation will involve until the baby has been properly assessed on the cardiac unit. Ideally, one or both parents should accompany the baby and most cardiac units now have good facilities for parents to stay with their children, and frequently midwifery input for the mothers as well.

Implications for practice

- An understanding of the normal post-natal changes in circulation is vital to allow the neonatal nurse to be aware of the important clinical signs which suggest that normal adaptation is not taking place.
- The neonatal nurse needs to have basic knowledge of the condition to be able to support parents and answer their potential questions.
- Parental support is crucial for all families whether the diagnosis has been made prenatally or post-natally.

Nursing care

The current treatment of a baby with a congenital heart disease aims to anticipate and treat heart failure so as to prevent permanent damage to the heart and lungs before definitive treatment is undertaken. This is done by monitoring vital signs, observing the baby, managing fluid balance, giving good nutrition and administering drug treatment to strengthen and stabilise circulatory function.

The baby should be weighed on admission so that drug doses, fluids and nutritional needs can be calculated on this weight. Baseline observations of heart rate, respiratory rate, oxygen saturation, central and peripheral temperature, and blood pressure should be taken. Continuous cardiorespiratory and saturation monitoring is usual and a blood pressure reading should be taken on each of the baby's limbs if possible as some conditions can cause upper and lower limb pressures to be different, depending on the site of the circulatory obstruction. Regular blood gas analysis is also crucial to assess the efficacy of resuscitation and stabilisiation.

Babies remaining on the neonatal unit are generally those with other congenital malformations, e.g. gastroschisis, or where the problems of prematurity outweigh or preclude the need for definitive cardiac treatment. These latter infants may need to be 'grown', sometimes on prostaglandin treatment, until they are sufficiently large or mature enough for more interventional management. These babies will need careful attention to their nutritional and developmental needs in addition to their cardiac care.

Observation and monitoring of anticipated cardiac failure

Heart failure occurs when the heart is unable to pump sufficient blood to meet the metabolic requirements of the body. This needs prompt treatment to prevent damage to other organs such as the kidneys, brain and gut, which function poorly or fail when blood supply is diminished. The baby's condition should be carefully monitored and attention paid to the following areas:

Tachycardia

Tachycardia indicates that the heart is beating faster in an effort to pump sufficient blood round the body to meet its metabolic requirements. This itself can use up valuable energy.

Perspiration

The baby may perspire excessively, especially with feeding,

Core/toe temperature gap

Cool extremities may indicate a reduced cardiac output. The core and toe temperatures should be monitored, as a difference of more than 3°C may suggest incipient collapse. To ensure the baby's comfort, even when the core temperature is satisfactory, bootees and mittens should be worn.

Cyanosis

Congenital heart disease is divided conventionally into acyanotic and cyanotic lesions. Cyanosis is the result of blood shunting from the right side of the heart to the systemic circulation without having been reoxygenated by the lungs, or of mixing of oxygenated blood with deoxygenated blood. In acyanotic conditions the lung perfusion and blood oxygenation may not be affected.

True cyanosis is 'central' and the baby may be very pale with blueness of the gums and mucous membranes. This can be confirmed by pulse oximetry. Saturations may be lower in the feet than the hands when the duct is patent and shunting right to left, e.g. in severe coarctation, so it is important to assess upper *and* lower limb saturations. Some newborn babies have blueness of the palms of the hands and soles of the feet (with normal saturations), called acrocyanosis, which clears spontaneously and has no cardiac implications.

Respiratory effort

Increased respiratory effort may be the result of pulmonary congestion, either from increased blood flow to the lungs or obstructed venous return from them, as well as from respiratory disease. The baby may be tachypnoeic with intercostal or subcostal recession, sternal or suprasternal retraction on inspiration and reduced air entry on auscultation. Mechanical ventilation may be necessary to stabilise oxygenation and ventilation and to maintain normal blood gases. Diuretics may be given to relieve pulmonary congestion and oedema. If the baby is not ventilated, breathing may be easier if the incubator mattress is raised at the head end.

Raised oxygen requirements

Oxygen can be very useful but there are also significant risks associated with its use, particularly in infants with cardiac disease: In duct dependent lesions high arterial oxygen concentrations promote ductal closure, so high inspired oxygen levels can sometimes be life-threatening under these conditions. It can also lead to pulmonary vasodilatation which may encourage left to right shunting and pulmonary oedema. Oxygen requirements are monitored using pulse oximetry or transcutaneous monitoring. Acceptable pulse oximetry readings for babies with cardiac problems, where there is mixing of oxygenated and deoxygenated blood, will be much lower than for a baby with a normal heart. Readings below 80% saturated arterial oxygen may be accepted if the baby is well perfused, not distressed or tachypnoeic and not acidotic on blood gas analysis.

Oedema

It may be necessary to restrict fluids in babies with pulmonary oedema but in general a certain amount of fluid is necessary to provide the nutritional or calorific requirements needed by the infant, so diuretics are used to remove 'excess water'. An accurate fluid balance should be kept and urinary output monitored to check for fluid retention or anuria. If the baby is producing less than 1 ml/kg per hour, the urine is concentrated (as shown by a high specific gravity on ward testing), or there are signs of oedema, then renal function is poor. Reduced renal function is a reliable indicator of reduced cardiac function because a diminished cardiac output causes renal failure. Daily weighing is necessary to accurately assess fluid management.

Nutritional problems

The high metabolic rate seen in infants with cardiac disease means that the baby has a higher energy or calorie requirement and even if fluids are not restricted weight gain may be slow unless additional calorie supplements are added to the feeds. Tube feeding may be required as the babies may be unable to feed (ventilated) or too exhausted to feed. If the baby will tolerate oral feeds, breast-feeds or expressed breast milk can be given. However, care is needed as a reduced cardiac output and an increased work of breathing impairs gastric performance, causing slower emptying and frequent vomiting or gastro-oesophageal reflux. If intravenous parenteral nutrition is used the baby should have a central line, and high energy fluids which include fats, proteins and glucose should be used.

Implications for practice

Other than the parents the neonatal nurse has the greatest 'hands on' contact with the infant and should perform careful nursing observations and be alert to subtle changes in an infant's condition.

Medical treatment of cardiac problems

The medical management of cardiac failure is aimed at maintaining an adequate circulation for the baby's metabolic needs. The exact balance depends on the underlying pathology but relies on a combination of cardiac support drugs and diuretics. Commonly used cardiac drugs include:

- Prostaglandin E_1
- Adrenaline
- Dopamine
- Dobutamine

- Furosemide
- Spironolactone
- Captopril
- Digoxin
- Indomethacin
- Nitric oxide
- Propranolol
- Adenosine

Prostaglandin E_1

Many congenital heart defects depend on the patency of the ductus arteriosus to keep the circulation intact. Prostaglandin E_1 is given as a continuous infusion to keep the duct open while diagnosis and assessment of the defect is taking place (see Table 11.5). Prostaglandins are endogenously produced lipids that have a variety of effects in the body. Artificial prostaglandin E_1 acts on the smooth muscle of the duct to keep it open. It must be given as a continuous infusion because it is rapidly metabolised and as soon as the infusion stops the duct starts to close[44]. It is essential to give it through a large vein, peripherally or centrally, and to maintain the patency of the line. It is useful to have a second peripheral line ready for use in case one fails. It can be given orally but needs then to be given each hour.

Prostaglandin has the potential to cause apnoea, particularly at higher doses and in more preterm infants, and all babies should have

Table 11.5 Congenital heart defects for which prostaglandin E_1 is used.

- Transposition of the great arteries

Duct dependent pulmonary flow (left to right shunt through duct)
- Pulmonary atresia
- Severe pulmonary stenosis
- Tetralogy of Fallot with severe pulmonary stenosis

Duct dependent systemic blood flow (right to left through duct)
- Interrupted aortic arch
- Coarctation of the aorta
- Hypoplastic left heart syndrome
- Aortic stenosis

continuous ECG and oxygen saturation monitoring and intermittent blood gas analysis while receiving this treatment. If there are adverse effects such as apnoea, the baby may need to be ventilated but the drug must not be stopped, as closure of the duct could cause death. Other side effects to watch for include flushing and fever, blood pressure fluctuations (due to vasodilatation), hypoglycaemia, gastrointestinal disturbances and renal insufficiency[45].

Frusemide

Frusemide acts by preventing the reabsorption of sodium in the kidneys and so prevents water retention (as water tends to follow sodium). It thus controls oedema and eases the load on the heart. It can cause electrolyte imbalance so serum electrolytes need at least daily assessment. It can be given by mouth or intravenously.

Spironolactone

This is another (weaker) diuretic which acts on a different part of the kidney from frusemide and tends to cause potassium retention. This is useful to counteract the potassium loss from frusemide so both drugs are often given together but blood biochemistry still needs to be monitored.

Captopril

This is an angiotensin converting enzyme inhibitor which is given to treat heart failure. It is a peripheral vasodilator and hence diverts blood away from the lungs, improving renal blood flow and reducing pulmonary oedema. It can cause severe hypotension and renal failure and needs to be started at very low doses and increased gradually in babies on diuretic treatment. Like spironolactone, it causes potassium retention so spironolactone should be stopped if a baby is started on captopril. Serum electrolytes should be checked daily while the dose is being escalated, and the blood pressure monitored very carefully.

Digoxin

This is a cardiac glycoside which slows some arrhythmias and may improve cardiac function. It is given in divided doses orally or intravenously. Digoxin can reach toxic levels in the blood very easily, especially if renal function is reduced, which may precipitate fatal arrythmias, so serum levels must be monitored carefully. It also causes slowing of the normal heart rythmn so if the heart rate falls below an acceptable level (usually around 120 bpm) the next dose is omitted and the level checked.

Indomethacin

This is used to close the ductus arteriosus and can be given intravenously or orally. It blocks the actions of naturally circulating prostaglandins, which help to keep the duct open, by inhibition of prostaglandin synthesis. Electrolyte imbalance and hypoglycaemia, gastrointestinal bleeding and renal damage are side effects.

Nitric oxide

This is an inhaled drug which is used to reduce pulmonary vascular resistance and can be life saving. It can cause toxicity by accumulation of toxic metabolites and these should be monitored with the blood gases, and in general inhaled concentrations of > 20 ppm should be avoided. It can be given through standard ventilation circuits although some units do use special ventilators with scavenging for the exhaust.

Adenosine

This is a very short acting drug as it is metabolised by all living cells. It is extremely useful to treat some tachyarrythmias, but has to be given very quickly via a large vein and flushed through quickly afterwards. A small dose is given first and then incremental dose increases are given until effective. The baby may flush or breath rapidly as it takes effect and the heart may actually stop briefly, which is unnerving but short-lived. Adenosine should only be given with continous ECG monitoring attached and preferably a paper recording running so the traces can be checked afterwards by a cardiologist as they may contain valuable information which would otherwise be lost.

Propranolol

This is a beta blocker. It can be used to slow or stabilise the heart rate for some arrythmias. It also relaxes cardiac muscle and can be useful for severe cyanotic spells in babies with Tetralogy of Fallot, and for some babies with severe hypertrophic cardiomyopathy and infants of diabetic mothers.

Parents

Many cardiac defects carry a significant mortality and morbidity risk even with surgery and this should be clearly explained to the parents. If the baby has a major chromosome or other congenital abnormality this may also have a bearing on the risks of treatment and the baby's suitability for it (e.g. in trisomy 13 or 18). In some cardiac conditions the likelihood of a good long-term outcome is so poor that parents may opt for palliative care rather than surgery and this will need to be carefully discussed. Nurses will necessarily bear the brunt of any decision and may find working with the parents in this situation difficult.

Most neonatal units transfer babies who are to have cardiac surgery to their regional cardiac unit where there is the appropriate mix of medical and nursing skills[46]. Many are discharged home directly from there, but some may return to the neonatal unit after surgery for longer term care or preparation for discharge. Careful handover in both directions is critical to minimise the disruption for both baby and parents.

Investigation techniques

Radiology

A chest X-ray often gives clues to the diagnosis although heart changes may occur as a result of a traumatic delivery such as birth asphyxia[47]. Some heart shapes may be diagnostic, such as the boot-shaped heart of Fallot's tetralogy; the oval, egg shaped heart of transposition of the great vessels; or the square shape of tricuspid atresia[48].

Electrocardiogram (ECG)

This is a tracing of the heart's activity. The normal ECG consists of a series of waves (see above).Usually a 12 lead (or as close as possible) ECG is obtained, especially when rythmn abnormalities are suspected.

Cardiac ultrasound (echocardiography)

Echocardiography is the mainstay of modern cardiac diagnosis and management. It is non-invasive and can be performed at the baby's bedside. Cross-sectional studies provide a two-dimensional picture of the heart, while Doppler echocardiography uses the principle that moving objects alter the frequency of sound waves. This can be colour coded for speed and direction of blood flow through valves and septal defects (abnormal holes), and extrapolations made about pressure in the various cardiac chambers. Newer machines also allow increasingly rapid and sophisticated techniques for assessment of cardiac function and some even allow real-time three-dimensional reconstruction of valves and other structures. The diagnostic accuracy of echocardiography has taken away the need for cardiac catheterisation in many cases.

Cardiac catheterisation

Cardiac catheterisation can be used as a diagnostic tool or as part of interventional management. It is a major invasive procedure for a new-born baby especially if small or sick and necessitates the use of a general anaesthetic.

As a diagnostic tool, cardiac catheterisation enables the cardiologists to measure pressures within the cardiac chambers and great vessels, obtain blood samples to analyse their oxygen content and inject radio-opaque dye to visualise the anatomy and function of the heart, great vessels and coronary circulation. A radio-opaque catheter is inserted into the femoral vein either by venipuncture or by cut-down. The catheter is then threaded up into the heart under X-ray guidance so that the four chambers of the heart can be visualised.

Cardiac catheterisation is principally now used for interventional procedures. Success rates are good and indications for such procedures generally increasing. In neonates these mainly include balloon septostomy or Rashkind's procedure. A balloon catheter is advanced across the foramen ovale into the left atrium, the balloon is inflated and then pulled across the foramen ovale into the right atrium to create a larger atrial septal defect. This procedure is essential in an infant with transposition of the great arteries to facilitate mixing of oxygenated and deoxygenated blood. Balloon atrial septostomy is now frequently performed at the bedside on the neonatal intensive care unit, as the positioning of the balloon can be monitored by ultrasound alone, but most catheters are still performed in a specialised X-ray laboratory and hence require the baby to be transferred as for surgery. Additional uses of balloon catheters are to treat narrowings or blockages of the pulmonary and aortic valves.

Cardiac surgery

Congenital heart disease is a lifelong disease and cardiac surgery can rarely offer a complete cure; even patients who have had VSDs closed need long-term follow-up and may need further treatment in the future. Risks of surgery are generally less after three months of age as by this time the pressures within the systemic and pulmonary circulations should have stabilised and the brain is also more mature. However, preliminary surgery is often necessary to help stabilise the circulations and allow the infant to grow before more definitive surgery is performed. Some babies will need definitive surgery in the first few days or weeks of life. However, generally (except for balloon septostomy which needs to be done very promptly) these procedures can be planned and the infant maintained on Prostin until the operation. This allows time for the transition from foetal to post-natal state to stabilise, for the pulmonary vascular resistance to begin to fall and initial post-natal feeding and parental bonding to become established. This is particularly important for prenatally diagnosed babies.

Initial procedures include interventional catheterisation, balloon atrial septostomy, aortopulmonary shunts and pulmonary artery banding. These do not require cardiopulmonary bypass. Aortopulmonary shunts are tubes of Gore-Tex® (usually), placed between either the aorta or proximal upper limb arteries and the pulmonary artery and provide a replacement for the arterial duct to allow the baby to go home and grow before more definitive surgery is undertaken. Pulmonary artery banding is performed in babies with large ventricular defects or functionally single ventricles with unrestricted pulmonary blood flow, to reduce the pulmonary artery flow and pressure either until the baby is large enough for definitive closure of the VSD or for the next stage of long-term palliation.

Cardiopulmonary bypass is a highly invasive technique used during some forms of cardiac surgery. It is a technique used to temporarily replace the patient's own heart and lungs with a mechanical system, thus permitting complex surgery to be undertaken on the heart or great vessels without interference from cardiac movement or bleeding. It requires full anticoagulation and also sometimes periods of complete circulatory arrest, albeit with the patient profoundly cooled (to around 18°C). Hence there are considerable risks, especially to the neonatal brain, and neonatal bypass surgery is therefore only performed where there is no other realistic alternative. The length of circulatory arrest during bypass is directly related to the likelihood of neurological abnormalties later on[49]. The commonest procedure to utilise cardiopulmonary bypass is the arterial switch operation for transposition of the great arteries, which needs to be done in the first few weeks of life because otherwise the left ventricle becomes too weak to readily support the systemic circulation after surgery. Most other neonatal bypass procedures are also those where major rearrangements/reconstruction of the great vessels are required for the baby to survive without long-term damage to the pulmonary circulation. These include repair of a common arterial trunk (truncus arteriosus), the Norwood procedure for hypoplastic left heart, and repair of interrupted aortic arch. Sometimes critical aortic stenosis also needs neonatal bypass surgery but in general cardiac catheterisation treatment is preferred first.

Common defects seen in the neonatal unit

The lesions which account for 80% of all cases are listed below in order of commonest incidence:

- Patent ductus arteriosus
- Ventricular septal defect
- Atrioventricular septal defects
- Fallot's tetralogy
- Pulmonary stenosis/atresia
- Coarctation of the aorta
- Aortic stenosis
- Transposition of the great arteries
- Hypoplastic left heart syndrome

Acyanotic heart disease

Non-duct-dependent

The most common heart problems in the neonatal unit are caused by left-to-right shunting of the blood through the heart. The most common of these defects are patent ductus arteriosus, ventricular septal defect, atrial septal defect and atrioventricular canal. These are not dramatic or life-threatening conditions and often do not need surgery in the immediate neonatal period but they may cause a degree of heart failure needing treatment.

Patent ductus arteriosus
See below.

VSD
This is the most common form of congenital heart defect and is responsible for 20–25% of

babies with congenital heart defects. It is often associated with other problems, e.g. coarctation of the aorta. There is a gap in the ventricular septum caused by imperfect septal division during early foetal development. It may vary in size from a small hole which causes no problems to a complete absence of the septum (see Figure 11.7).

Clinical presentation
A small ventricular septal defect does not cause any problems of growth or development. A moderate one will cause tachypnoea, poor feeding, failure to thrive and repeated chest infections. A large defect may cause congestive heart failure and will usually be repaired in infancy. Congestive cardiac failure can develop at about 4–6 weeks in babies with larger defects because blood will shunt from the left ventricle into the right ventricle and into the pulmonary circulation causing pulmonary hypertension. Increased pressure in the right ventricle, resulting from shunting and increased pulmonary resistance, can cause the right ventricle to hypertrophy and the right atrium to enlarge to accommodate the increased work.

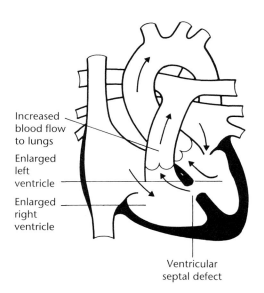

Increased blood flow to lungs

Enlarged left ventricle

Enlarged right ventricle

Ventricular septal defect

Figure 11.7 Diagram of a ventricular septal defect.

Diagnosis
A murmur will be heard on chest auscultation and a chest X-ray will reveal cardiomegaly of varying degree with enlargement of the right atrium. Echocardiography will provide an accurate diagnosis of the position and size of the defect.

Medical treatment
Some 30–40% of small ventricular septal defects close naturally in the first year of life and moderate ones tend to become smaller as the baby grows.

Surgical treatment
In a very large VSD palliative banding of the pulmonary artery may be needed to reduce the volume and pressure of pulmonary blood flow to the lungs and to relieve congestive cardiac failure. If the congestive cardiac failure does not respond to medical treatment and right ventricular pressure remains elevated then surgical closure (on cardiopulmonary bypass) is usually performed after about three months of age. If heart failure is well controlled and right ventricular pressure is low then surgery can be deferred until around a year of age as some defects will have closed spontaneously given enough time.

Atrioventricular septal defects (canal)
This defect accounts for 2% of cardiac defects and occurs in approximately 30% of Down's syndrome babies. There may be only an atrial communication and there may even be almost complete absence of the ventricular septum. The mitral and tricuspid valves are essentially joined so that this condition appears as a cleft or canal through the middle of the heart (see Figure 11.8).

Clinical presentation
The baby may become blue on crying (right to left shunting through the atrial component of the defect), or there may be failure to thrive and repeated chest infections. Murmurs are frequently absent or soft if the defect is large. Congestive heart failure generally occurs at 1–2 months of age except in some babies with Down's syndrome who may have persistent elevation of the pulmonary vascular resistance.

Diagnosis
The ECG shows an abnormal cardiac axis, there may be a murmur heard and the chest X-ray generally shows an enlarged heart with increased pulmonary vascular markings. Echocardiography will reveal the extent of the defect and the degree of atrioventricular valve leakage.

Medical treatment
Medical treatment is used to control heart failure as for ventricular septal defects.

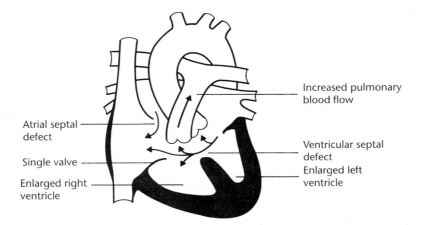

Figure 11.8 Diagram of a complete atrioventricular defect (AV canal).

Surgical treatment

Some babies may need palliative banding of the pulmonary artery to decrease the blood flow to the lungs but this can exacerbate leakage of the atrioventricular valves so in general is rarely undertaken. Complete repair using cardiopulmonary bypass is generally carried out bewteen 3 and 6 months of age as the atrioventricular valves are more robust at this stage. The surgery is more complicated than standard VSD surgery, mainly because of the bivalvar abnormalities. During surgery the septal defects are closed and a valvoplasty performed to make the atrioventricular valves as competent as possible . Further surgery may be needed later to replace an incompetent mitral valve.

Left heart obstruction

This is a range of defects, mainly involving narrowing of the aortic (or more rarely the mitral) valve, or of the aorta itself. Milder cases are acyanotic, but more severe cases (and hypoplastic left heart syndrome) rely on patency of the arterial duct to support the systemic circulation and hence are effectively cyanotic until the duct closes. Then the infant suffers overwhelming circulatory collapse and will die quickly unless the duct can be reopened.

Coarctation of the aorta

The term coarctation describes a constriction of the aorta (see Figure 11.9) which leads to an obstruction to left ventricular outflow. Over half of the patients with a coarctation of the aorta have other lesions such as ventricular septal defects, mitral valve abnormalities and aortic stenosis. Initial survival depends on a patent ductus arteriosus to maintain the systemic circulation.

Clinical presentation

Symptoms usually begin between the second to tenth day of life when the ductus arteriosus starts to close and blood flow to the body becomes compromised. The initial symptoms may include poor feeding, irritability and signs

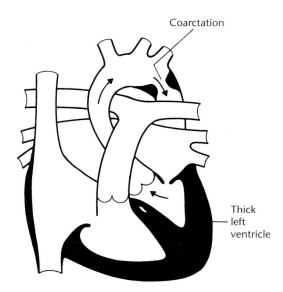

Figure 11.9   Diagram to illustrate the coarctation of the aorta.

suggestive of infection. The signs will include poor peripheral pulses and a systolic heart murmur. The femoral pulses will be reduced in volume (when compared to the brachial) or absent and in severe cases the brachial pulses will disappear as the systemic circulation fails. A four limb blood pressure is often requested, although in isolation this is not very predictive. However, blood pressure in the upper limbs that is > 10–15 mmHg higher than that in the lower limbs may be suggestive of a coarctation.

Diagnosis

A provisional diagnosis may have been made antenatally in severe cases and the definitive diagnosis is made echocardiographically.

Medical treatment

A prostaglandin infusion should be commenced to reopen or keep the duct open to ensure circulation to the lower half of the body while the baby is prepared for surgery. Ventilatory support and correction of acidosis and electrolyte imbalance are essential. Inotropic support may also be required as the blood supply to the kidneys may be poor, resulting in renal failure. Balloon dilatation can be used but in general surgery is preferred.

Surgical treatment
The coarctation is usually repaired by excision of the narrow segment and ligation of the duct (end-to-end repair), but longer narrowings may also be patched with a flap of arterial wall taken from the left subclavian artery. If the aortic arch is also small an extended repair may require cardiopulmonary bypass. Whatever the choice of operation, there is a risk of either residual narrowing or recurrent narrowing with time, but this is generally amenable to balloon dilatation.

Hypoplastic left heart syndrome
Hypoplastic left heart syndrome (HLHS) is one of the commonest congenital heart defects after VSD and ASD, but a significant proportion are now diagnosed (and 30–50% terminated) before birth. The condition and its associated cardiac defects were considered fatal until the last 15–20 years, but improvements in knowledge and technology have led to effective management strategies which offer a chance of long-term survival,

although the mortality rate is still high and the long-term prognosis uncertain.

In the most severe form there is atresia of the aortic valve, a rudimentary left ventricle and atresia or hypoplasia of the mitral valve and ascending aorta. The left atrium empties through the foramen ovale into the right atrium and ventricle causing mixing of oxygenated and deoxygenated blood (see Figure 11.10). As these babies have only one effective ventricle they depend on the patency of the ductus arteriosus for their systemic and coronary circulation (see Table 11.6).

Clinical presentation
A provisional diagnosis may have been made antenatally and a post-natal plan discussed with the cardiologists and cardiac surgeons but some infants still present post-natally. These infants are well at birth and mothers may have taken their babies home before any symptoms appear. Problems arise when the ductus arteriosus begins to close. The blood supply to the aorta comes from the pulmonary artery via the ductus arteriosus and as the duct begins to close the systemic circulation begins to fail (in a similar way to severe coarctation of the aorta). Initially,

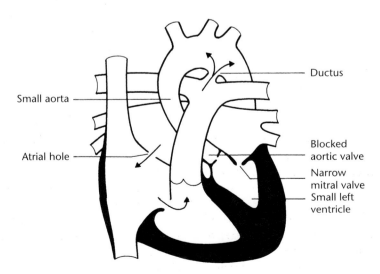

Figure 11.10   A schematic diagram of a hypoplastic left heart.

Table 11.6 Primary defects in hypoplastic left heart syndrome.

Diminutive aorta, sometimes aortic atresia
Mitral valve stenosis
Aortic valve stenosis
Mitral valve atresia
Hypoplastic left ventricle

the baby becomes breathless and blue on feeding before suddenly deteriorating as the duct closes fully. Symptoms include:

- Poor systemic perfusion
- Tachycardia
- Tachypnoea
- Respiratory distress
- Decreased peripheral pulses
- Decreased urinary output with cool extremities and mottling
- Enlarged liver

Diagnosis
The diagnosis of HLHS may be suspected on examination when the peripheral pulses are found to be absent or faint and the blood pressure equal but low on all limbs. Chest X-ray shows an enlarged globular heart outline with variable pulmonary vascular markings. The diagnosis is confirmed on echocardiography which demonstrates the small left ventricular cavity and ascending aorta and the nature of both the mitral valve and aortic valves.

Medical treatment
A prostaglandin infusion should be commenced to reopen the duct/maintain ductal patency while treatment options are considered. Surgical repair utilises the one effective ventricle as the systemic pumping chamber by a series of staged operations. The initial surgery is extremely difficult as the aorta has to be reconstructed and joined to the pulmonary artery, whilst the branch pulmonary arteries are disconnected from the main pulmonary artery, repaired and then resupplied with blood via a systemic to

pulmonary arterial shunt. Results are improving all the time but 10–30% of babies may not survive the first stage. At least two further operations are needed to establish a stable long-term circulation (the right ventricle pumps the blood to the aorta, the systemic veins are connected directly to the pulmonary arteries; the 'Fontan' circulation) and the long-term prognosis remains uncertain. Cardiac transplantation is not available for this condition in the neonatal period although it may be an option later, but still requires lifelong drug treatment and probably only lasts around 20 years. Hence some parents may decline surgery for their babies, and 'comfort care' remains a valid option for this condition.

Cyanotic congenital heart disease

These are defects with outflow obstruction to the right side of the heart with right to left shunting across a VSD or the foramen ovale or an ASD. They include:

- Tetralogy of Fallot
- Pulmonary atresia (or severe stenosis)

Although mild forms may not be duct dependent, in more severe forms the pulmonary circulation may be supplied from the aorta via the arterial duct.

Fallot's tetralogy
This is a defect causing a right ventricular outflow obstruction (see Figure 11.11). The condition usually consists of four linked anatomical defects. These are:

- Ventricular septal defect
- Aorta that overrides the ventricular septal defect, thus getting its supply from both ventricles
- Valvar, subvalvar or supravalvar pulmonary artery obstruction
- Right ventricular hypertrophy

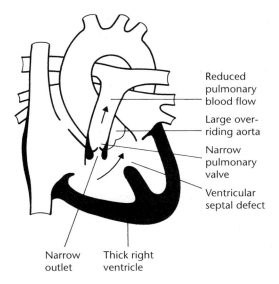

Reduced pulmonary blood flow

Large over-riding aorta

Narrow pulmonary valve

Ventricular septal defect

Narrow outlet

Thick right ventricle

Figure 11.11 Diagram illustrating Fallot's tetralogy.

The severity of this lesion depends on the degree of obstruction to the right ventricular outflow tract.

Clinical presentation
Infants with Fallot's tetralogy are often subclassified into 'pink' Fallots who have a mild degree of pulmonary stenosis and 'blue' Fallots who have a more severe degree of stenosis. If blood is unable to pass up through the pulmonary artery because of a severe pulmonary stenosis it shunts across the VSD and up the aorta. This is a right-to-left shunt and the degree of shunting will determine the degree of cyanosis at presentation (and hence duct dependency). The hypertrophy of the right ventricle occurs secondary to the associated pulmonary stenosis. Paroxysmal hypoxic or cyanotic 'spells' typically start at about two months of age and occur as a result of episodes of an increase in the right-to-left shunting. The baby will have a period of rapid deep breathing followed by a prolonged bout of irritable crying. There will be increasing cyanosis during this time and decreased heart sounds. A severe attack may cause limpness, unconsciousness, cerebrovascular accident or even

death. Management includes methods of non-pharmacologically increasing the systemic vascular resistance (knee-elbow positioning) to reverse the shunt or pharmacological management. Cyanotic 'spells' are an indication for surgery.

The chronic arterial desaturation seen in these patients may result in the development of finger clubbing and polycythaemia, which increases the risk of strokes. Bacterial endocarditis is also associated with Tetralogy of Fallot, so surgical repair is now generally performed much earlier than previously to avoid such complications.

Diagnosis
A provisional diagnosis may have been made antenatally and the definitive diagnosis will be also be made by echocardiography. Cardiac catheterisation may be required, particularly to define the coronary artery relationships prior to surgery, but increasingly surgery can be planned following echocardiography alone. Balloon dilatation of the pulmonary valve may also be helpful for extended palliation in some infants.

Medical management
Medical treatment is mainly the use of propranolol to reduce the incidence of cyantic spells in smaller infants.

Surgical management
The timing of surgical treatment is governed by the degree of pulmonary valve stenosis and the size of the pulmonary arteries[50]. Duct dependent babies and small infants with severe cyanosis or spells will generally require an initial arterio-pulmonary shunt (usually a Gore-Tex® tube between the subclavian/innominate artery and the right pulmonary artery), although some surgeons will now undertake primary repair in the neonatal period. Most babies will now undergo definitive repair before a year of age but very complex cases may require longer initial palliation. The VSD is closed on cardiopulmonary bypass and the pulmonary valve and muscle below it opened out to relieve the stenosis. Long-term survival is excellent although it is increasingly recognised

that replacement of the pulmonary valve may be required many years after surgery.

Isolated pulmonary valve stenosis (or indeed atresia; complete blockage) is generally present in a similar way to Tetralogy of Fallot in the newborn period, with cyanosis +/- collapse. Milder forms may simply be detected as a murmur later on. Most are treated with balloon dilatation of the pulmonary valve in the catheterisation laboratory, where a balloon catheter is guided through an artery in the groin up to the heart. When it reaches the stenosed area it is inflated to dilate the valve. Radio frequency energy catheters can be used to burn a hole through a completely blocked valve which can then be stretched up the same way. Hence, very few babies with this condition require surgical valvotomy now, and results are generally very good if the right ventricle is a reasonable size. Babies with very severe pulmonary stenosis/atresia may have very small right ventricles. These may never grow enough to support the circulation even if the pulmonary valve can be successfully opened up and these babies need an arteriopulmonary shunt and subsequent staged operations to achieve a Fontan circulation, similar to those for hypoplastic left heart syndrome.

Implications for practice

Infants with non-duct dependent lesions are less likely to require urgent admission to the NNU due to the CHD.

Other duct dependent problems

These include:

- Transposition of great arteries
- Tricuspid atresia

Transposition of the great arteries (TGA)

TGA is a life-threatening condition in which the aorta arises from the right ventricle and the pulmonary artery from the left ventricle. The left and right sides of the heart function as two parallel circuits (see Figure 11.12). Mixing of blood between the pulmonary and systemic circulations occurs *in utero* through the ductus arteriosus and foramen ovale but when these close, there is effectively no mixing of the two circulations unless there is an associated VSD (see Figure 11.7). When the diagnosis is suspected a prostaglandin infusion should be started to reopen the duct or keep it open.

Clinical presentation
This condition is less frequently diagnosed before birth and if not diagnosed antenatally, the baby generally presents soon after birth with deepening cyanosis which does not improve with oxygen administration. This is an emergency as even if the duct is open mixing may be inadequate without an urgent balloon septostomy. Definitive diagnosis is made by echocardiography.

Medical treatment
Most centres perform an early balloon septostomy to improve the mixing of blood, followed by an operation to revert the circulatory systems a week later. The surgery most preferred is the arterial switch procedure which was first used by Gaiters in 1975. The aorta and pulmonary artery are 'switched' back and correct implantation of the coronary arteries made. The most common complication following the switch procedure is pulmonary artery stenosis, which can be improved by balloon dilatation. Initial research results of the 'switch' operation found this operation was successful and gave a good quality of life to children of eight years of age who had had surgery in infancy[51], and the vast majority of children are now expected to survive long term, although there is a theoretical risk of longer term problems as well, especially with the coronary arteries.

Tricuspid valve atresia

This is a cyanotic lesion that is often associated with other anomalies such as ventricular septal defect, atrial septal defect or hypoplastic

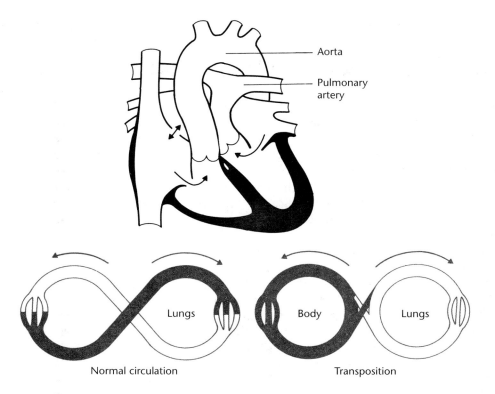

Aorta

Pulmonary
artery

Lungs

Body   Lungs

Normal circulation   Transposition

Figure 11.12   Schematic diagram of simple transposition of the great vessels without VSD.

right ventricle. Blood supply to the lungs is poor and if the atresia is complete, there is no outlet from the right atrium except through the ASD (see Figure 11.13). Survival depends on the size of the ASD or VSD and a patent ductus.

Clinical presentation
Like hypoplastic left heart syndrome, this is frequently diagnosed antenatally and the baby started on prostaglandin from birth. If not, the baby may present with severe cyanosis in the neonatal period if there is no VSD and/or if the pulmonary stenosis is very severe and the ductus arteriosus starts to close. Respiratory distress may be present with hypoxic episodes and poor feeding ability.

Medical treatment
A prostaglandin infusion should be commenced to keep the duct open if there is severe pulmonary/subpulmonary stenosis. A balloon

septostomy may also be required if the atrial septal communication is restrictive. The blood flow to the lungs needs to be adequate but not excessive and either arteriopulmonary shunting or pulmonary artery banding may be required depending on the precise anatomy. Since the tricuspid valve cannot be created, even if there is a good sized right ventricle filled from a VSD, long-term palliation is also achieved with the Fontan circulation.

Implications for practice

- Infants with duct dependent lesions will usually present within the first hours after birth.
- A prostaglandin (prostin) infusion will maintain ductal patency.
- Prostin may cause apnoea at higher doses and ventilatory support should be available.

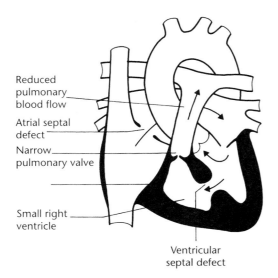

Reduced
pulmonary
blood flow

Atrial septal
defect

Narrow
pulmonary valve

Small right
ventricle

Ventricular
septal defect

Figure 11.13 Schematic diagram of tricuspid atresia.

The future outlook for those with congenital heart disease

The successful treatment of congenital cardiac defects means that many people who would have died or had their lives severely restricted by their condition can now live relatively active lives. Many conditions require extensive follow-up and some need long-term medication. Life span is likely to be reduced and late re-interventions may be required As babies who are born with cardiac defects increasingly survive into adulthood, they now present a different challenge to cardiologists in the medical and psychosocial aspects of the effects of the defect on adult health. As a result of modern paediatric cardiology a new and growing section of adults need life-long medical care and treatment to maintain their health[52].

Persistent ductus arteriosus

Embryology and physiology of the ductus arteriosus

The ductus arteriosus is an essential component of the foetal circulation (see Chapter 3).

It connects the proximal end of the left pulmonary artery to the top of the descending aorta just below the origin of the left subclavian artery and is one of three cardiovascular 'shunts' that are essential to maintain foetal circulation. Following the birth of the infant the ductus arteriosus closes as a result of contraction of smooth muscle within its wall. The major physiological factor influencing this process is the rise in oxygen tension. In addition, a reduced pulmonary vascular resistance and increased systemic vascular resistance results in reversal of the flow through the ductus from right to left in foetal life to left to right in neonatal life. On a molecular level there is a fall in the concentration of prostaglandin E_2 which is a potent ductal vasodilator in the foetus, associated with a rise in vasoconstrictors such as bradykinins.

Functional closure of the ductus arteriosus starts within hours of birth and is usually complete by 48 hours of age in the term infant. Complete anatomical closure may take several days to a few weeks and eventually all that is left is the ligamentum arteriosum.

Clinical relevance of the ductus arteriosus

There are four main situations when persistence of the ductus arteriosus is clinically important:

(1) Duct-dependent congenital heart disease: in these situations a pDA is necessary for survival to support either pulmonary or systemic blood flow and if it begins to close prostaglandin needs to be commenced urgently.
(2) Persistent pulmonary hypertension of the newborn (see Chapter 8): this may accompany clinical situations such as meconium aspiration syndrome or hypoplastic lungs. These infants will have increased *right to left* or *bidirectional* transductal shunting of blood, due to a failure of the pulmonary

vascular resistance to drop and an increased pulmonary vascular pressure.

(3) Idiopathic persistent ductus arteriosus: this refers to a ductus arteriosus that has failed to close for no obvious reason.

(4) The preterm infant: a patent ductus arteriosus is common in preterm infants and this is discussed in detail below.

Idiopathic persistent ductus arteriosus.

The incidence of an isolated persistent ductus arteriosus in the term infant may vary from 1 in 500 for the 'silent' pDA, to 1 in 2000 for 'symptomatic' pDAs. The term 'silent pDA' refers to a pDA that is anatomically patent and may be clinically apparent on examination but has not become 'symptomatic'. The clinical symptoms and signs will depend on the size of the duct and the size of any left to right shunt and they are likely to reach a maximum at three months of age which is when the pulmonary vascular resistance has reached its lowest point. The signs may include:

- Incidental murmur: this murmur has classically been described as a machinery murmur, which is heard throughout the cardiac cycle (systole and diastole)
- Bounding pulses: this term refers to pulses that are easily palpable, peak and then fall away quickly
- Active praecordium: this reflects the palpable activity of the left ventricle
- Evidence of pulmonary oedema and left ventricular volume overload: this occurs when the extent of the left to right shunt has led to left sided heart failure

Closure will be recommended even in asymptomatic ducts in view of the risk of endocarditis secondary to the turbulent blood flow through the duct. Methods of occlusion include the use of transcatheter devices that are threaded up through the femoral vein and surgical closure.

Persistent ductus arteriosus in the preterm infant

Anatomy and physiology

A pDA is a common finding in preterm infants and could be considered a normal anatomical occurrence in all preterm infants < 28 weeks gestation; these infants were expecting to be *in utero* for a further three months and they lack the smooth muscle to facilitate efficient ductal closure. One of the challenges of neonatal care in these situations is assessing whether the pDA is haemodynamically significant (HSDA) and whether the risks of closure are less than the risks of the HSDA itself[53].

Implication for practice

- PDA may be an associated feature of congenital heart disease and the presence of congenital heart disease must be considered even in the preterm infant.
- PDA is common in preterm infants, especially those of lower birthweight and gestational age.

Pathophysiology

In an unventilated moderately preterm infant with mild respiratory distress syndrome the pulmonary resistance will remain relatively high following delivery. This will occur because the lungs will not have completely opened up. As the lungs recover and they start to produce surfactant the pulmonary vascular resistance will fall and the difference between the systemic and pulmonary pressures will facilitate left to right blood flow through the duct if it has remained open.

The introduction of artificial surfactant and more effective ventilation techniques over the last 10 to 15 years has complicated this situation. One of the main aims of early neonatal management of the preterm infant is to normalise lung aeration as much as possible and so reduce the potential for lung injury through factors such as oxygen toxicity and trauma from positive pressure ventilation. A complication of this is that optimal ventilation and the use of surfactant will also lower the pulmonary resistance of the lung and this facilitates the early development of a left to right shunt which may become haemodynamically significant (HSDA). Patency does not necessarily imply pathophysiological impact. The term HSDA may be used to differentiate between a ductus arteriosus that is anatomically patent but does not have significant clinical effects (pDA) and one that has haemodynamic consequences[54].

The pathophysiological consequence of a HSDA in the preterm infant may be a significant blood flow from the systemic circulation (left) to the pulmonary circulation (right) with two main consequences:

- Increased flow to the pulmonary circulation and left ventricular volume and pressure overload
- Decreased flow to the systemic circulation with reduced perfusion of the brain, kidneys and gastrointestinal system (steal phenomenon)

Implications for practice

- The term pDA should be reserved for a patent duct that is not haemodynamically significant.
- A haemodynamically significant ductus should be referred to as HSDA.

Clinical features of a PDA in the preterm infant
The main clinical features of a HSDA can be summarised as:

- Signs of the duct itself
- Those resulting from a consequence of the altered pattern of blood flow:
  ○ Features of pulmonary oedema and left ventricular overload
  ○ Hypoperfusion of systemic organs

The severity of symptoms and signs of a duct primarily depend on the size of the shunt. This in turn is influenced by factors such as the size of the duct, systemic and pulmonary vascular resistance and underlying disease states.

Signs of pDA
The most commonly mentioned sign is a murmur. In the early stages this is often just systolic and loudest over the pulmonary area. As things progress clinically the murmur can develop into a continuous murmur heard throughout systole and diastole. It is heard over the praecordium and radiates to the left axilla.

Pulmonary oedema
- Increased pulmonary blood flow will contribute to an increased work of breathing such that the infant will show increasing respiratory distress, such as tachypnoea, sternal and intercostal recession
- An increasing incidence of apnoeas in the otherwise well preterm infant can also be associated with an underlying HSDA

Left ventricular overload
- An active praecordium is the result of the increased return of blood from the lungs to the left ventricle
- Easily palpable or 'bounding' peripheral pulses are the result of the increased systolic function of a volume loaded left ventricle and the lower diastolic component due to the quick run off as blood flows away from the aorta into the pulmonary circulation

Hypoperfusion of systemic organs
- Invasive arterial blood pressure monitoring may show a widened pulse pressure gap between the systolic and diastolic components. There may also be an overall lowering of both, leading to hypotension in the first 48–72 hours of life indicative of *relative* systemic hypovolaemia. This reflects the inability of the immature myocardium to increase its stroke as a means to augment cardiac output.
- Complications of the reduced blood flow in the descending aorta include metabolic acidosis, renal impairment and an increased susceptibility to necrotising enterocolitis (NEC). A further significant complication is intraventricular haemorrhage, which can be associated with significant neurodevelopmental morbidity.

One of the main concerns of an HSDA is that it may affect the ability of an extreme preterm infant to wean from the ventilator. The nurse caring for these infants may report that the saturation levels are consistently 'swinging' and that the infant is tachycardic. This variation in peripherally measured oxygen saturations occurs secondary to episodes of right to left shunting which may be occurring through an open duct or at an intrapulmonary level and does not respond to an increase in FiO_2. In an infant that has been extubated there may be a deterioration in respiratory parameters with tachypnoea and increased respiratory distress. The presence of an HSDA is associated with an increased risk of chronic lung disease and pulmonary haemorrhage.

Over time, as the heart struggles to maintain an effective systemic circulation the infant will show signs of cardiac failure with pulmonary oedema and peripheral oedema, an increased oxygen requirement, low blood pressure, poor colour and mottling, prolonged capillary refill time, reduced urine output and poor growth. Blood gas analysis may demonstrate a respiratory acidosis +/− a metabolic component. As these signs may also be suggestive of sepsis, it is imperative that this is ruled out.

The main long-term morbidity associated with a persistent HSDA is an increased risk of chronic lung disease, but otherwise there is no evidence it has any other significant long-term impact, despite its undoubted association with short-term morbidity.

Implications for practice

- An HSDA causes clinical features that occur as a result of increased pulmonary blood flow and decreased systemic blood flow.
- Signs and symptoms of an HSDA may be similar to those associated with sepsis, which should be excluded.
- A definitive diagnosis of a HSDA requires echocardiography.

Echocardiographic features

Echocardiography has now become accepted as an essential part of the evaluation of the significance of the ductus arteriosus in the premature infant on the neonatal unit. The most important measurements are the size of the duct itself, the characteristics of the flow pattern across the duct, evidence of systemic hypoperfusion and evidence of volume overload to the left side of the heart (LA:Ao ratio). This is done using 2D echocardiography with colour wave Doppler.

A short axis left parasternal view allows direct measurement of the size of the duct. The additional use of colour wave signals helps with this measurement and also enables direct observation of the shunt direction. In infants less than 1500 g birthweight a duct size of greater than 1.5 mm diameter is usually significant whilst a diameter greater than 2.0 mm has been shown to equate to twice as much pulmonary blood flow as systemic[55].

Continuous wave Doppler of the descending aorta is used to identify evidence of systemic hypoperfusion. Flow down the aorta should be continuously in a forward direction. As the shunt through the duct increases the diastolic component of the Doppler signal will reduce, eventually becoming negative, indicating a reversal of flow (retrograde flow) due to the steal phenomenon. This may clinically equate to an infant in whom there is feeding intolerance or a deterioration in renal function. M mode (motion mode) echocardiography has been used to measure the diameters of the aortic root (Ao) and left atrium (LA) in diastole. From these an LA:Ao ratio is calculated which is an indirect measure of the degree of shunting through the ductus and hence its haemodynamic significance. A ratio of greater than 1.4:1.0 is suggestive of a significant ductus shunt. However, these measurements are subjective and potentially influenced by a number of factors such as other shunts (including VSDs and PFOs), intravascular volume, use of diuretics and underlying disease severity. The LA:Ao ratio cannot be considered as a reliable measure of duct significance in isolation.

Studies in recent years have shown that a haemodynamically significant duct can be detected by echocardiography at least 48–72 hours before it becomes clinically apparent[56]. As a result there is an increasing move toward early echocardiographic measurements to guide treatment decisions. In determining haemodynamic significance it should be noted that no one measure is on its own reliable and most authors recommend combining 2D echocardiography with Doppler wave studies and m-mode measurements to define the size and significance of the duct in the preterm infant more accurately.

What is a significant duct?

In the past a pDA has been referred to as either 'significant' or not. The significance was then sub-classified as clinically significant or echocardiographically significant and more recently it has been proposed that all preterm infants at risk of HSDA should have early and serially performed echocardiography to guide management decisions[57]. It has recently been proposed that the significance should be graded or staged using clinical and echocardiographic criteria, with the aim of more accurately predicting which infants need active management of their pDA[58]. This system recognises that there is a spectrum of severity which would seem to represent clinical reality more accurately.

Management decisions

The gold standard in management would be the ability to prevent the development of an HSDA and to promote ductal closure within the first few days of life. There may be some aspects of the management of the preterm infant that can reduce the risk of the development of an HSDA. These would include meticulous attention to detail in fluid balance (see Chapter 7):

- Avoiding overhydration: some neonatal units would advocate a mild degree of dehydration as long as systemic blood flow is maintained.

This is particularly relevant if non-steroidal anti-inflammatory therapy is being used (ibuprofen, indomethacin).
- Minimising fluid or bicarbonate boluses.
- Accurately recording the volume of flushes used in arterial lines or after medications.

Other supportive care for infants with a pDA includes:

- Temperature control: ensuring that the infant is nursed in a thermoneutral environment to reduce the risks of pulmonary vasoconstriction.
- Oxygenation and ventilation:
  ○ Avoiding hypoxia (SpO2 < 85%) or significant acidosis (pH < 7.2).
  ○ Hyperoxia should also be avoided and monitoring with transcutaneous monitors as well as oxygen saturation monitors may be useful.
  ○ Allowing a permissive hypercapnia, together with avoiding hyperoxia may maintain a slightly higher pulmonary vascular resistance which will help to minimise the transductal shunt.
- Management of hypotension: hypotension should be managed with inotropes which augment cardiac output, e.g. dobutamine. Treatments with vasoconstricting properties (e.g. dopamine) may increase left-to-right transductal shunt by elevating systemic vascular resistance.
- Management of anaemia: in the early correction of anaemia when transfusing infants with pDAs there is often the question of whether to give diuretic cover or not using frusemide. There is evidence indicating that frusemide can potentiate patency of the duct when given regularly and this is no longer recommended as part of any treatment regime for ducts. However, a blood transfusion represents a significant volume which may also encourage ducts to remain open.

The main treatment strategies are medical treatment (indomethacin or ibuprofen), surgical ligation or supportive expectant management waiting for spontaneous ductal closure.

Medical closure

The use of a prostaglandin inhibitor such as the non-steroidal anti-inflammatory medications, indomethacin or ibuprofen may promote ductal closure by causing constriction of the smooth muscle within the duct. The main area of controversy is whether to treat prophylactically, on echocardiographic evidence or clinical evidence. Large clinical trials have shown no benefit for prophylaxis and current evidence indicates that early targeted treatment on the basis of echocardiographic findings may be a more successful approach with fewer side effects with treatment being started within the first three days. However, the staging system already referred to may enable treatment to be targeted more accurately to those infants that need it, facilitate a more accurate appraisal of response to therapy and guide future trials of therapeutic intervention.

Side effects of prostaglandin inhibitors include:

- Bleeding due to reduced platelet adhesive properties: oozing from puncture sites, blood in gastric aspirates and stools, petechiae
- Decreased renal function: urine output < 1 ml/kg/day, increase in serum urea > 5 mmol/l and creatinine > 100 mmol/l
- Electrolyte disturbances: hyponatreamia and hypokalaemia due to water retention, hypoglycaemia
- Gastro-intestinal effects: NEC, intestinal perforations
- Hyperbilirubinaemia: due to displacement of bilirubin from binding sites

It is important that strict monitoring for these side effects takes place throughout the course and for at least 48 hours after completion. The two most commonly used dosage regimes of indomethacin are a low dose regimen over six days (0.1 mg/kg 12 hourly) or a high dose over three days (0.2 mg/kg 12 hourly). The administration of indomethacin may achieve functional ductal closure but until anatomical closure has been achieved the duct remains at risk of reopening with an altered clinical status. Ibuprofen is claimed to have less side effects than indomethacin but the evidence suggests there is no difference in efficacy. The most commonly used ibuprofen dosage regime is a single three-day course (10 mg $\times$ 1 dose; 5 mg $\times$ 2 doses).

If a medical regime is unsuccessful it may be worth considering a second course, but after 21 days of age the success rates for closure with medication diminish.

Surgical closure

Definitive closure may be achieved surgically by duct ligation or the occlusion of the duct using a surgical clip. The risks associated with surgery include:

- Risks of transferring an unstable infant to a cardiac centre, which may be at a different hospital
- General anaesthetic
- Haemorrhage
- Pneumothorax
- Clipping the wrong vessel
- Wound sepsis
- Phrenic nerve injury
- Post-ligation cardiac syndrome (PLCS) characterised by oxygenation failure and systolic hypotension secondary to left ventricular dysfunction

The decision to treat with medication or surgery can be a difficult one. Indomethacin and Ibuprofen given early have been shown to have a good success rate for closure and obviously reduce the need for surgical intervention. This is usually the treatment of first choice. In those infants that fail pharmacological treatment, or are deemed unsuitable, surgery is the next step.

Children outside the neonatal period, and adults, with patent ductus arteriosus are treated primarily with closure using occluding devices and 'coils' placed via a transcatheter route.

All of these strategies have an associated mortality and morbidities and treatment of a HSDA has not always shown an improvement in the measured outcomes of CLD or NEC. The improved classification of a HSDA and targeted treatment may facilitate enhanced decision making and improve outcome data.

Implications for practice

The neonatal nurse caring for infants receiving indomethacin should be aware of the potential side effects of indomethacin and any change in the infant's condition:

- Reduced urine output < 1 ml/kg.
- Bleeding from puncture sites.
- Blood in stools/gastric aspirates/poor toleration of feeds.
- Increase in jaundice level.
- Electrolyte disturbances.

Conclusion

This chapter has aimed to revise some of the important methods of cardiovascular assessment and to cover the three main areas of hypotension, congenital heart disease and the assessment and management of a pDA in the preterm infant. A clear understanding of the anatomy of the heart along with knowledge of the physiology of extra-uterine adaptation will facilitate the ability to nurse these challenging conditions effectively.

References

1. Sadler TW (1990) *Langman's Medical Embryology*, 6th edn. William and Wilkins, Baltimore, Maryland.
2. Crossland DS, Furness JC, Abu-Harb M, Sadagopan SN, Wren C (2004) Variability of four limb blood pressure in normal neonates. *Arch Dis Child Foetal Neonatal Ed*, **89** (4), F325–F327.
3. Gevers M, van Genderingen HR, Lafeber HN, Hack WW (1996) Accuracy of oscillometric blood pressure measurement in critically ill neonates with reference to the arterial pressure wave shape. *Intensive Care Med*, **22** (3), 242–248.
4. Gevers M, van Genderingen HR, Lafeber HN, Hack WW (1996) Accuracy of oscillometric blood pressure measurement in critically ill neonates with reference to the arterial pressure wave shape. *Intensive Care Med*, **22** (3), 242–248.
5. Crossland DS, Furness JC, Abu-Harb M, Sadagopan SN, Wren C (2004) Variability of four limb blood pressure in normal neonates. *Arch Dis Child Foetal Neonatal Ed*, **89** (4), F325–F327.
6. Fernandez E, Schrader R, Watterberg K (2005) Prevalence of low cortisol values in term and near-term infants with vasopressor-resistant hypotension. *J Perinatol*, **25** (2), 114–118.
7. Efird MM, Heerens AT, Gordon PV, Bose CL, Young DA (2005) A randomized-controlled trial of prophylactic hydrocortisone supplementation for the prevention of hypotension in extremely low birth weight infants. *J Perinatol*, **25** (2), 119–124.
8. Nuntnarumit P, Yang W, Bada-Ellzey HS (1999) Blood pressure measurements in the newborn. *Clin Perinatol*, **26** (4), 981–96, x.
9. Watkins AM, West CR, Cooke RW (1989) Blood pressure and cerebral haemorrhage and ischaemia in very low birthweight infants. *Early Hum Dev*, **19** (2), 103–110.
10. Watkins AM, West CR, Cooke RW (1989) Blood pressure and cerebral haemorrhage and ischaemia in very low birthweight infants. *Early Hum Dev*, **19** (2), 103–110.
11. Nuntnarumit P, Yang W, Bada-Ellzey HS (1999) Blood pressure measurements in the newborn. *Clin Perinatol*, **26** (4), 981–96, x.
12. Watkins AM, West CR, Cooke RW (1989) Blood pressure and cerebral haemorrhage and ischaemia in very low birthweight infants. *Early Hum Dev*, **19** (2), 103–110.
13. Nuntnarumit P, Yang W, Bada-Ellzey HS (1999) Blood pressure measurements in the newborn. *Clin Perinatol*, **26** (4), 981–96, x.
14. Watkins AM, West CR, Cooke RW (1989) Blood pressure and cerebral haemorrhage and ischaemia in very low birthweight infants. *Early Hum Dev*, **19** (2), 103–110.
15. Fernandez E, Schrader R, Watterberg K (2005) Prevalence of low cortisol values in term and near-term infants with vasopressor-resistant hypotension. *J Perinatol*, **25** (2), 114–118.

16. Efird MM, Heerens AT, Gordon PV, Bose CL, Young DA (2005) A randomized-controlled trial of prophylactic hydrocortisone supplementation for the prevention of hypotension in extremely low birth weight infants. *J Perinatol*, **25** (2), 119–124.

17. Finer NN, Powers RJ, Ou CH, Durand D, Wirtschafter D, Gould JB (2006) Prospective evaluation of postnatal steroid administration: a 1-year experience from the California Perinatal Quality Care Collaborative. *Pediatrics*, **117** (3), 704–713.

18. Ng PC, Lee CH, Bnur FL, *et al.* (2006) A double-blind, randomized, controlled study of a 'stress dose' of hydrocortisone for rescue treatment of refractory hypotension in preterm infants. *Pediatrics*, **117** (2), 367–375.

19. Gill AB, Weindling AM (1993) Randomised controlled trial of plasma protein fraction versus dopamine in hypotensive very low birth-weight infants. *Arch Dis Child*, **69** (3 Spec. No.), 284–287.

20. Osborn DA, Evans N (2004) Early volume expansion for prevention of morbidity and mortality in very preterm infants. *Cochrane Database Syst Rev* (2), CD002055.

21. Greenough A, Cheeseman P, Kavvadia V, Dimitriou G, Morton M (2002) Colloid infusion in the perinatal period and abnormal neurodevelopmental outcome in very low birth weight infants. *Eur J Pediatr*, **161** (6), 319–323.

22. Kavvadia V, Greenough A, Dimitriou G, Hooper R (2000) Randomised trial of fluid restriction in ventilated very low birthweight infants. *Arch Dis Child Foetal Neonatal Ed*, **83** (2), F91–F96.

23. CESDI, Project 27/28. (2003) *An Enquiry into the Quality of Care and its Effects on the Survival of Babies Born at 27–28 Weeks.* Maternal and Child Health Research Consortium, London.

24. Osborn DA, Evans N (2004) Early volume expansion for prevention of morbidity and mortality in very preterm infants. *Cochrane Database Syst Rev* (2), CD002055.

25. Greenough A, Cheeseman P, Kavvadia V, Dimitriou G, Morton M (2002) Colloid infusion in the perinatal period and abnormal neurodevelopmental outcome in very low birth weight infants. *Eur J Pediatr*, **161** (6), 319–323.

26) Kavvadia V, Greenough A, Dimitriou G, Hooper R (2000) Randomised trial of fluid restriction in ventilated very low birthweight infants. *Arch Dis Child Foetal Neonatal Ed*, **83** (2), F91–F96.

27. So KW, Fok TF, Ng PC, Wong W, Cheung KL (1997) Randomised controlled trial of colloid or crystalloid in hypotensive preterm infants. *Arch Dis Child Foetal Neonatal Ed*, **76** (1), F43–F46.

28. Alderson P, Schierhout G, Roberts I, Bunn F (2000) Colloids versus crystalloids for fluid resuscitation in critically ill patients. *Cochrane Database Syst Rev* (2), CD000567.

29. Subhedar NV, Shaw NJ (2003) Dopamine versus dobutamine for hypotensive preterm infants. *Cochrane Database Syst Rev* (3), CD001242.

30. Zhang J, Penny DJ, Kim NS, Yu VY, Smolich JJ (1999) Mechanisms of blood pressure increase induced by dopamine in hypotensive preterm neonates. *Arch Dis Child Foetal Neonatal Ed*, **81** (2), F99–F104.

31. Ng PC, Lee CH, Bnur FL, *et al.* (2006) A double-blind, randomized, controlled study of a 'stress dose' of hydrocortisone for rescue treatment of refractory hypotension in preterm infants. *Pediatrics*, **117** (2), 367–375.

32. Bourchier D, Weston PJ (1997) Randomised trial of dopamine compared with hydrocortisone for the treatment of hypotensive very low birthweight infants. *Arch Dis Child Foetal Neonatal Ed*, **76** (3), F174–F178.

33. Paradisis M, Osborn DA (2004) Adrenaline for prevention of morbidity and mortality in preterm infants with cardiovascular compromise. *Cochrane Database Syst Rev* (1), CD003958.

34. Wren C, Richmond S, Donaldson L (2000) Temporal variability in birth prevalence of cardiovascular malformations. *Heart*, **83** (4), 414–419.

35. Paul KE (1995) Recognition, stabilization, and early management of infants with critical congenital heart disease presenting in the first days of life. *Neonatal Netw*, **14** (5), 13–20.

36. Nieminen HP, Jokinen EV, Sairanen HI (2001) Late results of pediatric cardiac surgery in Finland: a population-based study with 96% follow-up. *Circulation*, **104** (5), 570–575.

37. Deanfield J, Thaulow E, Warnes C, *et al.* (2003) Management of grown-up congenital heart disease. *Eur Heart J*, **24** (11), 1035–1084.

38. Billett J, Majeed A, Gatzoulis M, Cowie M (2008) Trends in hospital admissions, in-hospital case fatality and population mortality from congenital heart disease in England, 1994 to 2004. *Heart*, **94** (3), 342–348.

39. Clur SA, Mathijssen IB, Pajkrt E, *et al.* (2008) Structural heart defects associated with an increased nuchal translucency: 9 years experience

in a referral centre. *Prenat Diagn*, **28** (4), 347–354.

40. Simpson LL, Malone FD, Bianchi DW, *et al.* (2007) Nuchal translucency and the risk of congenital heart disease. *Obstet Gynecol*, **109** (2 Pt 1), 376–383.

41. Wren C (1996) Foetal cardiography. *Current Paediatrics*, **6** (3), 145–149.

42. Browning Carmo KA, Barr P, West M, Hopper NW, White JP, Badawi N (2007) Transporting newborn infants with suspected duct dependent congenital heart disease on low-dose prostaglandin E1 without routine mechanical ventilation. *Arch Dis Child Foetal Neonatal Ed*, **92** (2), F117–F119.

43. Browning Carmo KA, Barr P, West M, Hopper NW, White JP, Badawi N (2007) Transporting newborn infants with suspected duct dependent congenital heart disease on low-dose prostaglandin E1 without routine mechanical ventilation. *Arch Dis Child Foetal Neonatal Ed*, **92** (2), F117–F119.

44. Rikard DH (1993) Nursing care of the neonate receiving prostaglandin E1 therapy. *Neonatal Netw*, **12** (4), 17–22.

45. Rikard DH (1993) Nursing care of the neonate receiving prostaglandin E1 therapy. *Neonatal Netw*, **12** (4), 17–22.

46. Jonas RA (1995) Advances in surgical care of infants and children with congenital heart disease. *Curr Opin Pediatr*, **7** (5), 572–579.

47. Kelnar, CJH, Harvey DR, Simpson C (2005) *The Sick Newborn Baby*, 4th edn. Baillière Tindall, London.

48. Paul KE (1995) Recognition, stabilization, and early management of infants with critical congenital heart disease presenting in the first days of life. *Neonatal Netw*, **14** (5), 13–20.

49. Jonas RA (1995) Advances in surgical care of infants and children with congenital heart disease. *Curr Opin Pediatr*, **7** (5), 572–579.

50. Allan L, Baker EJ (1993) Prenatal diagnosis and correction of congenital heart defects. *Br J Hosp Med*, **50** (9), 513–522.

51. Jonas RA (1995) Advances in surgical care of infants and children with congenital heart disease. *Curr Opin Pediatr*, **7** (5), 572–579.

52. Thorne S, Deanfield J (1996) Long-term outlook in treated congenital heart disease. *Arch Dis Child*, **75** (1), 6–8.

53. McNamara PJ, Sehgal A (2007) Towards rational management of the patent ductus arteriosus: the need for disease staging. *Arch Dis Child Foetal Neonatal Ed*, **92** (6), F424–F427.

54. McNamara PJ, Sehgal A (2007) Towards rational management of the patent ductus arteriosus: the need for disease staging. *Arch Dis Child Foetal Neonatal Ed*, **92** (6), F424–F427.

55. Evans N (2003) Current controversies in the diagnosis and treatment of patent ductus arteriosus in preterm infants. *Adv Neonatal Care*, **3** (4), 168–177.

56. Evans N (2003) Current controversies in the diagnosis and treatment of patent ductus arteriosus in preterm infants. *Adv Neonatal Care*, **3** (4), 168–177.

57. Evans N (2003) Current controversies in the diagnosis and treatment of patent ductus arteriosus in preterm infants. *Adv Neonatal Care*, **3** (4), 168–177.

58. McNamara PJ, Sehgal A (2007) Towards rational management of the patent ductus arteriosus: the need for disease staging. *Arch Dis Child Foetal Neonatal Ed*, **92** (6), F424–F427.

Chapter 12

NUTRITION OF THE TERM AND PRETERM INFANT

Lucy Hawkes and Michelle Paterson

Learning outcomes

After reading this chapter the reader will be expected to be able to:

- Categorise the basic nutrients required for growth and explain their role in the growth of the infant

- Explain the different methods of providing nutrients that can be used in both the preterm and term infant

- In preterm and term infants discuss:

  o The use of breast milk

  o The benefits of breast milk

  o The limitations of breast milk

  o The supplementation of breast milk

- Discuss the benefits and risks of parenteral nutrition

- Explain the advantages and disadvantages of available routes of parenteral nutrition administration

- Demonstrate the safe administration of parenteral nutrition

---

Introduction

Nutrition plays an essential role in the growth and development of both term and preterm infants. Breast milk remains the optimal nutrition for healthy term infants and term infants fed with breast milk have many advantages over those fed with formula; this includes protection against infection in the short term (essential in the developing world) and a reduced risk of the development of obesity in the long term as well as other probable benefits. The education and support of mothers in breast-feeding should be one of the aims of all professionals working in the perinatal specialities.

The provision of optimal nutrition for preterm infants and other low birthweight and sick infants forms an essential part of their management. In the short term, it may affect recovery from illness and in the longer term there is increasing evidence that early attention to their energy and growth requirements can have a profound effect on later outcome in terms of growth, intellectual and physical function.

These areas will be discussed in more detail within this chapter, together with the role of the neonatal nurse, who has an essential part to play both in feeding the infant and supporting the parents in feeding.

Nutritional requirements of term and preterm infants

The principle of good post-natal nutrition of the preterm infant is to provide the nutrients and energy to equal the growth rate of the age matched unborn foetus. During the last trimester of pregnancy there is a relatively large transfer and accumulation of nutrients, which includes 67% of a term newborn's mineral requirements as well as 36% of its body protein[1]. The average growth rate or weight gain during this time is 14–17 g a day[2], as the foetus lays down fat as an efficient energy store. An infant born before the last trimester will therefore be significantly disadvantaged regarding its nutrient and energy stores; for example an infant born weighing 1 kg has enough energy stores to survive for only four days without nutrition[3].

Nutrients can be divided into two groups, namely macronutrients and micronutrients. Macronutrients are energy-producing nutrients and include carbohydrates, fat and protein. Micronutrients refer to vitamins and minerals.

The nutritional requirements of term and preterm infants are summarised in Table 12.1. The following section explains this in more detail. It begins with the definition and function of each nutrient before briefly reviewing the situation *in utero*, in the term infant, and finally the preterm infant.

Energy

Energy is essential for basic functional requirements, maturation of the brain and other organs, and the growth of the infant. A term infant with increased energy expenditure will have an increased energy requirement and if this is not met and persists, the growth of the infant will be poor. Some causes of high energy expenditure are listed below:

- Hypothermia
- Increased temperature (hyperthermia)
- Infection
- Respiratory distress
- Congenital heart disease

Due to poor nutrient and energy stores, the energy requirements of preterm infants are much

Table 12.1 Nutritional requirements of preterm infants compared to term infants4 (Department of Health. Report on Health and Social Subjects No. 41 (1991) *Dietary Reference Values for Food Energy and Nutrients for the United Kingdom*. The Stationery Office, London).

Nutrients	ELBW ~ (< 27/40) After day 7 (growing phase)	VLBW # (27–31/40) After day 7 (growing phase)	Term
Energy (Kcal/kg)	130–150	110–130	100–115
Protein (g/kg)	3.8–4.4	3.2–3.8	2.1
Fluid (ml/kg)	160–220	135–190	150
Sodium (mmol/kg)	3–5	3–5	1.5
Potassium (mmol/kg)	2–3	2–3	3.4
Calcium (mmol/kg)	2.5–5.5	2.5–5.5	2.1
Phosphate (mmol/kg)	1.9–4.5	1.9–4.5	2.1
Iron (mg/day)	2–4	2–4	1.7
Zinc (mg/day)	1–3	1–3	0.9
Selenium (µg/day)	1.3–4.5	1.3–4.5	1.6
Vitamin A (IU/day)	700–1500	700–1500	580
Vitamin D (IU/day)	150–400*	150–400*	340
Vitamin E (IU/day)	6–12	6–12	2.2

~ ELBW – extremely low birthweight (<1kg)
# VLBW – very low birthweight (1–1.5 kg)
* Aim for a maximum of 400 IU/day

higher than those born at term, with extremely low birthweight infants having a 15–35% higher energy requirement than infants with a very low birthweight as seen in Table 12.1.

Protein

Proteins can be defined as a group of complex macromolecules that contain carbon, hydrogen, oxygen, nitrogen and usually sulphur. Proteins are made up of a chain of smaller molecules, called amino acids. Each protein has a characteristic structure, which is dependent on the order of amino acids and the manner in which the chain folds in space. This structure determines the function of the protein: transport function (haemoglobin transports oxygen by way of the blood), defence against micro-organisms (antibodies), hormonal activity (insulin, adrenalin, etc.), activation of biochemical reactions within cells (enzymes), and many others. Proteins are essential in the diet for the growth and repair of tissue and can be obtained from foods such as milk, fish, eggs, meat and legumes.

Term infants require 2.1 g of protein per kilogram. Premature infants have lower reserves and increased growth requirements and require between 3.2 and 4.4 g of protein per kilogram depending on their prematurity.

Fluid

Fluid balance refers to the concept of equilibrium between the amount of fluid lost from the body and the amount of fluid taken in (see Chapter 7). To maintain normal body fluid composition the following factors need to be taken into account:

- Insensible losses: significant amounts of fluid may be lost through trans-epidermal water losses (see Chapters 6 and 7)
- Sensible losses: urinary output
- Additional ongoing losses: losses from large aspirates, vomiting, diarrhoea or from exposed lesions such as open gastroschisis exomphalos (see Chapter 9), spina bifida

- Necessary fluid restrictions: renal failure, heart failure and patent ductus arteriosus

Most term infants require 150 ml/kg per day of fluids to meet their energy requirements and to ensure growth and development. Term infants who are on a neonatal unit may often be fluid restricted due to their medical status. Long-term fluid restriction may lead to poor weight gain and a more energy-dense feed will be required.

Most preterm infants require 150–200 ml/kg per day of fluids to meet their increased energy requirements. Very preterm infants are usually on parenteral nutrition (PN) for the first week of life while enteral feeds are being introduced and increased. PN is decreased as enteral feeds are increased. Once the preterm infant has reached and tolerates full enteral feeds (150 ml/kg/day), the fluid volume may be increased further to ensure nutritional adequacy from enteral feeds.

Micronutrients

A micronutrient is a substance, such as a vitamin or mineral, that is essential in very small amounts for the adequate growth and metabolism of a living organism. A term infant receiving full enteral feeds usually meets its micronutrient requirements except in the specific circumstances mentioned below. Micronutrient requirements are increased in premature infants as they have fewer reserves, as described above.

Minerals
Sodium
Sodium chloride (salt) is essential for life. Sodium (Na^+) and chloride (Cl^-) are the principal ions in the fluid outside cells (extracellular fluid), which includes blood plasma. They play critical roles in a number of life-sustaining processes like maintenance of membrane potential, nutrient absorption and transport, as well as maintenance of blood volume and blood pressure.

Term infants require about 1.5 mmol of sodium per kilogram per day. Preterm infants require between 3 and 5 mmol of sodium per kilogram per day due to high sodium losses from their immature kidneys. In preterm infants who have had bowel surgery, the sodium requirements may be even higher than the above recommendation.

Calcium and phosphate

Calcium is one of the most important micronutrients in the diet because it is a structural component of bones, teeth and soft tissues, and is essential in many of the body's metabolic processes. Calcium is used to regulate the permeability and electrical properties of biological membranes (such as cell walls), which in turn control muscle and nerve functions, glandular secretions, and blood vessel dilation and contraction. Calcium is also essential for blood clotting. Most dietary calcium is absorbed in the small intestine.

Phosphorus is an essential mineral that is required by every cell in the body for normal function. The majority of the phosphorus in the body is found as phosphate. Dietary phosphorus is readily absorbed in the small intestine, and any excess is excreted by the kidneys. Inadequate phosphorus intake leads to hypophosphataemia. The effects of hypophosphataemia may include anaemia, muscle weakness, rickets, osteopenia and increased susceptibility to infection.

Preterm infants' calcium and phosphate requirements are increased due to poor stores. Breast milk fortifier and all preterm formula feeds meet the requirements for calcium and phosphate if given at 150 ml/kg per day or higher.

Iron

Iron stores are acquired during the last trimester of pregnancy. During development, iron is needed for erythropoiesis (production of blood cells), brain development, muscle function and cardiac function. Infants born at term should have enough iron stores to ensure a good iron status until solids are started at six months of age.

Premature infants have poor iron stores and it has been shown that their iron stores become depleted at about eight weeks of age[5]. An iron

supplement is usually started between 4–6 weeks of age (unless the infant is on a preterm formula that contains adequate iron supplementation) and continued until the infant is on a varied diet or about one year of age.

Trace elements

Trace elements are chemical elements required in minute quantities by an organism to maintain proper physical functioning. Some studies have shown the following benefits: protein synthesis, antioxidant effects, immune function, muscle function, cognitive function and bone function. The most important trace elements for infants are: selenium, zinc, copper and iodine. Although trace element levels are not routinely monitored, term infants should meet their minimum requirements via enteral feeds. Infants who receive long-term parenteral nutrition are more at risk of trace element deficiencies.

Vitamins

Vitamins are nutrients required for essential metabolic reactions in the body. Vitamins are classified as either water soluble or fat soluble.

Water soluble vitamins

Water soluble vitamins are not stored and are eliminated in urine. Water soluble vitamins include vitamin B1, vitamin B2, vitamin B3, vitamin B6, vitamin B12, vitamin C, pantothenic acid, biotin and folate.

Term and preterm infants' requirements are usually met via their appropriate enteral feed. They can, however, easily be supplemented by a multivitamin supplement as these contain the major water soluble vitamins.

Fat soluble vitamins

Fat soluble vitamins dissolve in fat before they are absorbed in the bloodstream to carry out their functions. Excesses of these vitamins are stored in the liver. Because they are stored, they are not needed every day in the diet. These vitamins include vitamin A, vitamin D, vitamin E and vitamin K. Infants who have cholestasis or long-standing severe liver disease may require additional fat soluble vitamins as they have impaired absorption.

Vitamin A

Vitamin A plays an important role in the formation and maintenance of healthy skin, hair, and mucous membranes and is necessary for vision, growth and development, immunity and reproduction.

Preterm infants may require up to three times more vitamin A than an infant born at term. Most preterm infants are routinely supplemented with vitamin A via a multivitamin supplement.

Vitamin D

Vitamin D is essential for maintaining normal calcium metabolism. It can be synthesised by humans in the skin upon exposure to ultraviolet-B (UVB) radiation from sunlight, or it can be obtained from the diet.

Vitamin D requirements are only slightly higher in preterm infants when compared to term infants, but vitamin D remains an important nutrient to prevent rickets. The maximum recommended dose for vitamin D is 400 IU/day as there has been no benefit shown in infants receiving higher doses[6]. These requirements are usually met via appropriate enteral feeds.

Vitamin E

The main function of vitamin E in humans appears to be that of an antioxidant. Severe vitamin E deficiency results mainly in neurological symptoms, including impaired balance and coordination (ataxia), injury to the sensory nerves (peripheral neuropathy), muscle weakness (myopathy), and damage to the retina of the eye (pigmented retinopathy).

Infants with a birthweight of 1.5 kg or more are able to maintain their vitamin E status much better than smaller birthweight infants. Vitamin E deficiency in preterm infants could increase the risk of retinopathy of prematurity. Vitamin E requirements are usually met via appropriate enteral feed.

Long chain poly-unsaturated fatty acids (LCPs)

The n-3 and n-6 fatty acids linolenic acid and linoleic acid are precursors of the n-3 and n-6 LCPs. In the past, infant formula only contained the fatty acid precursors of the LCPs and controversy still exists over whether LCPs are also essential nutrients in infancy, improving growth, visual and cognitive development.

Maternal diets can be very varied but similar amounts of LCPs are found in all breast milk[7]. There are currently no specific recommendations made for LCPs, but now all term, preterm and nutrient-enriched post-discharge formulas have LCPs added.

Nucleotides

A nucleotide is defined as a cellular constituent that is one of the building blocks of ribonucleic acids (RNA) and deoxyribonucleic acid (DNA). Breast milk is a good source of nucleic acid and nucleotides[8].

In term infants the advantages of nucleotides are improved growth, reduced diarrhoea and support of the immune system[9]. Due to lack of evidence there are currently no recommendations for supplementation of nucleotides in preterm formula but all preterm and term formula do have nucleotides added.

Prebiotics

Prebiotics are non-digestible carbohydrates, which encourage the growth of friendly bacteria in the gut and in turn support the natural immune system. Breast milk naturally contains prebiotics and some of the term and preterm formulas (Milupa and Cow & Gate) now also have prebiotics added to them.

Implications for practice

- Infants born prematurely have poor stores of macronutrients and micronutrients.
- Preterm infants have higher requirements than term infants due to poor stores.

Part I

Enteral feeding: term infant

Breast milk

Breast milk is the optimal source of nutrition for term infants and in addition it provides the following benefits:

- Immunological
  - Colostrum contains immunoglobulins, which help protect the infant against infections
  - Infants fed breast milk have less incidence of respiratory and/or gastrointestinal infections[10]
- Nutritional and gastrointestinal
  - Breast milk is nutritionally complete for healthy term infants; this may be due to the fact that nutrients in breast milk are more bioavailable than those in formula milk
  - Lactoferrin is contained within breast milk and binds to iron, which improves iron absorption, and therefore there is less iron available for bacterial growth in the gut
  - Breast milk contains LCPs, which are likely to help with brain and retinal development

The composition of breast milk varies considerably throughout lactation and within each feed. Colostrum is the early milk that is rich in protein and is produced in small volumes immediately following delivery. Colostrum contains leukocytes, lactoferrin, lysozyme, and all of the immunoglobulins: IgA, IgD, IgE, IgG and IgM. These components together protect against bacteria, viruses and yeast.

Milk production can be variable immediately after birth irrespective of the length of gestation. One study in women giving birth at term reported a mean quantity of 37.1 g (range 7–122.5 g) colostrum in the first 24 hours after birth. There is usually a rapid increase in milk production at 30–40 hours post-partum[11]. If the mother has decided to breast-feed, the infant

should be given a breast-feed as soon as possible after birth (ideally within 30 minutes) to promote the production of colostrum. If the infant is on the neonatal unit and requiring nasogastric feeds, the mother should be encouraged to begin expressing as soon as possible, ideally within 4–6 hours after the birth.

Foremilk is the watery milk that is seen first, when breast-feeding or expressing breast milk. This is low in fat and not very energy dense. Hindmilk is the more energy dense milk that follows after foremilk has been expressed. Hindmilk contains more fat, which increases the energy content. Emptying of the breast when breast-feeding or expressing ensures that the energy dense hindmilk is given to the infant, which in turn satisfies the infant for longer and aids weight gain.

Term infants should be offered breast-feeds from birth if there are no contraindications to enteral feeds. A healthy term infant should thrive on breast milk alone until six months of age. If the maternal diet is good, the infant should not require any additional feeds before then.

Implications for practice

- Health care professionals play an important role in helping mothers to initiate and establish breast-feeding.
- Breast milk has many benefits, especially the colostrum.
- Hindmilk is energy dense and mothers should be encouraged to empty breasts when feeding or expressing milk.

Enteral feeding: preterm infant

Breast milk

Preterm infants fed on breast milk have been shown to have a decreased risk of mortality due to their reduced risk of infection[12]. It is important that mothers should be aware of the benefits of breast milk in these infants and encouraged to breast-feed or express breast milk. Some neonatal units also have access to donor or banked milk.

It is important to encourage mothers to start expressing soon after the birth and to continue to express regularly, aiming for a minimum of 6 times per 24 hours within the first few days. Premature infants generally receive expressed breast milk via a nasogastric or orogastric tube until their suck-swallow reflex is present at 32–34 weeks gestation. It is especially important in preterm infants that all the hindmilk (energy dense) is expressed to ensure the infant meets their energy requirements.

The protein content of breast milk can be variable, depending on the stage of lactation and the volume of milk expressed. The protein content does fall as lactation increases and therefore protein may need supplementing if the infant is not growing well.

Breast milk may not meet the iron, calcium and phosphate needs of the growing preterm infant. Many of the vitamins are dependent on the maternal diet. Fat soluble vitamins are dependent on the maternal body stores. Premature infants have an increased requirement, especially for the fat soluble vitamins and these are routinely supplemented.

Supplementation of breast milk

The term 'growth' not only refers to an increase in weight but to an increase in length and head circumference. In preterm infants it is not always possible to measure an accurate length, which is why many centres have not been routinely performing these measurements. Head circumference is used more commonly as an indicator of growth in preterm infants as it is reported to be more accurate.

Breast milk should only be supplemented if the infant is tolerating the maximum volume of milk but shows insufficient growth. Commercial fortifier is added to expressed breast milk to provide extra protein, sodium, calcium and phosphate as well as some other vitamins and minerals. Fortifier does not contain any iron.

Preterm infants on breast milk alone should routinely be supplemented with a multivitamin like Abidec® or Dalivit®, until they are eating a varied solid diet. Ideally, the multivitamin should be started once the infant is tolerating full enteral feeds. Individual infants may need vitamin D, phosphate and/or calcium supplements. Iron is routinely supplemented in all preterm infants and prescribed from 4–6 weeks of age. Iron should not be given at the same time as phosphate or calcium as they will form an insoluble salt and therefore not be absorbed[13,14].

Implications for practice

- If growth is poor, increase to maximum tolerated volume of feed before commercial fortifiers are added.
- All preterm infants should receive iron supplementation, starting at 4–6 weeks of life.
- Preterm infants, who are on breast milk alone, should be started on a multivitamin supplement.
- Extra calcium, phosphate and vitamin D should be given on an individual basis.

Storage of breast milk

It is important that mothers who are expressing milk have sterile and sealed containers to store the expressed breast milk in. Freshly expressed breast milk can be stored in the fridge for up to 48 hours. It can also be frozen and kept for three months in the freezer. The milk should be thawed overnight in a refrigerator and is then safe in the refrigerator for 24 hours but cannot be refrozen. When expressed breast milk is used as a continuous feed, it should not be hung or left at room temperature for more than four hours.

These storage guidelines should be adhered to as milk that has been frozen has lost some of the immune properties that inhibit bacterial growth in fresh refrigerated milk.

Problems experienced with breast- feeding or expressing breast milk

Privacy is essential in establishing breast-feeds and expressing breast milk. Women who have privacy to breast-feed are three times more likely to continue and breast-feed their infants on discharge[15]. It is tiring to have a baby on the neonatal unit and regular breast feeding or expressing is needed to sustain lactation. In some cases mothers can be prescribed domperidone, which may increase milk supply in the short term[16].

Feeding routes

Non-nutritive sucking occurs *in utero* and premature infants can suck intermittently on a pacifier as early as 27–28 weeks gestation. The suck-swallow-breath coordination is not developed before 32–34 weeks gestation so infants born before this age will usually be fed via a gastric tube.

Orogastric and nasogastric tubes are passed routinely in infants admitted to a neonatal unit. It is important to use an appropriate size tube for the size of the infant. The tube position should be checked by confirming the cm reading of where the tube enters the nose and by obtaining the pH of the aspirate. The pH should be checked before each feed and/or medication. If the pH is 5 or less, the tube position is in the stomach and feed can be administered. If a higher pH is obtained it may mean that the tube has migrated to the duodenum or has been passed into the lungs rather than the stomach. In some cases where it is not possible to obtain an aspirate or the aspirate pH is high, it may be worthwhile confirming the tube position with an X-ray.

Minimal enteral nutrition (MEN)

MEN (also referred to as trophic feeds or gut priming) is defined as the early introduction of low volume feeds. MEN is used on most neonatal units to promote feed tolerance and has also been found to reduce the number of days until the infant tolerates full feeds and reduce the length of stay in hospital. A recent Cochrane Review has shown that the effect of MEN on major clinical outcomes, including NEC and death, remains uncertain[17].

Increasing feeds

After MEN is completed, feeds should be increased with caution in very premature infants and those weighing less than 1.5 kg. Some studies have recommended that feeds should be increased by a maximum of 20 ml/kg/day (e.g. an increase in 1 ml every 24 hours in an infant fed hourly weighing 1.2 kg) as there was a higher risk of NEC seen in infants receiving greater volumes[18]. However, in other studies infants receiving larger daily increments of 30 ml/kg/day (e.g. an increase of 1 ml every 24 hours in an infant fed hourly weighing 800 g) reached full feeds earlier and had a shorter hospital stay[19]. Each neonatal unit should have their own policy on increasing enteral feeds, and infants should be monitored for feed tolerance.

Once on full volume of feeds and tolerating them well, the frequency of feeds can be gradually decreased. Many infants when discharged will demand feed as frequently as 2–3 hourly. In some circumstances, i.e. where the infant has gastro-oesophageal reflux, the infant may tolerate two-hourly feeds better as a smaller volume is administered. Breast or bottle feeds can be started once the suck-swallow reflex is present and may be offered at 1–2 feeds per day to start with and increased as tolerated by the infant.

If the mother wishes to breast-feed exclusively, the infant can be offered oral feeds via a cup until breast-feeds are established. This is because giving bottles too early in breast-fed infants may undermine the establishment of breast-feeding although evidence for this is unclear. Studies comparing premature infants during bottle feedings and during breast-feeding have shown that breast-feeding is actually less stressful as the infant's breathing and heart rate are more stable during feeds at the breast; they have more control over the milk flow and can establish a more regular rhythm of sucking, swallowing and breathing[20].

Continuous vs. bolus feeds

Most infants seem to tolerate bolus feeds better than continuous feeds. The benefits of bolus feeds include reduced bacterial contamination and reduced loss of fat from adherence to tubing, and therefore an increased total energy intake[21,22]. Continuous feeds could be used with certain infants who do not tolerate bolus feeds. In infants prone to respiratory instability, it may be more beneficial to feed continuously[23].

Implications for practice

- MEN should be considered from day one of life and breast milk should be used where possible.
- Feeds should be increased slowly in very premature infants.
- Bolus feeds should be used routinely.
- Continuous feeds can be used for infants not tolerating bolus feeds.

Formula feeds

Whey dominant term formula feeds (SMA Gold, C & G Premium, Aptamil First)

Term formulas are used for term infants and preterm infants with a birthweight above 2 kg, when the mother is unable to express milk, or breast-feed, or wishes to formula feed. Whey protein is digested more easily than casein and is therefore more appropriate for newborn infants. There is little variation in nutritional composition of different brands of term formula and most provide 67 kcal/100 ml and 1.5 g protein/100 ml. Term formulas should not be used routinely in preterm infants weighing less than 2 kg, as they will not meet their nutritional requirements.

Preterm formula feeds (Nutriprem 1, SMA LBW, Pre-Aptamil)

Preterm formulas are usually used when breast milk is not available. The protein and energy content of these formulas are higher than that of term formula. They all contain LCPs, most contain nucleotides and some contain prebiotics. All preterm formulas contain sufficient vitamins and minerals to meet the needs of the growing preterm infant more closely. They also have additional calcium, phosphate, iron, selenium and zinc.

Specialist formula

Specialist formulas can be divided into feeds that have partially hydrolysed protein (e.g. Nutramigen, Pepti-Junior, Prejomin, Pregestimil) and feeds that consist of extensively hydrolysed protein (e.g. Neocate). Partially and extensively hydrolysed feeds are absorbed more easily via the gut and are usually used where breast milk is not available and there is some degree of feed intolerance, e.g. malabsorption or short-bowel-syndrome.

Additives

If infants are on the maximum volume of feed tolerated and still not gaining weight appropriately, products such as Duocal, Polycal or Calogen can be added to increase the energy content of feeds. These may be particularly indicated in infants with a high energy requirement, such as infants with chronic lung disease. When these products are added, the osmolarity of the milk is increased and the infant requires monitoring for tolerance. Signs of intolerance may include diarrhoea, vomiting, bilious aspirates or abdominal distension. These products do not contain any protein but do provide additional energy in the form of fat and/or carbohydrate. These products should therefore only be added to feeds that are higher in protein, i.e. breast milk with fortifier, nutrient enriched preterm formula, nutrient enriched post-discharge formula, nutrient enriched term formula. They should not be added to any of the standard term formulas as the protein-energy ratio will be too low and therefore not aid weight gain.

Implications for practice

In an infant experiencing high stoma losses, a change in formula to a hydrolysed feed could reduce high stoma output. This could improve growth.
Case study:
An infant was diagnosed with NEC and needed to have surgery. Fourteen days post-surgery the surgeons agreed to start enteral feeds; the infant was started on nutrient enriched preterm formula, as there was no breast milk available. A few days after enteral feeds were started, the infant was having high stoma losses, which increased as the feed was increased and the infant started to show poor weight-gain. The feed was changed to a partially hydrolysed feed. Stoma losses decreased thereafter and subsequently led to improved growth.

Assessing growth and nutrition in term infants

Weight

Most term infants experience a weight loss during the first 10–14 days of life, which is due to a loss of excess extracellular fluid. Infants should be weighed at birth and on a regular basis thereafter to monitor their growth. Ideally, weight gain should be determined over a period of seven days. In term infants a weight gain of 200 g per week or 30 g per day is aimed for. Changes to a feed regimen should not be made based on an individual measurement; it is essential to look at the pattern of growth over a period of time and to make appropriate changes thereafter.

Length

Length is a better indicator of growth, but is difficult to obtain accurately and two individuals are needed to take the measurement. Infants should be measured at birth and every two weeks thereafter until discharged from hospital. Healthy term infants grow about 1 cm per month in the first few months of life.

Head circumference

Head circumference is a useful measurement in infants, especially when it is difficult to obtain an accurate length measurement. The head circumference can be used as a valuable measurement to monitor nutritional status as long as conditions that affect head circumference, e.g. hydrocephalus, are not present. Head circumferences should be measured at birth and repeated on a weekly basis until discharged. If conditions present that affect the head circumference, it may be useful to repeat the measurements more frequently.

Assessing growth and nutrition in preterm infants

Weight

There is some debate about whether weight loss after birth in preterm infants reflects catabolism of protein stores and lean body mass rather than fluid shifts, as in term infants. It is thought that this may be due to premature infants having less fat stores; thus, protein stores are more likely to be used to meet metabolic demands[24].

Preterm infants should be weighed at birth and at least once a week thereafter. It may be useful to weigh daily in the first few weeks of life, as their weight can fluctuate from day to day, most commonly due to changes in fluid balance. Weight measurement techniques should follow the same procedures as described for term infants. In preterm infants the aim is to match the *in utero* growth rate. Infants weighing less than 2 kg should aim for a weight gain of 15–20 g/kg/day and in preterm infants greater than 2 kg should aim for a weight gain of 25–30 g/day.

Length

In preterm infants it is even more difficult to obtain an accurate length than in term infants. Preterm infants should be measured at birth, then weekly until 40 weeks post-conception and thereafter every two weeks until discharged from hospital.

Head circumference

As in term infants, head circumference can be a useful measurement in preterm infants, especially when it is difficult to obtain an accurate length measurement. The head circumference can be used as a valuable measurement to monitor nutritional status in a similar way as with term infants. Head circumference should be measured without any hats or caps on, or it will not be accurate enough for interpretation.

Implications for practice

- Weight, head circumference and length should be measured regularly and plotted on an appropriate centile chart.
- Do not make changes to the feed based on individual measurements.

Intrauterine growth retardation (IUGR) in term and preterm infants

Many studies have now shown that the infant with IUGR will show catch-up growth at some stage in life and this is not dependent on an increased energy intake as an infant. Some research has even shown that there is an increased risk of obesity later in life if excessive weight is gained as an infant[25]. It is important to ensure the infant gains weight and is following its centile, then catch-up growth can be expected in later years.

Steroids

Steroids (e.g. dexamethasone) are occasionally given to premature infants who have developed chronic lung disease. Dexamethasone leads to increased catabolism and increased protein breakdown, which results in a raised serum urea. Growth is restricted while the infant is on steroids and increasing the energy or protein content of the feed will lead to extra stress on the infant. Therefore, during periods when the infant is treated with steroids, growth should be monitored. Feed changes, to aid catch-up growth, should be made once steroids have been discontinued.

Post-discharge feeding interventions

Nutrient enriched post discharge formula (NEPDF)

There is currently one NEPDF (Nutriprem II) available in the UK. It contains some extra protein, energy, vitamins and minerals and is usually used where an infant is thought to need further catch-up growth. Some studies have shown that NEPDF improves growth but this is usually only seen in the first two months, with no additional benefit thereafter[26]. Therefore NEPDF should only given to individual infants who require further catch-up growth and are monitored closely while on NEPDF.

Nutrient enriched formula (NEF) designed for term infants

There are currently two prescription nutrient enriched formulas (Infatrini and SMA High Energy) available in the UK, but they have not specifically been designed for preterm infants. Although they can be used for preterm infants, e.g. when on a strict fluid restriction, they do not meet the nutritional requirements for preterm infants and some may need additional calcium, phosphate, zinc and iron.

Implications for practice

- NEPDF can be used for preterm infants who need to show further catch-up growth.
- NEF for term infants is not suitable for preterm infants.

Part II

Parenteral nutrition

Indications for parenteral nutrition

Following birth and the initial cardiorespiratory adaptation to post-natal life, survival of the term neonate depends on the successful transition from *in utero* parenteral nutrition via the placenta, to *ex utero* enteral nutrition. Parenteral nutrition should be considered when full enteral nutrition is contraindicated such as in the term infant with a surgical diagnosis or in the preterm infant (see Table 12.2).

In preterm infants, respiratory and gastrointestinal immaturity may preclude tolerance of enteral feeds in the first days or weeks of life. In practice all neonates who are unlikely to establish full enteral feeding within one week of birth are usually started on PN.

The decision to start PN should not be taken lightly; it is far safer and simpler and more beneficial for the infant to provide nutrition via the enteral route where this is an option. Infants fed

parenterally require venous access, often central, facilities for intensive monitoring and the support and expertise of a multidisciplinary team that may necessitate transfer of the infant to an alternative unit.

Controversy exists around the optimum time to start PN and further studies are required to confirm any significant benefit of early aggressive PN. However, recent guidelines suggest that when indicated, PN incorporating protein, carbohydrate and fat, should be started soon after birth, and preferably on day one of life, particularly for premature infants[27,28].

Where PN is used as the sole nutrition source to support normal growth it is referred to as total parenteral nutrition (TPN). PN may also be used to supplement sub-optimal enteral nutrition while milk feeds are gradually introduced (supplemental parenteral nutrition). Even where TPN is required, minimal enteral nutrition should also be considered as soon as clinically possible in order to stimulate post-natal development of the gastro-intestinal system, prevent gut atrophy and reduce the risk of PN associated liver dysfunction[29-32].

Benefits of parenteral nutrition

The objective of using PN is to maintain optimal nutritional status and achieve satisfactory post-natal growth until adequate enteral nutrition can be established. Supplemental PN may also have benefits in allowing enteral feeds to be more cautiously introduced in preterm and sick infants. PN must be used and monitored appropriately so that the possible benefit of prolonged survival is accompanied by appropriate growth, development and quality of life.

Relative contraindications

There are very few absolute contraindications to PN. In infants with acute, severe sepsis it may be preferable to achieve clinical stability with antibiotics before starting PN. In infants with severe acidosis an attempt should be made to

Table 12.2 Indications for parenteral nutrition in the infant.

Enteral feeding contraindicated	Enteral feeding inadequate
Congenital malformations of gastrointestinal tract (pre-operatively): • Gastroschisis • Tracheoesophageal fistula	• Immature gut function – extreme prematurity, VLBW infants • Severe fluid restriction • Difficulty maintaining enteral access
• Intestinal atresias • Post-gastrointestinal surgery where gut requires resting in the short or long term • Congenital diaphragmatic hernia (peri-operatively) • Necrotising enterocolitis requiring gut rest • Severe respiratory distress syndrome	• Severe gastroesophageal reflux disease with feed intolerance • Intractable diarrhoea • Short gut syndrome

correct blood gases before PN is commenced, as PN itself may worsen the metabolic acidosis (see complications, below).

Implications for practice

- Use PN in infants where enteral feeding is contraindicated or inadequate to meet nutritional needs.
- PN can be used to provide the total nutritional requirements (TPN) or to supplement poor enteral intake.
- When PN is indicated it should be started soon after birth and be accompanied with minimal enteral nutrition.

Composition of parenteral nutrition solutions

PN solutions consist of sources of protein, carbohydrate and fat (macronutrients), and electrolytes, vitamins, minerals and trace elements (micronutrients). PN is either tailor-made daily to meet individual patient needs or pre-prepared as standard bags (containing fixed quantities of macronutrients and micronutrients) which are then run at different rates to meet the infants' requirements. Neonatal PN is usually supplied in two discrete containers (2 in 1 admixtures). This is the two-compartment system:

- Protein, carbohydrate, electrolytes, trace elements, minerals and water
- Fat and vitamins

The energy requirements that need to be met by the provision of TPN, or of PN in combination with enteral feeds, are calculated for each infant on a regular basis and vary depending on the infant's nutritional status, medical condition, age, weight and previous exposure to enteral or parenteral feeds. Infants generally require fewer calories when fed parenterally, than when fed enterally[33]. Average daily total parenteral energy intakes (including energy from protein) are shown in Table 12.3.

Table 12.3 Average daily total parenteral energy requirements (from Koletzko *et al.*, 2005 [34]).

Age	kcal/kg/day
Preterm infant	110–120
0–1 years	90–100

Fat, protein and carbohydrate are introduced simultaneously over several days with the aim of achieving the optimum energy intake and correct ratios of macronutrients within three to five days of starting parenteral nutrition. The PN solution is usually administered over a 24-hour period each day.

Protein

Protein is given as amino acids and manufactured solutions are produced to match the amino acid profile of either cord blood or the profile of a normally growing breast-fed infant. A minimum of 1.25 g/kg/day of protein should be provided on the first post-natal day to prevent loss of body protein stores[35,36], and this should be increased to a target maximum of 3.3–3.85 g/kg/day protein in preterm and low birthweight infants, and 2.5–3 g/kg/day in term infants[37,38]. In the first days of life the neonate's fluid requirements may restrict the rate of protein administration. Where this is not the case, there seems to be no evidence to support the gradual introduction of protein[39]. Early (day 1–2) introduction of total protein requirements is tolerated even in VLBW infants[40,41].

Carbohydrate

Carbohydrates and fats are used to provide the necessary non-nitrogen energy to enable the protein source to be utilised for growth and new tissue production. Carbohydrate should supply ~60–75% of these non-protein calories[42].

Glucose is used to provide the carbohydrate. The infant's response to intravenous glucose maintenance infusions (blood sugars, urinalysis) can be used as a guide to the total amount of glucose required in their first bag of PN. On day one of PN between 8.6 and 11.5 g/kg/day glucose is appropriate and the quantity is gradually increased, according to response, over the following few days to a maximum of 18 g/kg/day[44,45].

Fat

The lipid (fat) component of parenteral nutrition is energy dense and provides essential fatty acids (EFA). Fat should provide 25–40% of non-protein calories in fully PN fed infants[46]. A 20% lipid emulsion is routinely used as it is better tolerated than the 10% solution by neonates[47–49]. A minimum of 0.5 g–1 g/kg/day lipid, started within the first three days of life, is required to prevent EFA deficiency[50,51]. Lipid can be started on the first day of life even in preterms[52,53]. The quantity of lipid can be increased daily in a step-wise approach to a maximum of 3–4 g/kg/day fat[54–57], and although recent guidelines suggest this step-wise practice does little to improve fat tolerance, increments of 0.5–1 g/kg/day may facilitate monitoring for hypertriglyceridaemia[58,59]. Tolerance of lipid by preterms is improved by giving a continuous 24-hour infusion rather than an intermittent regime[60,61].

Electrolytes

The infant's blood and urine chemistry determine the amount of electrolytes that are to be added to each day's PN solution. The electrolytes added include sodium, potassium, calcium, phosphate and magnesium. Calcium phosphate can form precipitates as the pH of the PN solution approaches neutral[62]. The desired calcium and phosphate combination may need to be modified in this situation to avoid precipitates and to achieve stability.

Vitamins, minerals and trace elements

Water and fat soluble vitamins, minerals and trace elements are added to the PN solution to prevent deficiency. However, the optimal parenteral vitamin requirements for neonates have not yet been established.

The addition of fat and water soluble vitamins to the lipid solution improves their stability. The fat reduces vitamin loss from photo-degradation (breakdown by light) and adherence to plastic tubing during administration. The vitamins can also help protect the lipid solution from peroxidation (oxidative degradation of lipid with production of free radicals). Lipid is also prone to photo-degradation and it is good practice to protect the lipid compartment from light using aluminium foil or amber syringes. This is particularly important if the infant (and, therefore, the lipid infusion line) is exposed to phototherapy.

Trace elements and minerals are added to the amino acid glucose solution. The trace elements added do not routinely include iron, molybdenum, or chromium but these may be added in those infants on long-term PN (usually > 4 weeks). Parenterally fed infants do not routinely require iron supplements until they reach 4–6 weeks old unless they were VLBW.

Implications for practice

- PN consists of macronutrients (fat, protein, carbohydrate) and micronutrients (electrolytes, vitamins, minerals and trace elements).
- Protein, glucose and fat can all be started on the first day of life.
- PN stability may limit the quantity of micronutrients that can be added.

Preparation and storage

PN solutions are ideal media for microbial growth so must be prepared under strict aseptic conditions by trained staff. Due to increased stability of the tried and tested formulations, standard bags have longer shelf-lives than tailor-made bags. Hospitals providing tailor-made PN may also stock a limited number of standard bags for use in unforeseen circumstances and outside pharmacy operating hours.

Although prepared under strict aseptic conditions, PN bags have a limited shelf-life and must be refrigerated at 2–8°C before use to minimise the risk of microbial growth. Care should be taken during PN administration to ensure that only the minimum length of delivery circuit should be inside the incubator and consequently exposed to the incubator heat.

Implications for practice

- Your patient's PN may be tailor-made to meet their own requirements, or be run from a standard bag at a rate calculated to suit their needs.
- PN must be refrigerated at 2–8°C before use.
- Avoid exposing PN to high incubator temperatures.

Administration of parenteral nutrition

Route of infusion

Parenteral nutrition can be delivered in the following ways:

- Via short peripheral cannulae
- Via central lines:
  - Umbilical venous catheters (UVC)
  - Peripherally inserted central venous catheter (PICC), also called a 'long line', where a subcutaneous vein is used as the entry site to reach the central vein
  - Central venous catheter (CVC) directly inserted via the subclavian, jugular or femoral vein
  - Surgically inserted tunnelled CVC (Broviac®, Hickman®) introduced through one of the deep veins. These tunnelled CVCs are used in infants requiring long-term PN, or where venous access has become particularly difficult to obtain.

Both peripherally and centrally administered PN have inherent hazards and complications associated with the route of administration. Where peripheral PN is used, the composition of the PN is limited by osmolarity. Subcutaneous infiltration of hypertonic, irritant PN can result in skin ulceration, secondary infection and scarring[62,63]. As a result, dilute solutions of PN must be used when given peripherally, which limits their usefulness in fluid restricted infants. It may be difficult to achieve administration of the required amounts of energy from glucose, fat and protein solution for optimal growth. For this reason central venous access is required in infants receiving PN for more than a few days and further discussion will refer to centrally-administered PN.

Where central access (UVC, PICC or CVC) is used for PN administration, the osmolarity of the solution is not restricted because the tip of the catheter enters the bloodstream in a large vessel with high blood flow (usually just above or below, but not into, the right atrium), so the PN solution is rapidly diluted out into the blood, making the risk of damage to the blood vessel minimal. As a result, the PN can be concentrated to provide more calories in a relatively low volume of fluid. The main risks from central venous PN are associated with misplacement, thrombosis and sepsis (see complications).

Implications for practice

- PN can be given peripherally or centrally.
- Risks of peripheral administration of PN are associated with irritation and extravasation.
- Risks of central administration of PN are associated with misplacement, thrombosis and infection.

Administrative procedure

To reduce the risk of catheter related sepsis, strict, aseptic, non-touch technique should be used when setting up and administering PN, and when changing the bags, syringes, filters and giving sets, and scrupulous cleaning and care of the line exit site is essential.

PN must be delivered via a rate-controlled infusion pump to maintain constant, accurate delivery of small volumes and to prevent free flow, and must be monitored carefully as for any intravenous infusion. Line pressure should be monitored: High pressures may indicate blockage of the line or extravasation. The line entry site should also be inspected regularly to ensure the line has not been displaced and to check for signs of thrombophlebitis.

Parenteral nutrition solutions should be filtered during administration to reduce infusion of particulate matter and reduce thrombophlebitis[64]. With appropriate 0.22 micrometre filters the life of the administration set may be extended but the chemical and microbial stability of the PN solution being infused may be less than 48 hours and advice should be sought from the manufacturer or your pharmacist on an individual basis.

Ideally, PN should be administered via a dedicated central IV line through which no other fluids or drugs are run, and through which blood samples are not taken. This is to reduce the number of times the line is broken into in an attempt to reduce rates of infection, and to reduce the risk of interactions between drugs and PN. The stability of PN may be adversely affected by changes in pH caused by the presence of other fluids and drugs in the line. A resulting precipitant may form which can cause line occlusion or embolisation. Alternatively, the reaction between the PN and drugs may create chemical instability or inactivation of the drug. Where use of the dedicated PN line for the administration of other drugs is unavoidable, always consult the drug product literature and the hospital pharmacist for further advice and try to time drug administration to coincide with other procedures that will involve breaking into the line (e.g. the daily change of PN bag).

Where a double lumen CVC has been inserted, one lumen should be dedicated to PN use only. The second lumen can be considered as a separate line through which drugs and other fluids may be administered without significant interaction with the PN solution.

Implications for practice

- Strict aseptic non-touch technique must be followed when using PN.
- Line entry sites should be regularly inspected.
- Ideally, one line should be dedicated for PN use only, and the number of line breaks minimised.
- Drugs and other fluids may interact with PN.

Monitoring

The PN composition should be adjusted in response to changes in the infant's biochemistry and anthropometry in order to provide optimal macronutrients, micronutrients and electrolytes. Monitoring is also used to ensure early recognition of potential complications of PN such as sepsis, acidosis and cholestatic jaundice (see complications).

Suggested monitoring and justification are shown in Table 12.4. A balance must be made between the risks and costs of repeated blood-sampling and the need for biochemical information to ensure the safe use of PN. Generally, biochemical monitoring will be required more frequently in the first week or so of PN, whilst macronutrients are being gradually titrated, with a reduction in frequency once stability is achieved. The monitoring intervals will depend on the infant's clinical status, underlying pathophysiology, current treatments and duration on PN.

Implications for practice

- Without adequate monitoring PN is a hazardous treatment.
- Adjust the frequency of monitoring to the needs of your patient; don't take unnecessary samples in a stable infant.

Complications of parenteral nutrition

PN associated complications can broadly be categorised as catheter-related (infectious, thrombotic,

Table 12.4 Suggested monitoring of infants receiving PN.

Suggested monitoring	Justification
Body weight, length, head circumference (anthropometry), serum albumin, urea	To ensure PN is meeting nutritional requirements and promoting normal development
Blood urea, creatinine and sodium. Urinary sodium, osmolarity, fluid input/output	Enable adjustments in volume of PN prescribed to maintain fluid balance
Blood sodium, potassium, calcium, phosphate, magnesium, urinary electrolytes	Enable adjustments to electrolyte content of PN to maintain homeostasis of blood chemistry
Blood glucose, urinary glucose	Determine suitable glucose content of PN, monitor for hyper- and hypo-glycaemia as a complication of PN; detection of possible sepsis secondary to PN
Plasma triglycerides	Determine lipid clearance and adjust fat content as necessary
Blood chloride and blood gases	To detect developing metabolic acidosis and hyperchloridaemia
FBC, WCC, platelets, CRP, body temperature, core-peripheral temperature gap, respiratory rate, heart rate	Detection of developing sepsis secondary to PN, e.g. central line infection
LFTs (including GGT), total and conjugated bilirubin, clotting	To detect adverse hepatic effects of PN, prevent kernicterus
Vitamin and trace element blood levels (long-term PN only)	To detect and correct any deficiencies
Venous access site	To detect any developing phlebitis, extravasation of PN

mechanical), metabolic, and those involving other organ systems.

Catheter-related complications

PN-associated infection

Catheter-related bloodstream infection is one of the most common complications of central venous access and is potentially life-threatening[65], with a prevalence of up to 45%[66]. Bacteria most commonly originate from the outer surface of the line, with organisms coming from the skin at the time of line insertion, or from the line lumen if bacteria enter the catheter hub during connection and disconnection[67,68]. Line infections must always be considered when an infant receiving PN shows signs of infection or their condition seriously deteriorates.

Preventative measures include aseptic manufacture of PN; strict aseptic non-touch technique during line insertion and PN administration[69]; skin exit site location compatible with meticulous cleaning; proper care of the site, connections and tubing; limiting the frequency with which the line is broken; avoiding using the line for blood sampling and drug administration wherever possible; using lines with the minimum number of lumens and hubs required for the management of the patient; regular staff education[70]; and the use of in-line filters.

Venous thromboembolism

Approximately 70% of neonatal thromboses are associated with CVC use and may result in severe morbidity or death[71]. At-risk infants tend to be those receiving PN for several weeks or more.

Mechanical – line occlusion

Central venous lines can become occluded by a blood clot or occasionally by precipitation of drugs or PN given via the line. Blood clots and precipitation can be reduced by using central lines as described above and by flushing lines well with sodium chloride 0.9% before and after every use, using a syringe no smaller than 10 ml. In-line filters will also help trap debris.

Mechanical – line kinks
Hypoglycaemia can develop rapidly if a kink in the line occurs, so it is essential to monitor the hourly delivered volume, set and monitor pump pressure alarms, and to identify mechanical pump failures as soon as possible.

Mechanical – central line malposition
Rare complications associated with PN infused via malpositioned central lines include pleural and pericardial effusion, cardiac tamponade, ascites, pericarditis, erosion into pulmonary vessels and diaphragmatic paralysis[72]. CVCs should be X-rayed to confirm the line tip position before use.

Mechanical – accidental removal or damage
Central venous lines are easily dislodged or damaged if not secured adequately with tapes and dressings[73]. Splints and looping of the line beyond the exit site may give added security. Potentially fatal bleeding can occur from damaged or displaced CVCs and from loose connections, so an experienced practitioner should be alerted to any concerns about the line immediately.

Implications for practice

- Catheter-related infection should be considered in neonates with a central line in situ.
- Reduce the risk of central line sepsis with the use of strict aseptic non-touch technique and line filters. Dedicate the line for PN use only and where this is not possible time drug administration to minimise the number of breaks made into the line.
- Do not use central lines for blood sampling.
- Flush central lines with 0.9% sodium chloride before and after every drug administration.
- Do not give PN via a central line until you are sure the correct position has been confirmed by X-ray.

Metabolic complications

Metabolic acidosis
Chloride loads in excess of 6 mmol/kg/day result in increased incidence of hyperchloraemia (plasma chloride > 115 mmol/l). Hyperchloraemia is one of the many causes of metabolic acidosis in preterm infants[74]. The partial replacement (up to 6 mmol/kg/day) of the sodium and potassium chloride in neonatal PN with sodium and potassium acetate (which in turn is metabolised in the body to bicarbonate), can reduce the incidence of hyperchloraemia, metabolic acidosis and requirement for bicarbonate infusions[75,76].

Hyperglycaemia and glycosuria
The risk of hyperglycaemia and glycosuria increase with decreasing gestation and decreasing birthweight. Preterms have an increased risk of hyperglycaemia, possibly due to saturation of insulin receptors, insulin insensitivity and immaturity of the hepatic and pancreatic response[77]. If hyperglycaemia limits glucose administration such that adequate calorie delivery and weight gain cannot be achieved, insulin infusion may be necessary to facilitate additional glucose delivery[78]. Insulin use requires close infant monitoring to prevent hypoglycaemia.

Hypoglycaemia may be caused by the sudden cessation of PN[79]; PN should be weaned gradually as an alternative source of glucose is introduced.

Lipid intolerance
PN associated hypertriglyceridaemia is often secondary to uncontrolled hyperglycaemia or excessive lipid delivery[80]. Sepsis also reduces lipid clearance[81]. Where hyperglycaemia and hypertriglyceridaemia co-exist an attempt to normalise blood glucose should initially be attempted[82], before lipid delivery is reduced. If plasma triglyceride levels exceed 2.8 mmol/l lipid intake may need to be reduced, although the upper acceptable limit for plasma triglycerides

remains unresolved and it is not clear at what triglyceride level adverse effects may occur[83,84].

Decreased clearance (results in increased plasma triglycerides) and decreased utilisation (results in increased plasma free fatty acid concentrations) of fat is more common in ELBW, preterm and IUGR infants.

Implications for practice

- Chloride in PN solutions can contribute to metabolic acidosis.
- Monitor blood sugar regularly in infants on PN.
- If PN is no longer required, wean gradually and ensure an alternative glucose source is provided to prevent hypoglycaemia.

Complications affecting other organs

Hepatobiliary complications

Most hepatobiliary complications of PN are moderate and reversible, but more severe consequences including cholestasis, biliary sludging, gallstones, cirrhosis, hepatic decompensation and death can occur.

PN associated cholestatic jaundice is thought to occur in 15–67% neonates receiving PN[85]. One small neonatal study found that cholestasis occurred rarely and mildly in neonates on PN for less than two weeks, but occurred universally and more severely in those on PN for more than six weeks[86]. A raised serum bilirubin is often the first noticeable change in the blood chemistry. The infant's skin may take on a waxy appearance and become tinged a khaki-grey colour.

In most affected patients cholestasis exists for as long as PN is administered and jaundice and abnormal liver enzymes improve when PN is withdrawn and enteral feeding is re-established[87]. Ursodeoxycholic acid, a bile acid, may be useful in reducing the duration of cholestasis[88,89], but is limited to use in infants where the enteral route is available. The progression of PN associated cholestasis to biliary cirrhosis and liver failure is more common in infants than adults. Cholestatic

jaundice progresses to overt liver failure (which may be fatal) in approximately 25% of neonates receiving PN after intestinal resection[90].

Jaundice

PN should not be withheld from infants with, or at risk of, hyperbilirubinaemia but serum triglyceride and bilirubin levels should be monitored, particularly whilst lipid volumes are being increased, and lipid rates then reduced if necessary[91].

Implications for practice

- Infants on PN for > 2 weeks are at increased risk of hepatobiliary complications.
- Unless contraindicated, give minimal enteral feeds alongside PN to reduce the risk of liver disease.
- Ursodeoxycholic acid may be useful in infants with PN associated cholestasis.
- Lipid cycling or restriction may be trialled in severe cholestasis.

Transition to enteral feeds

When the enteral route becomes available enteral feeds should be gradually introduced and increased as tolerated and the PN gradually reduced. During this transition period blood sugars must be monitored to avoid hypoglycaemia. Central access should be maintained until the infant is receiving at least 75% of their nutritional requirements enterally. The line should then be removed as soon as possible to reduce risk of infection. At this stage weaning the infant off PN is the priority and the method of enteral feeding can be adjusted to a more practical, physiologic method later as required.

Implications for practice

- Wean PN gradually as enteral feeds are increased, with close monitoring of blood sugars.
- In PN fed infants the priority is to establish full enteral feeding. Once this target is achieved the method of enteral feeding can be fine-tuned.
- Remember to remove the central line when it is no longer required.

Conclusion

One of the main challenges of neonatal intensive care is to meet the nutritional requirements of the sick term infant and the preterm and extremely preterm infant. This chapter has summarised the nutritional requirements of the term and preterm infant and the two main ways in which these requirements can be delivered: enteral and parenteral. In the first section the benefits of breast milk have been discussed, as well as the nutritional composition of formula feeds. The second section concentrated on parenteral nutrition and its delivery, an important way of providing nutrition on a neonatal intensive care unit. An improvement in clinical knowledge within these areas will facilitate the nutritional care of the vulnerable infants that require intensive care. There is no doubt that optimising nutrition can aid recovery from illness and surgery and improve neurodevelopmental outcome in the preterm infant.

References

1. Picciano MF (2003) Pregnancy and lactation: physiological adjustments, nutritional requirements and the role of dietary supplements. *J Nutr*, **133** (6), 1997S–2002S.
2. Crawford DM (1994) *Neonatal Nursing*. Chapman & Hall, London.
3. Heird WC, Driscoll JM, Schillinger JN, Grebin JN, Winters RW (1972) Intravenous alimentation in pediatric patients. *J Pediatr*, **80** (3), 351–372.
4. Tsang RCU, Koletzko RB, Zlotkin SH (eds) (2005) *Nutrition of the Preterm Infant: Scientific Basis and Practical Guidelines*, 2nd edn. Digital Educational Publishing, Cincinnati, OH.
5. Olivares M, Llaguno S, Marin V, Hertrampf E, Mena P, Milad M (1992) Iron status in low-birth-weight infants, small and appropriate for gestational age. A follow-up study. *Acta Paediatr*, **81** (10), 824–828.
6. Backstrom MC, Maki R, Kuusela AL, *et al.* (1999) Randomised controlled trial of vitamin D supplementation on bone density and biochemical indices in preterm infants. *Arch Dis Child Foetal, Neonatal Ed*, **80** (3), F161–F166.
7. Koletzko B, Thiel I, Abiodun PO (1992) The fatty acid composition of human milk in Europe and Africa. *J Pediatr*, **120** (4 Pt 2), S62–S70.
8. Schlimme E, Martin D, Meisel H (2000) Nucleosides and nucleotides: natural bioactive substances in milk and colostrum. *Br J Nutr*, **84** (Suppl. 1), S59–68.
9. Pickering LK, Granoff DM, Erickson JR, *et al.*(1998) Modulation of the immune system by human milk and infant formula containing nucleotides. *Pediatrics*, **101** (2), 242–249.
10. Quigley MA, Kelly YJ, Sacker A (2007) Breastfeeding and hospitalization for diarrheal and respiratory infection in the United Kingdom Millennium Cohort Study. *Pediatrics*, **119** (4), e837–e842.
11. Arthur PG, Smith M, Hartmann PE (1989) Milk lactose, citrate, and glucose as markers of lactogenesis in normal and diabetic women. *J Pediatr Gastroenterol Nutr*, **9** (4), 488–496.
12. Quigley MA, Kelly YJ, Sacker A (2007) Breastfeeding and hospitalization for diarrheal and respiratory infection in the United Kingdom Millennium Cohort Study. *Pediatrics*, **119** (4), e837–e842.
13. Peters T Jr, Apt L, Ross JF (1971) Effect of phosphates upon iron absorption studied in normal human subjects and in an experimental model using dialysis. *Gastroenterology*, **61** (3), 315–322.
14. Cook JD, Dassenko SA, Whittaker P (1991) Calcium supplementation: effect on iron absorption. *Am J Clin Nutr*, **53** (1), 106–111.
15. Bolling K, Grant C, Hamlyn B, *et al.* (2007) *Infant Feeding Survey 2005: Early Results*. The Information Centre, Government Statistical Service, London.
16. da Silva OP, Knoppert DC, Angelini, MM (2001) Effect of domperidone on milk production in

mothers of premature newborns: a randomized, double-blind placebo-controlled trial. *Canadian Med Ass J*, **164** (17–21), 106–111.

17. Tyson JE, Kennedy KA (2000) Minimal enteral nutrition for promoting feeding tolerance and preventing morbidity in parenterally fed infants. *Cochrane Database Syst Rev* (2), CD000504.

18. Book LS, Herbst JJ, Jung AL (1976) Comparison of fast- and slow-feeding rate schedules to the development of necrotizing enterocolitis. *J Pediatr*, **89** (3), 463–466.

19. Caple J, Armentrout D, Huseby V, *et al.* (2004) Randomized, controlled trial of slow versus rapid feeding volume advancement in preterm infants. *Pediatrics*, **114** (6), 1597–6000.

20. Meier P (1988) Bottle- and breast-feeding: effects on transcutaneous oxygen pressure and temperature in preterm infants. *Nurs Res*, **37** (1), 36–41.

21. Doolittle G, Mills M (1992) Continuous drip feedings in the very low birth weight infant. *Neonatal Netw*, **11** (3), 33–35.

22. Brennan-Behm M, Carlson E, Meier P, Engstrom J (1994) Caloric loss from expressed mother's milk during continuous gavage infusion. *Neonatal Netw*, **13** (2), 27–32.

23. Blondheim O, Abbasi S, Fox WW, Buthani VK (1993) Effect of enteral gavage feeding rate on pulmonary functions of very low birth weight infants. *J Pediatr*, **122** (5 Pt 1), 751–755.

24. Denne SC (2001) Protein and energy requirements in preterm infants. *Semin Neonatol*, **6** (5), 377–382.

25. Stettler N, Zemel BS, Kumanyika S, Stallings VA (2002) Infant weight gain and childhood overweight status in a multicenter, cohort study. *Pediatrics*, **109** (2), 194–199.

26. Lucas A, Fewtrell MS, Morley R, *et al.* (2001) Randomized trial of nutrient-enriched formula versus standard formula for postdischarge preterm infants. *Pediatrics*, **108** (3), 703–711.

27. ASPEN (The American Society for Parenteral and Enteral Nutrition) Board of Directors (2002) Guidelines for the Use of Parenteral and Enteral Nutrition in Adult and Pediatric Patients. *JPEN*, **261** (1), 1SA–138SA.

28. Koletzko B, Goulet O, Hunt J, Krohn K, Shamir R (2005) 1. Guidelines on Paediatric Parenteral Nutrition of the European Society of Paediatric Gastroenterology, Hepatology and Nutrition (ESPGHAN) and the European Society for Clinical Nutrition and Metabolism (ESPEN), Supported by the European Society of Paediatric Research (ESPR). *J Pediatr Gastroenterol Nutr*, **41** (Suppl. 2), S1–87.

29. ASPEN (The American Society for Parenteral and Enteral Nutrition) Board of Directors (2002) Guidelines for the Use of Parenteral and Enteral Nutrition in Adult and Pediatric Patients. *JPEN*, **261** (1), 1SA–138SA.

30. Koletzko B, Goulet O, Hunt J, Krohn K, Shamir R (2005) 1. Guidelines on Paediatric Parenteral Nutrition of the European Society of Paediatric Gastroenterology, Hepatology and Nutrition (ESPGHAN) and the European Society for Clinical Nutrition and Metabolism (ESPEN), Supported by the European Society of Paediatric Research (ESPR). *J Pediatr Gastroenterol Nutr*, **41** (Suppl. 2), S1–87.

31. Hay WW Jr, Lucas A, Heird WC, *et al.* (1999) Workshop summary: nutrition of the extremely low birth weight infant. *Pediatrics*, **104** (6), 1360–1368.

32. Andorsky DJ, Lund DP, Lillehei CW, *et al.* (2001) Nutritional and other postoperative management of neonates with short bowel syndrome correlates with clinical outcomes. *J Pediatr*, **139** (1), 27–33.

33. Koletzko B, Goulet O, Hunt J, Krohn K, Shamir R (2005) 1. Guidelines on Paediatric Parenteral Nutrition of the European Society of Paediatric Gastroenterology, Hepatology and Nutrition (ESPGHAN) and the European Society for Clinical Nutrition and Metabolism (ESPEN), Supported by the European Society of Paediatric Research (ESPR). *J Pediatr Gastroenterol Nutr*, **41** (Suppl. 2), S1–87.

34. Koletzko B, Goulet O, Hunt J, Krohn K, Shamir R (2005) 1. Guidelines on Paediatric Parenteral Nutrition of the European Society of Paediatric Gastroenterology, Hepatology and Nutrition (ESPGHAN) and the European Society for Clinical Nutrition and Metabolism (ESPEN), Supported by the European Society of Paediatric Research (ESPR). *J Pediatr Gastroenterol Nutr*, **41** (Suppl. 2), S1–87.

35. Koletzko B, Goulet O, Hunt J, Krohn K, Shamir R (2005) 1. Guidelines on Paediatric Parenteral Nutrition of the European Society of Paediatric Gastroenterology, Hepatology and Nutrition (ESPGHAN) and the European Society for Clinical Nutrition and Metabolism (ESPEN), Supported by the European Society of Paediatric Research (ESPR). *J Pediatr Gastroenterol Nutr*, **41** (Suppl. 2), S1–87.

36. Ibrahim HM, Jeroudi MA, Baier RJ, Dhanireddy R, Krouskop RW (2004) Aggressive early total parental nutrition in low-birth-weight infants. *J Perinatol*, **24** (8), 482–486.

37. ASPEN (The American Society for Parenteral and Enteral Nutrition) Board of Directors (2002) Guidelines for the Use of Parenteral and Enteral Nutrition in Adult and Pediatric Patients. *JPEN*, **261** (1), 1SA–138SA.

38. Koletzko B, Goulet O, Hunt J, Krohn K, Shamir R (2005) 1. Guidelines on Paediatric Parenteral Nutrition of the European Society of Paediatric Gastroenterology, Hepatology and Nutrition (ESPGHAN) and the European Society for Clinical Nutrition and Metabolism (ESPEN), Supported by the European Society of Paediatric Research (ESPR). *J Pediatr Gastroenterol Nutr*, **41** (Suppl. 2), S1–87.

39. Shulman RJ, Phillips S (2003) Parenteral nutrition in infants and children. *J Pediatr Gastroenterol Nutr*, **36** (5), 587–607.

40. Ibrahim HM, Jeroudi MA, Baier RJ, Dhanireddy R, Krouskop RW (2004) Aggressive early total parental nutrition in low-birth-weight infants. *J Perinatol*, **24** (8), 482–486.

41. Thureen PJ, Melara D, Fennessey PV, Hay WW Jr (2003) Effect of low versus high intravenous amino acid intake on very low birth weight infants in the early neonatal period. *Pediatr Res*, **53** (1), 24–32.

42. Koletzko B, Goulet O, Hunt J, Krohn K, Shamir R (2005) 1. Guidelines on Paediatric Parenteral Nutrition of the European Society of Paediatric Gastroenterology, Hepatology and Nutrition (ESPGHAN) and the European Society for Clinical Nutrition and Metabolism (ESPEN), Supported by the European Society of Paediatric Research (ESPR). *J Pediatr Gastroenterol Nutr*, **41** (Suppl. 2), S1–87.

43. ASPEN (The American Society for Parenteral and Enteral Nutrition) Board of Directors (2002) Guidelines for the Use of Parenteral and Enteral Nutrition in Adult and Pediatric Patients. *JPEN*, **261** (1), 1SA–138SA.

44. Koletzko B, Goulet O, Hunt J, Krohn K, Shamir R (2005) 1. Guidelines on Paediatric Parenteral Nutrition of the European Society of Paediatric Gastroenterology, Hepatology and Nutrition (ESPGHAN) and the European Society for Clinical Nutrition and Metabolism (ESPEN), Supported by the European Society of Paediatric Research (ESPR). *J Pediatr Gastroenterol Nutr*, **41** (Suppl. 2), S1–87.

45. Jones MO, Pierro A, Hammond P, Nunn A, Krouskop RW (1993) Glucose utilization in the surgical newborn infant receiving total parenteral nutrition. *J Pediatr Surg*, **28** (9), 1121–1125.

46. Koletzko B, Goulet O, Hunt J, Krohn K, Shamir R (2005) 1. Guidelines on Paediatric Parenteral Nutrition of the European Society of Paediatric Gastroenterology, Hepatology and Nutrition (ESPGHAN) and the European Society for Clinical Nutrition and Metabolism (ESPEN), Supported by the European Society of Paediatric Research (ESPR). *J Pediatr Gastroenterol Nutr*, **41** (Suppl. 2), S1–87.

47. Shulman RJ, Phillips S (2003) Parenteral nutrition in infants and children. *J Pediatr Gastroenterol Nutr*, **36** (5), 587–607.

48. Cairns PA, Wilson DC, Jenkins J, McMaster D, McClure BG (1996) Tolerance of mixed lipid emulsion in neonates: effect of concentration. *Arch Dis Child Foetal Neonatal Ed*, **75** (2), F113–F116.

49. Haumont D, Richelle M, Deckelbaum RJ, Coussaert E, Carpentier YA (1992) Effect of liposomal content of lipid emulsions on plasma lipid concentrations in low birth weight infants receiving parenteral nutrition. *J Pediatr*, **121** (5 Pt 1), 759–763.

50. Shulman RJ, Phillips S (2003) Parenteral nutrition in infants and children. *J Pediatr Gastroenterol Nutr*, **36** (5), 587–607.

51. Gutcher GR, Farrell PM (1991) Intravenous infusion of lipid for the prevention of essential fatty acid deficiency in premature infants. *Am J Clin Nutr*, **54** (6), 1024–1028.

52. Koletzko B, Goulet O, Hunt J, Krohn K, Shamir R (2005) 1. Guidelines on Paediatric Parenteral Nutrition of the European Society of Paediatric Gastroenterology, Hepatology and Nutrition (ESPGHAN) and the European Society for Clinical Nutrition and Metabolism (ESPEN), Supported by the European Society of Paediatric Research (ESPR). *J Pediatr Gastroenterol Nutr*, **41** (Suppl. 2), S1–87.

53. Ibrahim HM, Jeroudi MA, Baier RJ, Dhanireddy R, Krouskop RW (2004) Aggressive early total parental nutrition in low-birth-weight infants. *J Perinatol*, **24** (8), 482–486.

54. ASPEN (The American Society for Parenteral and Enteral Nutrition) Board of Directors (2002) Guidelines for the Use of Parenteral and Enteral Nutrition in Adult and Pediatric Patients. *JPEN*, **261** (1), 1SA–138SA.

55. Koletzko B, Goulet O, Hunt J, Krohn K, Shamir R (2005) 1. Guidelines on Paediatric Parenteral Nutrition of the European Society of Paediatric Gastroenterology, Hepatology and Nutrition (ESPGHAN) and the European Society for Clinical Nutrition and Metabolism (ESPEN), Supported by the European Society of Paediatric Research (ESPR). *J Pediatr Gastroenterol Nutr*, **41** (Suppl. 2), S1–87.

56. Haumont D, Richelle M, Deckelbaum RJ, Coussaert E, Carpentier YA (1992) Effect of liposomal content of lipid emulsions on plasma lipid concentrations in low birth weight infants receiving parenteral nutrition. *J Pediatr*, **121** (5 Pt 1), 759–763.

57. Hilliard JL, Shannon DL, Hunter MA, Brans YW (1983) Plasma lipid levels in preterm neonates receiving parenteral fat emulsions. *Arch Dis Child*, **58** (1), 29–33.

58. ASPEN (The American Society for Parenteral and Enteral Nutrition) Board of Directors (2002) Guidelines for the Use of Parenteral and Enteral Nutrition in Adult and Pediatric Patients. *JPEN*, **261** (1), 1SA–138SA.

59. Koletzko B, Goulet O, Hunt J, Krohn K, Shamir R (2005) 1. Guidelines on Paediatric Parenteral Nutrition of the European Society of Paediatric Gastroenterology, Hepatology and Nutrition (ESPGHAN) and the European Society for Clinical Nutrition and Metabolism (ESPEN), Supported by the European Society of Paediatric Research (ESPR). *J Pediatr Gastroenterol Nutr*, **41** (Suppl. 2), S1–87.

60. Koletzko B, Goulet O, Hunt J, Krohn K, Shamir R (2005) 1. Guidelines on Paediatric Parenteral Nutrition of the European Society of Paediatric Gastroenterology, Hepatology and Nutrition (ESPGHAN) and the European Society for Clinical Nutrition and Metabolism (ESPEN), Supported by the European Society of Paediatric Research (ESPR). *J Pediatr Gastroenterol Nutr*, **41** (Suppl. 2), S1–87.

61. Shulman RJ, Phillips S (2003) Parenteral nutrition in infants and children. *J Pediatr Gastroenterol Nutr*, **36** (5), 587–607.

62. Ainsworth SB, Clerihew L, McGuire W (2004) Percutaneous central venous catheters versus peripheral cannulae for delivery of parenteral nutrition in neonates. *Cochrane Database Syst Rev* (2), CD004219.

63. McGuire W, Henderson G, Fowlie PW (2004) Feeding the preterm infant. *BMJ*, **329** (7476), 1227–1230.

64. Bethune K, Allwood M, Grainger C, Wormleighton C (2001) Use of filters during the preparation and administration of parenteral nutrition: position paper and guidelines prepared by a British pharmaceutical nutrition group working party. *Nutrition*, **17** (5), 403–408.

65. Hodge D, Puntis JW (2002) Diagnosis, prevention, and management of catheter related bloodstream infection during long term parenteral nutrition. *Arch Dis Child Foetal Neonatal Ed*, **87** (1), F21–F24.

66. Puntis JW, Holden CE, Smallman S, Finkel Y, George RH, Booth IW (1991) Staff training: a key factor in reducing intravascular catheter sepsis. *Arch Dis Child*, **66** (3), 335–337.

67. Hodge D, Puntis JW (2002) Diagnosis, prevention, and management of catheter related bloodstream infection during long term parenteral nutrition. *Arch Dis Child Foetal Neonatal Ed*, **87** (1), F21–F24.

68. Puntis JW, Holden CE, Smallman S, Finkel Y, George RH, Booth IW (1991) Staff training: a key factor in reducing intravascular catheter sepsis. *Arch Dis Child*, **66** (3), 335–337.

69. Puntis JW, Holden CE, Smallman S, Finkel Y, George RH, Booth IW (1991) Staff training: a key factor in reducing intravascular catheter sepsis. *Arch Dis Child*, **66** (3), 335–337.

70. Puntis JW, Holden CE, Smallman S, Finkel Y, George RH, Booth IW (1991) Staff training: a key factor in reducing intravascular catheter sepsis. *Arch Dis Child*, **66** (3), 335–337.

71. Schmidt B, Andrew M (1995) Neonatal thrombosis: report of a prospective Canadian and international registry. *Pediatrics*, **96** (5 Pt 1), 939–943.

72. Cartwright DW (2004) Central venous lines in neonates: a study of 2186 catheters. *Arch Dis Child Foetal Neonatal Ed*, **89** (6), F504–F508.

73. Chowdhary SK, Parashar K (2000) Central venous access in neonates through the peripheral route. *Curr Opin Clin Nutr Metab Care*, **3** (3), 217–219.

74. Peters O, Ryan SW, Matthew L, Cheng K, Lunn J (1997) Randomised controlled trial of acetate in preterm neonates receiving parenteral nutrition. *Arch Dis Child Foetal Neonatal Ed*, **77** (1), F12–F15.

75. Peters O, Ryan SW, Matthew L, Cheng K, Lunn J (1997) Randomised controlled trial of acetate in preterm neonates receiving parenteral nutrition. *Arch Dis Child Foetal Neonatal Ed*, **77** (1), F12–F15.

76. Ekblad H, Kero P, Takala J (1985) Slow sodium acetate infusion in the correction of metabolic acidosis in premature infants. *Am J Dis Child*, **139** (7), 708–710.

77. ASPEN (The American Society for Parenteral and Enteral Nutrition) Board of Directors (2002) Guidelines for the Use of Parenteral and Enteral Nutrition in Adult and Pediatric Patients. *JPEN*, **261** (1), 1SA–138SA.

78. ASPEN (The American Society for Parenteral and Enteral Nutrition) Board of Directors (2002) Guidelines for the Use of Parenteral and Enteral Nutrition in Adult and Pediatric Patients. *JPEN*, **261** (1), 1SA–138SA.

79. ASPEN (The American Society for Parenteral and Enteral Nutrition) Board of Directors (2002) Guidelines for the Use of Parenteral and Enteral Nutrition in Adult and Pediatric Patients. *JPEN*, **261** (1), 1SA–138SA.

80. ASPEN (The American Society for Parenteral and Enteral Nutrition) Board of Directors (2002) Guidelines for the Use of Parenteral and Enteral Nutrition in Adult and Pediatric Patients. *JPEN*, **261** (1), 1SA–138SA.

81. ASPEN (The American Society for Parenteral and Enteral Nutrition) Board of Directors (2002) Guidelines for the Use of Parenteral and Enteral Nutrition in Adult and Pediatric Patients. *JPEN*, **261** (1), 1SA–138SA.

82. ASPEN (The American Society for Parenteral and Enteral Nutrition) Board of Directors (2002) Guidelines for the Use of Parenteral and Enteral Nutrition in Adult and Pediatric Patients. *JPEN*, **261** (1), 1SA–138SA.

83. Koletzko B, Goulet O, Hunt J, Krohn K, Shamir R (2005) 1. Guidelines on Paediatric Parenteral Nutrition of the European Society of Paediatric Gastroenterology, Hepatology and Nutrition (ESPGHAN) and the European Society for Clinical Nutrition and Metabolism (ESPEN), Supported by the European Society of Paediatric Research (ESPR). *J Pediatr Gastroenterol Nutr*, **41** (Suppl. 2), S1–87.

84. Shulman RJ, Phillips S (2003) Parenteral nutrition in infants and children. *J Pediatr Gastroenterol Nutr*, **36** (5), 587–607.

85. Btaiche IF, Khalidi N (2002) Parenteral nutrition-associated liver complications in children. *Pharmacotherapy*, **22** (2), 188–211.

86. Zambrano E, El-Hennawy M, Ehrenkranz RA, Zelterman D, Reyes-Mugica M (2004) Total parenteral nutrition induced liver pathology: an autopsy series of 24 newborn cases. *Pediatr Dev Pathol*, 7 (5), 425–432.

87. Quigley EM, Marsh MN, Shaffer JL, Markin RS (1993) Hepatobiliary complications of total parenteral nutrition. *Gastroenterology*, **104** (1), 286–301.

88. Heubi JE, Wiechmann DA, Creutzinger V, *et al.* (2002) Tauroursodeoxycholic acid (TUDCA) in the prevention of total parenteral nutrition-associated liver disease. *J Pediatr*, **141** (2), 237–242.

89. Chen CY, Tsao PN, Chen HL, Chou HC, Hsieh WS, Chang MH (2004) Ursodeoxycholic acid (UDCA) therapy in very-low-birth-weight infants with parenteral nutrition-associated cholestasis. *J Pediatr*, **145** (3), 317–321.

90. Sondheimer JM, Asturias E, Cadnapaphornchai M (1998) Infection and cholestasis in neonates with intestinal resection and long-term parenteral nutrition. *J Pediatr Gastroenterol Nutr*, **27** (2), 131–137.

91. Koletzko B, Goulet O, Hunt J, Krohn K, Shamir R (2005) 1. Guidelines on Paediatric Parenteral Nutrition of the European Society of Paediatric Gastroenterology, Hepatology and Nutrition (ESPGHAN) and the European Society for Clinical Nutrition and Metabolism (ESPEN), Supported by the European Society of Paediatric Research (ESPR). *J Pediatr Gastroenterol Nutr*, **41** (Suppl. 2), S1–87.

Chapter 13

NEONATAL STABILISATION AND TRANSPORT

Robert Bomont and Lynda Rafael

Learning outcomes

After reading this chapter the reader will be expected to be able to:

- Compare and contrast inter and intra-hospital transfers

- Discuss the type of equipment necessary to transfer an acutely unwell neonate safely

- Describe the essential information that should be communicated to the transport team and receiving hospital from the referral hospital

- Justify the need for obsessive clinical re-evaluation at all stages of the transfer

- Discuss the need for a high standard of verbal and written communication in the transfer of acutely unwell infants

- Consider how to design a course that addresses the training needs of staff involved in transport

---

Introduction

The transfer of neonates from one location to another is a common occurrence for which all staff should be adequately prepared. This chapter considers this in the following sections:

- Type of transfer
- Personnel and training
- Equipment
- Recognition and referral
- Transport and stabilisation
- Documentation

Type of transfer

Inter-hospital

Following the introduction of managed clinical networks within the UK and the resultant regionalisation of neonatal intensive care (see Chapter 1), babies requiring specialist or tertiary level care frequently have to undergo inter-hospital transfer. About 3% of all infants will require this specialist or tertiary level of care[1], with approximately 1.3% of all infants requiring transfer to a different centre[2]. *In utero* transfers have better clinical outcomes, but are not always possible for reasons which include maternal ill-health, imminent labour or the unavailability of maternity beds. Unfortunately *ex utero* transport has been shown to be associated with an increase in morbidity and mortality[3,4].

Ex utero inter-hospital transfers may be further subclassified with respect to the degree of urgency for the transfer to occur. This is dictated by the clinical status of the infant.

- Time-critical: this category of transfer is very unusual. Some infants require treatment that is so specialised, such as ECMO (extracorporeal membrane oxygenation), that there is nothing that can be done to improve their clinical status without it. Therefore, delaying transfer with prolonged periods of stabilisation is counterproductive. For this kind of transfer the potential benefits of the treatment available at the receiving centre outweigh the risk of immediate transfer.

- Emergency: this category is for infants who require transfer to meet their ongoing care needs, such as intensive care or urgent surgery. For these transfers it is necessary and safe to ensure that the infant's clinical status is optimised prior to transfer.

- Elective or back-transfer: this category is for infants who are clinically stable. They would not be compromised if their transfer did not occur within a particular timeframe.

Implications for practice

There is some evidence that early post-natal transfer of the preterm infant is associated with an increase in morbidity which is why *in utero* transfer should be encouraged where possible.

Intra-hospital

Babies are frequently transferred within their own hospitals, for example from delivery suite to the neonatal unit, or from the neonatal unit to theatre and back. These transfers should not be considered as less important than those between hospitals and must be adequately prepared for and handled in a similar way.

Personnel and training

The members of the clinical team required for a transfer are dependent upon the clinical status of the baby and the nature of the journey to be undertaken. Each transfer requires at least one nurse. For transfers of all but the most clinically stable infants a second member of the team is required. Historically this was a more senior doctor, but more recently it has been demonstrated to be safe and practical to use advanced neonatal nurse practitioners in this role[5,6]. In other countries paramedics play a major clinical role in neonatal transfer teams, although this is not currently commonplace in the UK.

Both medical and nursing staff who transport neonates require specific transport related skills as well as a high level of clinical competence in neonatal intensive care. Each should have appropriate training in transport medicine, be familiar with their local organisational procedures and have an excellent working knowledge of their equipment. When adequately trained personnel are used as members of the transfer team, this can impact on the clinical status of the infant, with lower rates of in-transit deterioration and an improvement in clinical condition on arrival at the receiving unit.[7,8,9].

There are at present no agreed UK national competencies or standards for those working in transport teams. Local policies exist across some neonatal networks, which aim to streamline and standardise at least some areas of care. The STABLE©, PICCTs and PNeoSTaR courses have been developed and introduced to address some of the training needs.

Equipment

Equipment carried by the transport team should be adequate for the provision of neonatal intensive care in the transport environment. Box 13.1 outlines the broad categories of equipment required and a transport incubator is shown in Figure 13.1.

All transport team members should be trained in the use of the equipment and be able to 'trouble-shoot' if it malfunctions.

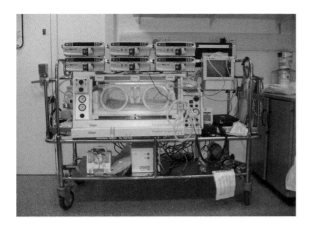

Figure 13.1 Transport incubator.

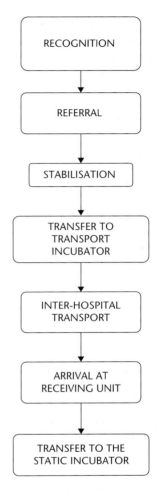

Figure 13.2 Suggested steps for inter-hospital transfer.

Box 13.1   Transport incubator

- Transport incubator with:
  - Multi-channel monitor, allowing heart rate, respiratory rate, invasive and non-invasive blood pressure, oxygen saturations and temperature
  - Neonatal ventilator and means to mask ventilate
  - Medical gases, often including nitric oxide
  - Suction apparatus
- Emergency drugs and those unavailable within the referring hospital
- Emergency equipment to allow for example reintubation, vascular access and drainage of tension pneumothorax
- Portable blood gas and glucose analysers

Implications for practice

The equipment necessary for the transport of a sick newborn infant should be that which allows the provision of a mobile intensive care unit.

Recognition and referral

Any transfer may be considered to comprise of several sequential steps. The flowchart in Figure 13.2 demonstrates the steps for inter-hospital transfer. It may be modified for intra-hospital transfers.

Each box in this figure is now considered in turn.

Recognition

The transfer process begins with the recognition that a particular infant may require ongoing intensive or specialist treatment unavailable at the referring unit. This may be obvious in the newborn with a congenital defect requiring surgery, such as a gastroschisis, or in an infant with cyanosis that may be due to cyanotic congenital heart disease or pulmonary hypertension, but may be more subtle in the intermittently grunting infant reviewed 60 minutes following delivery. This initial recognition of need and institution of appropriate care is of key importance and impacts on long-term outcome.

Referral

Knowledge of local referral procedures is important. Models differ among centres. Some units refer by telephone to their tertiary centres directly whilst others make a single contact with a central cot bureau. In this latter case the cot bureau in turn locate a suitable cot and notify the appropriate transfer team. This model has the advantage of reducing the administrative tasks of the referral unit, allowing them to concentrate on the clinical need. It does, however, necessitate basic clinical information being relayed to potential receiving units through a third party.

Box 13.2   Minimum information required at referral

- Name
- NHS number (if available)
- Date and time of birth
- Gestation
- Birthweight/current weight (if applicable)
- Name of referring consultant responsible for baby's care
- Antenatal history and reason for transfer
- Ventilation status and settings
- ET size and length
- Infective status of the baby
- Most recent blood gas
- Venous/arterial access
- Temperature
- Blood pressure
- Blood sugar
- Oxygen saturations
- Heart rate
- Inotropes/sedation/paralysis/antibiotics/other
- Fluid requirements – mls/kg/day (maintenance/boluses/enteral)

At referral the transport team will require a minimum set of information in order that they may accept the transfer and usually have standardised forms designed for this purpose (see Box 13.2).

This may seem unnecessarily time consuming when the referring team is often very busy, but it allows the transport team to prepare adequately and to offer informed advice regarding management.

On accepting the referral the transport team also accept joint responsibility for the infant's clinical care and should begin to work with the referring unit from this point onwards. As the transport progresses, the responsibility will gradually change from mostly that of the referring unit to primarily that of the transport team. In some situations the responsibility may be shared three ways if, for example, the infant is transferring to a specialist cardiac centre and an independent transport team is being utilised.

It is evident that clear and accurate communication, both written and oral, is of paramount importance at all times during the transfer. Members of each team should aim to update members of the other teams at frequent intervals. The transport team may, for example, offer guidance to the referring unit whilst in transit to collect the infant. Key points for communication are highlighted in Figure 13.3.

Stabilisation

As soon as the decision is made to move an infant the process of pre-transport stabilisation should commence. A period of stabilisation at the referring hospital has been demonstrated to significantly improve the clinical condition of a select group of infants, but one may envisage extrapolation to the wider population[10].

The aim of the stabilisation phase is to follow basic resuscitation measures and to prepare the infant for transfer. All remedial action should be completed prior to moving the baby in an attempt to pre-empt the need for intervention during the transfer.

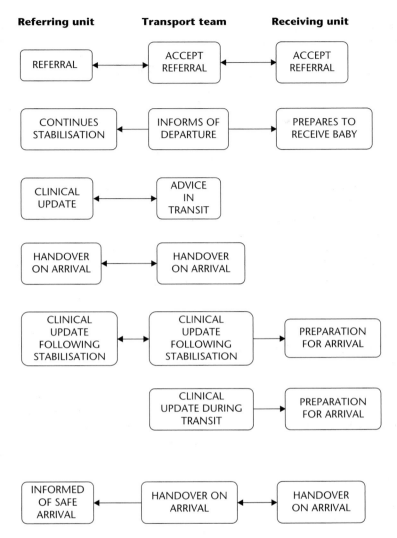

Referring unit   **Transport team**   **Receiving unit**

Figure 13.3 Key time points for communication.

It may be considered in two phases, as described below.

Initial stabilisation

This is from the moment a decision to transfer is made to the time that the transfer team arrives. Staff at the referring unit should be able to provide this care but may need to be guided by the transport team and specialist centre. The extent to which care may be given in this phase is dependent upon time before arrival of the transport team and the skills and availability of nursing and medical staff at the referral centres.

Preparation for transfer

This is from the time that the transfer team arrives to the time immediately prior to departure from the referring unit. During this phase the transfer team and the staff at the referring unit work together. Both teams share clinical knowledge, experience and skills to allow the most efficient stabilisation of the infant. The

Box 13.3 Key elements of the stabilisation process

- Airway and breathing
- Circulation
- Metabolic
- Thermal control
- Infection
- Comfort
- Counselling and communication with parents

- Apnoea
- Significant respiratory distress
- $FiO_2 > 50\%$
- Respiratory acidosis (rising $PaCO_2$)
- Severe metabolic acidosis
- Infants extubated for less than 48 hours
- Abdominal distension
- Preoperative surgical infants requiring significant opioid analgesia
- Cranio-facial abnormality

transfer team is working in an unfamiliar environment and may require assistance with seemingly routine tasks such as blood gas analysis and requesting laboratory investigations.

Implications for practice

Once a referral has been made the responsibility for the care of the infant is shared between the referral and receiving hospitals as well as the transport team; this can get complicated and clear lines of communication are essential.

The STABLE (S = sugar and safety, T = temperature, A = airway, B = blood pressure, L = laboratory results, E = emotional support) course was developed in the USA by Kris Karlsen to reinforce the knowledge and skills required in the stabilisation of the newborn (www.stable-program.org), particularly for those neonatal staff that work in peripheral neonatal units.

Airway and breathing

It is important to remember that one of the goals of stabilisation is to avoid the need for intervention during transfer. Intubation and ventilation should be considered in those infants that have not already been ventilated if further clinical deterioration is suspected. This is in order to safeguard the airway and these situations include:

Infants who are in the early phase of respiratory distress syndrome and likely to deteriorate further may also benefit from intubation and surfactant administration.

If an endotracheal tube is in situ it is of vital importance that this is securely fixed. The movement and vibration experienced during transfer may dislodge tubes, leading to a reintubation in a sub-optimal environment. There are many fixation techniques and local policy may determine which is used. Endotracheal tube tip position should be checked and noted in the transfer documentation.

Endotracheal intubation is not the only way of providing respiratory support during transfer[11]. Most teams will now consider the use of nasal CPAP during the transfer for a select group of infants, for example. CPAP delivery devices do often differ from those used in the static environment with most teams using the integral device on their transport ventilator.

Circulation

The goal is to ensure adequate perfusion of essential organs. This may be assessed using a combination of observations, clinical tests and physiological measurements. If the infant is volume depleted then appropriate volume replacement should be given. Most commonly this is in the form of 10 ml/kg aliquots of normal saline, but 4.5% human albumin solution (4.5% HAS) or blood products such as packed red cells or fresh frozen plasma may be indicated, depending upon the exact clinical scenario.

It may be appropriate to gain arterial access either by siting an umbilical arterial catheter or peripheral arterial line. Indications for this include:

- Hypotension or unstable blood pressure
- Inotrope dependence
- Need for frequent blood gas analysis

The lines must be securely fixed, whilst leaving the insertion site or limb exposed and easily accessible. Although this should be standard practice it is especially important prior to transfer. The line position should be checked, usually with X-ray, and noted in the transfer documentation. Lines should be transduced and infused with heparinised saline at low volume. Even if the transducer is not compatible with the monitoring system used by the transport team this should not preclude its use during the stabilisation phase as the transport team can change the transducer prior to transfer to enable monitoring during transit.

Adequate intravenous access should be obtained at an early stage. Frequently, in infants who are unwell, gaining access becomes more difficult as time passes. Two peripheral cannulae are the absolute minimum required for acute transport. Umbilical venous catheters which have been properly sited and secured provide a safe route for fluid and drug administration. They also provide a route by which to give inotropic support if required. Again, the catheter tip position should be checked and noted in the transfer documentation. Central venous access may also be secured by means of a percutaneous long line.

Metabolic

An important goal of metabolic stabilisation is to maintain normoglycaemia. Plasma blood sugar should be measured and normalised as a matter of urgency. Intravenous fluid containing dextrose should be commenced at rates dependent upon the clinical condition of the infant and local policy. Plasma blood sugar measurement should continue to be made at regular intervals following normalisation. The infant should not receive enteral nutrition prior to or during acute transfer to obviate the risk of respiratory aspiration but if feeds have been given the gastric contents can be withdrawn prior to transfer.

Many infants who are unwell develop metabolic acidosis. This can impact upon the physiological function of many organ systems, including respiratory, renal and cardiac. In most instances it is important to correct this acidosis. This is most commonly achieved by addressing the causative factor. For example, infants may become acidotic as a result of poor tissue perfusion, anaerobic metabolism and the consequent production of lactic acid. If the poor perfusion is as a result of hypovolaemia or abnormal fluid distribution (common in sepsis) then this should be corrected but it may be as the result of poor cardiac function, in which case inotropes are indicated. Infusion of sodium bicarbonate solution may also be indicated. There is at present no evidence to support the use of one approach in preference to the other in terms of reduction of morbidity or mortality[12].

Temperature

See Chapter 6. Strenuous efforts must be made to achieve and maintain thermoneutrality. This can often be particularly challenging during the period prior to transfer in view of the frequent episodes of prolonged handling which may be necessary during stabilisation of the baby. For example, intubation and gaining intravenous and intra-arterial access may require that incubator doors are opened for many minutes. Staff performing such procedures must do so in a planned and efficient manner, minimising cold stress. Infants must not be nursed on wet towels or clothing and should have hats put on at the earliest opportunity.

Attention should be paid to optimising and maintaining environmental temperature. The use of increased humidity may be appropriate, as may the use of chemical heating mattresses or plastic occlusive coverings.

Infection

Strict handwashing procedure must not be forgotten during this time when there may be a large number of people involved in the stabilisation, transfer and handover of the infant's care. In addition, there may be many clinical tasks to be completed in a short period of time and it is important to remember that the cause of the infant's illness may be infection, such as group B streptococcus. Ensure that appropriate antibiotics have been prescribed and administered promptly following collection of microbiological samples.

Comfort

Many clinical procedures and therapies are uncomfortable or painful. Non-pharmacological methods as well as pharmacological methods should be used to minimise the distress that these cause. Adequate chemical sedation is essential for those infants who are pharmacologically paralysed and unable to show physical signs of distress. Light and noise are also noxious stimuli and should be minimised where possible. Thought should also be given to the incubator environment during transit and the use of towels and blankets to provide physical support during the movement of the ambulance.

Implications for practice

There are very few reasons where a 'swoop and scoop' strategy is necessary (e.g. transposition of the great arteries) and time should be taken to stabilise the infant prior to transfer, utilising a structured approach to neonatal intensive care.

Counselling and communication with parents

Parents are understandably often very shocked and anxious when they are counselled about the need to transport their infant. Not only must they deal with the fact that their baby is in need of specialist care, but also that this will require transportation to a second unit. The unit may be many miles from their home, children and local support network and the staff and routines in the receiving unit will be different. Occasionally, the mother may be too unwell to be transferred at the same time, further compounding an already difficult situation.

Feedback from parents whose newborns had been transported identified their feelings of unpreparedness and their need to receive as much information as possible[13]. Parents must be informed of the need to transport their infant at the earliest opportunity and ideally this should be done by a senior member of the clinical team at the referring centre. As information becomes available this should be conveyed to the parents. As soon as is practicable, following their arrival, the transport team should meet and talk with the parents answering questions and outlining their management plan. Ideally, they should seek informed consent for transfer. Many transport teams carry parent information packs detailing their service, including directions for parents to use when travelling to the receiving unit and local arrangements for accommodation. Contact details for parents should be checked prior to departure, including mobile telephone numbers if available. It is good practice to inform parents of the team's imminent departure and also the safe arrival at the receiving unit. Families should be warned against the practice of following the ambulance, especially where blue light and/or siren facilitated transport is to be used. It is also important that they are made aware of the risks of transport.

Implications for practice

Ex utero transfer of their infant to another hospital is often a devastating situation for parents and the following are important considerations:
• The transport team should introduce themselves to parents where possible.

- Information about the receiving hospital should be communicated both verbally and in written form.
- The parents should not leave for the receiving hospital until after the ambulance has left the referring hospital at the earliest (in case the transfer is cancelled or the destination changed).

Transfer to the transport incubator

Transfer from the static incubator

Before transfer it is essential that all necessary stabilisation interventions have been completed. Prior to physically moving the infant the following checklist may be used.

Airway and breathing

Ensure continuing respiratory support is available, i.e.:

- ET tube, if present, is secure
- NCPAP, if present, is secure
- A satisfactory blood gas has been obtained prior to transfer
- Transport ventilator is set appropriately
- Bagging system is available

Circulation

Continuing circulatory support is available:

- Infusions, if practicable, should be disconnected from the pumps (not from the cannulae as this can cause confusion) prior to transfer into the transport incubator
- Inotropes should not be disconnected, or if this is unavoidable then for the briefest period only

Monitoring

- Ensure compatibility of monitoring probes with the transport system. If they are incompatible they should be changed prior to moving the infant.
- For all but the sickest infants all monitoring may be disconnected and then reconnected immediately before transfer.

- Ensure that the transducer and infusion fluids for invasive blood pressure monitoring are disconnected and that the catheter is securely locked in the 'off' position.
- Disconnect the temperature probe. It is commonly overlooked and can result in the infant not being 'freed' from the static incubator.

Thermal environment

Transport incubators are poorly insulated and the side door must be opened to allow access for the infant. The majority of transport incubators cannot be humidified. Therefore the incubator should be pre-warmed to a temperature greater than that of the static incubator.

The door should be opened for the shortest period possible. This is best achieved by an individual whose sole responsibility during the move from static to transport incubator is to open and close the door. Remember that chemical gel mattresses and plastic occlusive wrappings may be helpful when transporting preterm infants.

When the above checks have been completed a team leader should be identified who will then delegate tasks to the team of individuals required to move the infant. The team leader is the individual who will lift the infant from the static to the transport incubator. Most commonly this is the transport nurse. Each team member should be aware of their own individual responsibilities during the move and it is the responsibility of the team leader to ensure that this is the case and that all communications are clear and understood. Many teams find it helpful to practice their roles in real time during a mock move.

After being placed in the transport incubator respiratory support should be recommenced immediately, before commencing monitoring. Despite the earlier checks, ET tubes may be accidentally dislodged and therefore particular attention should be paid to the presence of chest movement and air entry on chest auscultation. Infusions may now be reconnected and commenced. The act of moving may in itself cause a period of instability in the infant's clinical status.

Before leaving the relative safety of the NICU, attempts should be made to re-optimise the condition of the baby. If ventilated, a blood gas should be measured following a period of transport incubator ventilation and any appropriate alterations made.

Inter-hospital transport

Choice of vehicle

Different vehicles may be used to transport neonates. The majority of transfers in the UK are made in road ambulances, although for transfers over water or large distances such as in rural Scotland specialised helicopters are used. In some regions there are dedicated neonatal ambulances that have been specially modified but in other regions standard ambulances are used. Knowledge of the vehicles and their equipment is necessary as it will dictate specific aspects of the transfer such as the volume and type of medical gases taken on the transport incubator. It is also important to be aware that there are mechanical or electrical lifts provided to lift the incubators up to the level of the ambulance floor. There should be no manual lifting of heavy equipment.

When secured, the transport incubator should be connected to the ambulance's power and medical gas supply. This is in order to preserve the incubator's battery power and gas. Although uncomfortable for the transport team it is often necessary to have the ambient temperature of the vehicle high in an attempt to maintain thermoneutrality for the infant. If possible it is good practice to prewarm the vehicle with all main doors closed until the incubator is ready to be loaded.

Safety during transfer

All transfers of neonates, however short the transfer time or small the distance, are potentially hazardous to both the infant and staff. Safety of the baby and the transport staff is a priority and neither should be exposed to greater risk than is absolutely necessary. Seat belts must be used whenever the ambulance is moving. If it is necessary for staff to leave their seats then the vehicle must be stationary. No effective restraint system is currently available for the infant in the incubator although there are a several methods currently used, which include the use of Velcro® straps. These may provide some restraint during transit but will not be effective during a significant deceleration force such as occurs during an accident. Excessive speed is dangerous and should be avoided. Lights and sirens are most safely used to allow movement through heavy traffic travelling at normal speeds.

There are many health and safety regulations which govern neonatal transport equipment, many of which in the past were overlooked. The European Committee for Standardisation (CEN) regulations define such particulars as overall weight of the transport system and their fixation systems within vehicles. It is worth remembering that any unsecured item, including personnel and equipment, in the back of an ambulance can act as a missile in the event of the ambulance driver having to brake sharply.

Arrival at the receiving unit

The receiving unit staff will have prepared appropriate equipment in order to support the infant in the static environment. Communication and regular updates between the transport team and the receiving unit permits this, even if the infant's clinical status has altered significantly since the referral was first accepted.

On arrival the transport team will connect the transport incubator to the NICU piped gas supply and plug into the electrical supply to preserve battery life. This ensures that the infant is not compromised should there be a delay in transferring from the transport to the static incubator.

A comprehensive verbal handover including all interventions made should then be provided by the transport team. In addition, written documentation from the referring hospital and from the transport team will be provided. It is also helpful to make available electronic or hard copies of recent relevant imaging such as X-rays and ultrasound scans.

Transfer to the static incubator

Using a system similar to that in Figure 13.4 the infant should be transferred to the static incubator.

Implications for practice

On arrival at the receiving hospital the infant's clinical condition should be thoroughly and systematically re-evaluated

Documentation

As with all clinical work it is important to keep clear and comprehensive documentation. This can be challenging when preparing a child for transfer as there are many differing pressures on time. In addition to photocopies of the clinical notes, drug and fluid charts and observation charts from the referral centre it is good practice to also include a nursing and medical handover letter in the documentation prepared for the transport team. Some transport teams provide referring units with standardised documentation to complete to ensure that the most important

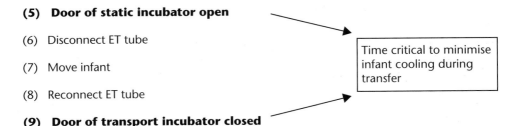

(1) Placing of transport incubator next to static incubator and setting temperature of

static incubator

(2) Preparation of additional heating measures: Transwarmer/bubble wrap

(3) Preparation of infant e.g.:

(a) Infusions

(b) Chest drain

(c) Monitoring[esl]

(4) Walk through practice run

(5) Door of static incubator open

(6) Disconnect ET tube

(7) Move infant

(8) Reconnect ET tube

(9) Door of transport incubator closed

(10) Reconnect:

(a) Infusions

(b) Chest drain

(c) Monitoring

Time critical to minimise infant cooling during transfer

Figure 13.4 An example of steps in a planned transfer from a transport incubator to a static incubator (Paediatric and Infant Critical Care Course (PICCTS) University Hospitals Leicester).

pieces of information are recorded and are easily accessible.

Transport teams in turn will complete their own documentation during the transfer. In addition to their clinical assessment they will document all interventions carried out. Frequency of recording observations during the transfer is to some extent dependent upon the clinical stability of the baby, but is not commonly greater than at 15-minute intervals.

Examples of documentation used by teams around the country may be found at http://www.neonatal.org.uk/

Conclusion

Neonatal transport nursing is an exciting field in which to work. Safety at all times is of prime importance. Adequately trained staff who are familiar with their equipment and the particular challenges of the transport environment are able to provide the best possible care to infants and their families. Communication between all parties involved in each stage of the transport process is a vital component of a successful transfer.

Useful texts

Advanced Life Support Group (2002) *Safe Transfer and Retrieval. The Practical Approach.* BMJ Books, Spain.

Barry P, Leslie A, Bohin S, *et al.* (2003) *Paediatric and Neonatal Critical Care Transport.* BMJ Books, Spain.

Karlsen K (2006) *The STABLE Program Learner Manual.* American Academy of Pediatrics, Utah.

References

1. Devane S (1999) Transport of ill infants. In: Rennie J, Roberton N (eds), *Textbook of Neonatology*, 3rd edn. Churchill Livingstone, Edinburgh.
2. Kempley S, Sinha A, on behalf of the Thames Perinatal Group (2004) Census of Neonatal Transfers in London and the South East of England. *Arch Dis Child – Fetal Neonatal Ed*, 89 (6), 521–526.
3. Costeloe K, Hennessy E, Gibson A, Marlow N, Wilkinson A, for the EPICure Study Group (2000) The EPICure Study: outcome to discharge from hospital for infants born at the edge of viability. *Pediatrics*, 106 (4), 659–671.
4. Shlossman P, Manley J, Sciscione A, Colmorgen G (1997) An analysis of neonatal morbidity and mortality in maternal (*in utero*) and neonatal transport at 24–34 weeks gestation. *Am J Perinatol*, 14 (8), 449–456.
5. Leslie A, Stephenson T (2003) Neonatal transfers by advanced neonatal nurse practitioners and paediatric registrars. *Arch Dis Child Fetal Neonatal Ed*, 88 (6), F509–F512
6. Leslie A, Bose C (1999) Nurse-led neonatal transport. *Semin Neonatol*, 4, 265–271.
7. Chance GW, Matthew JD, Gash J, *et al.* (1978) Neonatal transport: a controlled study of skilled assistance. *J Pediatr*, 93 (4), 662–666.
8. Leslie A, Stephenson T (1997) Audit of neonatal intensive care transport: closing the loop. *Acta Paediatr*, 86 (11), 1253–1256.
9. Hood JL, Cross A, Hulka B, *et al.* (1983) Effectiveness of the neonatal transport team. *Crit Care Med*, 11 (6), 419–423.
10. Bissaker S, Hindley H, Gauillar E, Shaw N (2004) Respiratory status of infants being transported with respiratory distress syndrome. The effect of pre-transport advice, stabilisation and the transport itself. *JNN*, 10 (3), 96–98.
11. Bomont RK, Cheema IU (2006) Use of nasal continuous positive airway pressure during neonatal transfers. *Arch Dis Child Fetal Neonatal Ed*, 91 (2, March), F85–F89. Epub 4 Oct 2005.
12. Lawn CJ, Weir FJ, McGuire W (2005) Base administration or fluid bolus for preventing morbidity and mortality in preterm infants with metabolic acidosis. *Cochrane Database Syst Rev* (2, 18 April), CD003215.
13. Frischer L, Gutterman DL (1992) Emotional impact on parents of transported babies. Considerations for meeting parents' needs. *Crit Care Clin*, 8 (3, 8 July), 649–660.

Chapter 14
NEONATAL NEUROLOGY

Eleri Adams and Marie Hubbard

Learning outcomes

By the end of the chapter the reader will be able to:

- Describe the main anatomical components of the brain; understand how the newborn brain develops and the main congenital neurological abnormalities that can occur

- Recognise the different types of intra and extra-cranial haemorrhage which may occur following birth trauma

- Recognise normal neurological patterns of behaviour in term and preterm infants

- Distinguish jitteriness from seizures and have knowledge of the immediate investigations and management that may be required

- Recognise features suggestive of neonatal abstinence syndrome

- Identify a baby who has moderate or severe encephalopathy and understand the principles of management of this condition

- Know the risk factors for development of preterm intraventricular haemorrhage and recognise symptoms and signs associated with raised intracranial pressure

---

Introduction

The development of the brain is a complex process beginning very early in foetal life and continuing to evolve throughout the neonatal period and beyond. Pathological processes affecting the newborn brain are varied and complex and this text is not designed to be exhaustive. It is hoped that this chapter will provide a sound understanding of the most common conditions and presentations of neurological abnormalities and it includes information on:

- Anatomy and embryology of the brain and the main congenital abnormalities (spina bifida and hydrocephalus)
- Birth trauma, including extracranial and intracranial haemorrhage
- Normal and abnormal findings in clinical neurological assessment

- Seizures
- Neonatal abstinence syndrome
- Hypoxic ischaemic encephalopathy
- Preterm brain injury – intraventricular haemorrhage and periventricular leucomalacia

Anatomy and embryology

Anatomy

The brain comprises 80% of the skull volume and consists of four main parts:

- Brain stem (midbrain, pons, medulla oblongata):
  - Relays motor and sensory impulses between the brain and spinal cord
  - Regulates heartbeat and breathing
- Cerebellum: responsible for muscle function, balance and movement
- Diencephalons (thalamus, hypothalamus, epithalamus, pineal gland):
  - relays sensory input to the cerebral cortex
  - provides basic appreciation for touch, pressure, pain and temperature
  - controls and regulates the autonomic nervous system and emotional and behavioural patterns
- Two cerebral hemispheres (each of which is divided into four lobes: parietal, frontal, occipital and temporal) and the corpus callosum (an important connection between the two hemispheres).

Each specific area is responsible for a specific function e.g. receptive speech (comprehension) or expressive speech (verbal language) and the cortex is responsible for 'higher' intellectual functions.

Embryology

Some of the concepts surrounding the development of the nervous system are useful for understanding important congenital brain malformations (see Table 14.1). Development of

Table 14.1 This table shows the embryological progression of specific areas of the brain to their final adult derivatives.

Foetus		Adult
Forebrain	Telencephalon	Cerebral hemispheres
	Diencephalon	Thalamus Hypothalamus Epithalamus
Midbrain	Mesencephalon	Colliculi Cerebral peduncles
Hindbrain	Metencephalon	Pons Cerebellum
	Myelencephalon	Medulla oblongata

the nervous system begins soon after conception and can be divided into six main stages:

- Dorsal induction (formation of the neural tube at 3–4 weeks' gestation): the brain develops from ectoderm which is the outermost of the three primary germ layers of ectoderm, mesoderm and endoderm. In the dorsal half of the embryo, the ectodermal layer folds inwards along the midline from head to tail. This eventually separates to form the neural tube. The cavity of the neural tube becomes the fluid filled ventricular system and its final shape is a reflection of the pressures induced by the growth of the different regions of the brain. In the roof of the ventricles some parts of the lining cells (the ependyma) become integrated with the highly vascular innermost covering of the brain (the pia mater) to become the choroid plexus. The choroid plexus is responsible for secreting cerebrospinal fluid into the ventricles, which then circulates to the subarachnoid space between the brain coverings.
- Ventral induction (5–6 weeks' gestation): this refers to the creation of the forebrain, thalamus, hypothalamus, cerebral hemispheres and basal ganglia.
- Neuronal proliferation (2–4 months' gestation): the first neurons are created within the first 100 days of gestation and they divide and multiply at a rate of 250,000 per minute. The adult human brain has around 100 billion neurons and these are responsible for all the information that is

Neonatal Neurology 245

processed through the central nervous system. Sensory neurons carry information towards the central nervous system and motor neurons carry information away. There are also interneurons, which carry information between the sensory and motor neurons. There are two periods in particular when there is a dramatic increase in the number of neurons; this is at 15–20 weeks gestation and then again at 30 weeks up to one year of age.

- Migration (3–5 months' gestation): neurons migrate to their final position in the cortex and this period is critical for the development of the cerebral cortex and deeper nuclear structures.
- Organisation (six months' gestation): the organisation of the brain that provides the basis for brain function begins at around six months' gestation.
- Myelination: this is necessary for rapid and efficient transmission of nerve impulses and is most prolific after birth and continues to adulthood[1,2,3]

Neurological assessment

General observations of posture, tone, movement, feeding and behaviour form the basis of the neurological assessment. The following provide a summary of some of the main observations. For a detailed neurological assessment please see Dubowitz et al.[4,5].

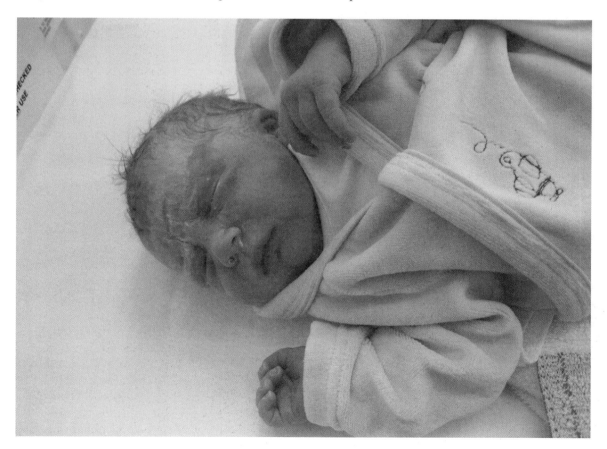

Figure 14.1 A term infant on day 1. The arms are well flexed and the hands are loosely clenched with the thumb curled over the fist.

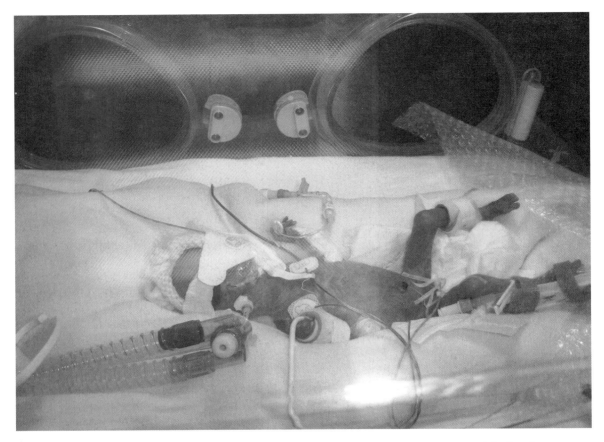

Figure 14.2 A preterm infant on day 7. The legs are abducted in the 'frog-like' posture and the hands are more open than the term infants above.

Implications for practice

- Careful observation elicits useful information about an infant's neurological and behaviour state.
- Knowledge of normal neurological behaviour at different gestations is useful to provide reassurance to parents.

Posture and muscle tone

Healthy term infants preferentially lie with arms and legs flexed and when supine (on their back) there is limited abduction of the hips (see Figure 14.1). The hands are generally loosely clenched with thumbs intermittently curled over the fist (persistent thumb adduction or excessive hand fisting is not normal). When pulled to sitting a healthy term infant will keep their arms slightly flexed at the elbow and the head only lags slightly behind the body.

More immature infants or those who are unwell lie in a more extended position with greater hip abduction, giving rise to the 'frog' posture (see Figure 14.2). Preterm infants may have a more open hand posture. When pulled to sitting, there is likely to be less or no flexion at the elbow and there may be significant head lag, so support for the head should be given when performing this manoeuvre on a preterm infant.

Movement and feeding

Intermittent spontaneous facial movements are usually seen. Normal infant limb movements are smooth, alternating and random. Jerky, rhythmic and/or unilateral movements are suspicious of convulsions. Many infants are jittery in the first 2–3 days[6], but this must be distinguished from fits (see seizures section later in this chapter). Most healthy term infants will develop good suck-swallow coordination within the first few days after birth. Suck swallow coordination in the preterm infant gradually develops from about 28 weeks' gestation, but sucking bursts are short-lived and good synchronisation with breathing becomes much improved from 32–34 weeks[7,8].

Behaviour

Term babies spend the majority of their time asleep, but have cycles of activity associated with different behavioural states both when asleep and awake9. They may cry intermittently but should be consolable. High pitched crying or inconsolability is not normal. Preterm babies also have cycles of activity but they are less well defined and occur more randomly10.

Implications for practice

- The preterm baby is more hypotonic than the term infant.
- Potentially abnormal signs which may indicate a neurological problem include:
  - Excessive wakefulness, persistent irritability, or high pitch crying
  - Poor sucking and feeding difficulties
  - Hyperexcitability and jitteriness
  - Generalised stiffness, back arching, excessive fisting and thumb adduction
  - Excessive floppiness ('frog' posture) and immobility
  - Jerky, asymmetric or rhythmical movements

Congenital abnormalities affecting central nervous system

The most common congenital abnormalities affecting the central nervous system are:

- Neural tube defects:
  - Anencephaly
  - Cranial meningocoele
  - Encephalocoele
  - Spina bifida
- Congenital hydrocephalus

Many of these defects, including the neural tube defects, can be detected antenatally at the 18–22 week anomaly scan. In addition, a high α-foetoprotein in the maternal blood and amniotic fluid is suggestive of an open neural tube defect (where neural tissue is in contact with the surrounding amniotic fluid)[11,12].

There has been a marked reduction in the incidence of CNS abnormalities over the last few decades and the reasons for this are not entirely clear[13]. Some of this is as a result of increased antenatal diagnosis and subsequent termination, but some reduction may be due to general improvements in women's diets (specifically improved folate intake).

Neural tube defects

Anencephaly
This term describes the situation where the posterior part of the skull bones fail to develop and close properly and the severely malformed brain protrudes through the bony defect. The outcome for this condition is universally poor and comfort care and support for the family should be provided. The incidence of neural tube defects and other brain malformations in subsequent offspring is increased and the parents should be offered genetic counselling[14].

Cranial meningocoele and encephalocoele
A rare defect in the skull bone results in protrusion of a skin or membrane-covered cystic

swelling containing CSF (meningocoele) or brain tissue (encephalocoele). These most commonly occur in the occipital region but can be of variable size and protrude from any part of the skull, including the nasal cavity. It can be difficult sometimes to differentiate meningocoele/encephalocoele from the more common but innocent skin-derived swellings. The diagnosis is important in view of the risk of meningitis if accidental rupture occurs, and needle aspiration should not be performed. An ultrasound can be helpful in determining whether a lesion only derives from skin or subcutaneous tissue. An MRI is needed if there is any uncertainty and is useful for diagnosing other neurological abnormalities which may be present.

Spina bifida

Spina bifida encompasses several lesions where there is separation of the vertebral arches. In the mildest form, spina bifida occulta, there is disruption of the vertebral arches only. Spina bifida occulta and meningocoele are *skin covered* lesions but there may be dimples, pits or hair growth at the level of the underlying lesion. Consequently, any midline skin abnormality or swelling (excluding pits in the natal cleft) should be investigated with an ultrasound and/or MRI of the spine[15]. This does not apply to sacral pits below the gluteal creases which are a common normal finding.

Implications for practice

Midline marks, pits, hairs or swellings over the spine (excluding pits in the natal cleft) should be investigated with an ultrasound scan in the first instance.

Meningomyelocoele is the most common form of spina bifida and neural tissue is exposed on the skin surface to form a neural plaque. The exact neurological deficit will depend on the level of the lesion and may include paralysis of the legs, inability to void urine spontaneously and paralysis of the perineal and rectal sphincter muscles. This can lead to dribbling incontinence and recurrent urinary infections and a patulous anus with either constipation or faecal incontinence. These babies require investigation for associated abnormalities of the renal tract and require long-term renal follow up. Early head circumference and cranial scans are useful to diagnose hydrocephalus and/or Chiari malformation (herniation of brain stem and cerebellum through bony defects into upper cervical spine).

Implications for practice

- Keep infant warm and comfortable in an incubator with spinal lesion covered with a non-adherent dressing until surgery can take place.
- Observe for signs of spontaneous leg movements that are not reflex in origin.
- Keep close eye on urine output – spontaneous voiding is unlikely and manual voiding may be required.

The parents should have received counselling in the antenatal period but further perinatal and post-natal counselling is also important. It is important to be aware that these infants are unlikely to require resuscitation unless complications occur during labour as their brainstem is intact. Following delivery the infant should be cared for according to the generic principles of neonatal care and the extent of the spinal lesion should be carefully assessed and covered with a non-adherent dressing. The infant should be examined carefully in order to document the associated findings, which may include lack of spontaneous leg movement and hydrocephalus.

The surgical defect is closed in the early neonatal period to reduce the risks of ascending neurological infection. Many babies will develop hydrocephalus after closure of the lesion, which may require a ventriculo-peritoneal shunt. In view of the multiple surgical procedures that these infants may have it has been advised that latex free gloves should be used in order to avoid the development of a latex allergy[16].

The prognosis for mobility and continence will depend on the level of the spinal lesion[17,18]. The intellectual outcome is related to the hydrocephalus and its complications.

> ### Implications for practice
>
> - Use latex free gloves when handling the infant – these babies are at high risk of developing latex allergy due to multiple exposures particularly during renal and orthopaedic procedures.
> - Head circumference and ventricular size (measured on ultrasound scan) should be documented regularly.
> - If hydrocephalus is suspected, watch for signs of raised intracranial pressure (see posthaemorrhagic hydrocephalus for details).

Congenital Hydrocephalus

Hydrocephalus occurs when the ventricular system becomes dilated as a result of excessive pressure from the cerebrospinal fluid. This can be due to:

- A restriction or blockage to flow through the ventricular system or spinal canal
- A reduced area of absorption through damage to the arachnoid villi
- Less commonly because of excess production of CSF

Congenital hydrocephalus is generally caused by restriction to the flow of CSF. It can occur in association with spina bifida (see above) or be associated with other congenital abnormalities such as aqueduct stenosis (narrowing of the connection between the third and fourth ventricle). Hydrocephalus can also occur after intraventricular haemorrhage, which is more common in the preterm infant (see below) or after subarachnoid haemorrhage or vitamin K deficiency bleeding in the term infant. Hydrocephalus may also be a late complication of viral and bacterial meningitis or encephalitis.

Congenital hydrocephalus may have been diagnosed antenatally on ultrasound scan but should be suspected post-natally in any baby with a disproportionately large head. Daily head circumference and cranial ultrasound are useful to see if there is rapid growth. Symptoms of raised intracranial pressure may occur, which include apnoea, seizures, irritability or feed intolerance. An MRI should be performed to provide anatomical detail to aid diagnosis and determine what neurosurgical intervention may be appropriate.

> ### Implications for practice
>
> - Hydrocephalus should be suspected if the head is large or there is a rapid increase in head circumference.
> - Symptoms of raised intracranial pressure include apnoea, seizures, irritability and feed intolerance.

Microcephaly

Microcephaly is defined as a head circumference that is two standard deviations below the average for the gestational age. Causes include the following:

- Congenital:
  - Genetic
  - Associated with TORCH infections (toxoplasmosis; other; rubella; cytomegalovirus; herpes)
- Maternal factors:
  - Maternal alcoholism, cocaine use
  - Maternal phenylalaninaemia
- Acquired:
  - Secondary to craniosynostosis
  - Secondary to cortical atrophy or underlying brain damage

Management includes monitoring growth (occipital frontal circumference (OFC), weight, length) and observing and reporting deviations from the normal. Imaging investigations may include X-rays (skull bones), ultrasound scan or MRI. The prognosis is dependent on the severity of the microcephaly, but most causes of microcephaly are associated with developmental delay.

Birth trauma

A traumatic delivery, including prolonged labour, instrumental intervention and malpresentation can lead to a number of neurological problems that range from having little or no consequence to being life-threatening, with adverse, long-term outcome. Intracranial and extracranial bleeds can occur as a result of birth trauma and the site of haemorrhage is important in guiding management and long-term prognosis. The sites of haemorrhage are described below.

Caput succedaneum

This term refers to oedema of the soft tissue of the scalp caused by pressure over the presenting part. It does not conform to the boundaries of the bone (a crucial point when differentiating from cephalohaematoma). No specific treatment is necessary and the swelling will subside in a few days.

Cephalohaematoma

This refers to a haematoma between the periosteum and the skull, caused by blood vessels rupturing during labour, particularly with an instrumental delivery. The bleeding does not extend beyond the area of the specific bone affected as the bleed is limited by the points at which the periosteum is fixed to the skull. A cephalohaematoma is usually unilateral but can be bilateral. There is usually little or no swelling at birth but the swelling increases in size by the second or third day. Blood loss is normally insignificant and treatment is rarely necessary. Resolution of the haematoma is often by two to three weeks of age but it is not uncommon for this to take some months. Very rarely, complications can occur which include hyperbilirubinaemia.

Subgaleal haemorrhage

Also known as a subaponeurotic haemorrhage, this is a rare but very important potentially life-threatening diagnosis to be aware of. It refers to bleeding into the subgaleal compartment (located beneath the galea aponeurosis) and is associated with instrumental delivery, particularly vacuum extraction[19]. The bleeding can be extensive because the subgaleal compartment can expand to accommodate large volumes of blood. The main signs to look out for are those of hypovolaemia and a rapidly increasing head circumference. If diagnosed, the infant will usually need urgent blood transfusion, followed by close monitoring and further neurological assessment. Serum bilirubin levels may also rise as a result of degradation of blood cells in the haematoma. If the infant survives the acute phase, recovery is usually within 2–3 weeks.

Subdural haematoma

Massive subdural haematoma is now a rare occurrence due to improved obstetric management. However, less severe subdural haematomas are now recognised more frequently because of improved imaging techniques. This traumatic injury most commonly occurs due to tearing of the large veins in the dural membrane, which separates the cerebrum from the cerebellum (tentorium cerebelli). They are associated with instrumental deliveries, particularly vacuum extraction [20], but may also occur with severe hypoxic ischaemic encephalopathy. Infants may appear well at birth, but lethargy, hypotonia and seizures can present within two to three days. There may also be unequal pupil reaction, with a dilated pupil on the side of the haematoma, apnoea or sighing respiration, fixed bradycardia and opisthotonus. Neuroimaging and a neurosurgical opinion should be sought as some cases may benefit from craniotomy and drainage[21,22]. There is a significant morbidity and mortality associated with this condition although almost half the survivors in one recent series had a normal outcome[22]

Subarachnoid haemorrahage

This can occur as a result of trauma, but can also be secondary to haemorrhage from another site and therefore can present in a preterm neonate secondary to an intraventricular haemorrhage. The bleeding is venous and usually small. Infants may be well initially, presenting with seizures around the second day of life. In preterm infants, there may be recurrent apnoea and hydrocephalus can occur. Unless the lesion is very large, most do not require surgical treatment and the prognosis for primary subarachnoid haemorrhage is good.

Cerebellar haemorrhage

A haemorrhage into the cerebellum most commonly follows traumatic breech delivery in a term infant. Symptoms include lethargy, fixed bradycardia, apnoea, falling haematocrit and blood stained CSF. Treatment is management of the symptoms, appropriate neuroimaging and neurosurgical opinion, as some cases respond to craniotomy and evacuation[23].Overall prognosis is dependent on the extent of the bleed, with a worse outcome associated with a larger bleed.

Seizures

A seizure is a sudden alteration in neurological function that may result in presenting clinical features that are:

- Motor
- Behavioural
- Autonomic

Seizures occur as a result of malfunctions in the brain's electrical system and occur more commonly in the newborn brain due to higher amounts of excitatory receptor sites and lower amounts of inhibitory neurotransmitters[24].

Commonest causes of seizures include:

- Hypoxic-ischaemic encephalopathy (HIE) in the term infant
- Intraventricular haemorrhage in the preterm infant

- Middle cerebral artery infarction in the well term infant[25]

Other causes of seizures include:

- Pre or post-natal infections e.g toxoplasmosis; CMV; herpes; hepatitis; meningitis
- Drug withdrawal following maternal illicit drug use
- Biochemical abnormalities, e.g. hypernatraemia/hyponatraemia; uraemia; hyperbilirubinaemia; hypocalcaemia; hypomagnesaemia; hypoglycaemia
- Inborn errors of metabolism
- Congenital malformations
- Haemorrhage, e.g. subdural or subarachnoid haemorrhage
- Benign familial seizures
- Idiopathic (no cause found)

Implications for practice

- Any unilateral or rhythmical movement should be carefully assessed.
- Blood glucose, blood gas and electrolyte measurements including Ca and Mg should always be done if seizures are suspected.
- Other investigations should be considered in light of the clinical history and include a full infection screen with lumbar puncture.

Diagnosis

Seizures can be focal, multifocal or generalised. There are four main types of seizures:

- *Tonic*: rigid extension or posturing which can affect limbs or trunk. There may be deviation of the head or eyes.
- *Clonic*: rhythmic jerking (approximately three per second) which usually has a fast component followed by a slower phase.
- *Myoclonic*: usually involves rapid spasm in the flexor muscle groups.

- *Subtle*: often overlooked; signs include rhythmic eye movement; eye deviation; staring; sucking or lip smacking; mouthing; cycling limb movements, apnoea and bradycardia.

Clinical seizures do not always coincide with electrical seizures seen on EEG – this is known as *electroclinical dissociation*.

It can be clinically important to identify the type of seizure. Myoclonic jerks which occur only during sleep are most likely to be benign neonatal sleep myoclonus. This diagnosis is important to make as reassurance can be given that it requires no treatment, has a good outcome and the movements will disappear by six months.

Jitteriness is very common in newborns and must be distinguished from seizures[26]. Tremors seen in jittery babies are usually occurring at a faster rate than clonic or myoclonic jerks and the movement is symmetrical and does not involve the face. Tremors are very sensitive to stimulation and will cease promptly if the affected area is held.

Implications for practice

- Seizures may be very subtle, involving only small facial or eye movements.
- Apnoea and/or bradycardia may be related to seizure activity – look carefully for signs indicative of possible seizure activity.
- It is important to be able to distinguish jitteriness (commonly seen in normal newborns) from seizure activity. Tremors seen in jittery babies are symmetrical movements which are very sensitive to stimulation and will cease promptly if the affected area is held.

Management

Treatment includes establishing and treating the cause and using anticonvulsants. Brief infrequent seizures are generally not treated unless there are multiple episodes. Seizures which last longer than a few minutes are treated until they clinically cease. There is no good evidence to support the treatment of seizures until they are electrically silent. Most neonatal units use phenobarbitone as a first-line drug for treating seizures. Drugs used as second-line therapy include clonazepam, phenytoin, lorazepam and midazolam.

Implications for practice

- An intravenous line is usually required to deliver anticonvulsants rapidly into the circulation.
- Respiratory depression is a common side effect of all anticonvulsants, so ventilatory support may be required.

Prognosis

Prognosis is largely dependent upon the cause of the seizures. Hypocalcaemia, familial seizures and neonatal sleep myoclonus have an excellent prognosis.

Neonatal abstinence syndrome

The use of any drug which has an effect on the neurological system of the foetus may result in the development of a withdrawal syndrome post-delivery. Withdrawal is most commonly seen with opiates although it can also occur with barbiturates, diazepam, tricyclic antidepressants and alcohol.

The diagnosis should be considered in any newborn that presents with poor feeding and excessive jitteriness and is also one of the differential diagnoses of seizures as described above. The signs can be classified as major or minor and the aim of management is to prevent the development of major signs but to tolerate minor ones.

Major signs

These include: seizures, increased or continuous tremors even when undisturbed, marked irritability even when undisturbed, rigid muscle tone, tachypnoea > 95 breaths per minute, profuse watery stools, profuse vomiting.

Minor signs

These include: mild irritability or jitteriness, tremors, shrill cry, poor sleep, sweating, poor feeding, vomiting, diarrhoea, weight loss, sneezing, yawning, hiccoughs, hyperthermia > 38°C.

These infants are often excessively alert, hyperactive and hypertonic. Jittery tremors are usually initiated by stimulation and are stopped by passive flexion of the involved limb (see above for distinguishing jitteriness from seizures). Although these infants may suck frantically on fingers or fists they may be poor at coordinating feeding. Most babies will present with symptoms in the first 2–3 days, although sometimes the interval is longer. This can occur with methadone and benzodiazepines where the onset of withdrawal symptoms may be delayed by up to 1–2 weeks. Not all babies exposed to drugs *in utero* will go on to develop neonatal abstinence syndrome and it should *never* be assumed that symptoms or signs are due to neonatal abstinence syndrome – other causes should be considered. Table 14.2 lists some of the neurological sequelae of commonly abused drugs[27–30].

Infants at risk of NAS should be assessed after feeds (when most likely to be settled). The aim is to prevent major signs and many units are no longer using scoring systems but are concentrating on the assessment of the infant as a whole and the use of non-pharmacological management where possible[31]. Individual units will have slightly different protocols but if high scores are demonstrated on two successive occasions using a scoring system, or major signs are observed, pharmacological treatment is usually indicated. Drug treatment varies but it is usual to give either oral morphine or oral methadone. The dose is titrated according to the infant's clinical condition and the baby may require treatment for some weeks. These babies are difficult

Table 14.2 Neurological sequelae of commonly abused drugs.

Substance	Sequelae
Cocaine	Perinatal brain lesions (cerebral infarctions), seizures, neuromotor deficits, impaired reflexes, abnormal EEG
Alcohol	Foetal alcohol syndrome (FAS) (dysmorphic facies, symmetrical growth retardation, mental retardation, congenital heart defect) chronic foetal hypoxia, CNS depression
Amphetamines/ methamphetamines	Similar to cocaine: perinatal brain lesions (haemorrhage; infarction), impaired reflexes, seizures
Heroin/methadone	Hyperirritability, CNS depression, autonomic dysfunction
Tobacco	Symmetrical growth restriction
Benzodiazepines	CNS depression
Barbiturates	Seizures
Marijuana	This can lead to an increase in FAS if used with alcohol

and demanding to nurse and need a calm quiet environment. There is evidence to suggest that swaddling may be helpful. The babies require frequent small feeds and may also benefit from use of a dummy. Maternal drug use is not usually a contraindication to breast-feeding, but advice should be sought on an individual basis if the mother is on high dose heroine. In addition, intravenous drug users are at increased risk of being HIV, hepatitis B or hepatitis C positive and this should have been checked antenatally (see Chapter 16). It is hoped that, in most cases, antenatal planning meetings with the appropriate multidisciplinary team will have occurred to facilitate discharge planning. In some cases post-natal meetings will also be held to determine the best options for care and support in the community.

Developmentally, many children who have had neonatal abstinence syndrome secondary to opiate withdrawal will do well. However, severe growth restriction, multiple exposure and particularly cocaine exposure increase the likelihood of sub-optimal developmental outcome[32]. There is also an increased incidence of sudden infant death syndrome in babies who have had neonatal abstinence syndrome[33].

Implications for practice

- Infants at risk of NAS or showing signs of withdrawal should be assessed for major and minor signs of withdrawal after feeds.
- Other causes of irritability or seizures should *always* be considered in infants at risk of withdrawal.
- The social situation and plan for discharge should be reviewed prior to discharge as some families may require support agencies.

Encephalopathy

Encephalopathy is a term that refers to pathology (opathy) of the brain (encephal) or a suppression of normal brain function, and the commonest cause in neonatal practice is hypoxic ischaemic encephalopathy. Other causes are:

- Maternal anaesthesia or drugs
- Meningitis or encephalitis
- Hypoglycaemia/hyponatraemia/hypocalcaemia
- Intracranial haemorrhage
- Congenital brain malformations
- Inborn errors of metabolism

Hypoxic ischaemic encephalopathy

Asphyxia occurring before, during or immediately after delivery can cause an encephalopathy in approximately 0.5–1 per thousand live births (higher in developing countries). Although hypoxic ischaemic injury can occur in the preterm population, the clinical presentation and pattern of injury described below is typically seen in term or near term infants.

Mechanism of brain injury

Extensive experimental studies have shown that there are two phases to neuronal injury[34–36]:

- *Primary neuronal injury*: intracellular energy failure occurs, resulting in immediate cell death by *necrosis*.
- *Secondary neuronal injury* occurs hours or days after the original insult.

Reperfusion injury: damage due to production of free radical metabolites and cell death by apoptosis, due to a lack of the complex signals required to maintain normal cell functioning, are some of the complex abnormal biochemical processes occurring following the hypoxic-ischaemic insult. It has been demonstrated that a significant proportion of the total cell death occurs during this phase.

Implications for practice

Understanding the mechanism of injury has been important for developing treatments which might limit the neuronal loss in the secondary phase with the potential to improve final neurological outcome in affected infants.

Diagnosis

Hypoxic ischaemia is the commonest cause of encephalopathy in the term newborn infant. However, it is important to consider other differential diagnoses in any infant with encephalopathy and it may be necessary to perform investigations that will exclude these.

The American Academy of Paediatrics provides a clear definition of HIE which is:

- Evidence of intrapartum hypoxia, e.g. profound metabolic or mixed acidaemia (pH < 7.00) in an umbilical artery blood sample or persistence of an Apgar score of 0–3 for longer than five minutes
  and
- Multiorgan involvement, e.g. neonatal neurologic sequelae (e.g. seizures, coma, hypotonia) or other organ involvement (e.g. kidney, lungs, liver, heart, intestines)

Clinical presentation

The asphyxial event affects the baby as a whole and is therefore a multi-system disease presenting as:

- Neurological depression, which can affect respiratory drive, necessitating respiratory support
- Cardiac hypoxia, which may result in poor myocardial contractility with resultant hypotension
- Renal hypoxia, which may cause acute renal failure with poor urine output
- High blood lactate levels, which cause acidosis
- High energy consumption, which results in hypoglycaemia

The encephalopathy can be clinically graded according to its severity and the most commonly used system is Sarnat and Sarnat (see Table 14.3).

Implications for practice

- Diagnosing hypoxic ischaemic encephalopathy requires evidence of perinatal asphyxia, *and* multiorgan dysfunction.
- Hypoxic ischaemic encephalopathy is a multi-system disease and the mainstay of treatment is supportive therapy.

Table 14.3 Modified Sarnat and Sarnat clinical grading system for hypoxic ishaemic encephalopathy [37, 38].

	Grade I (mild)	Grade II (moderate)	Grade III (severe)
Clinical features	Irritable, hyperalert, staring	Lethargic	Comatose
	Mild hypotonia	Moderate hypotonia arms > legs	Severe hypotonia
	Poor suck	Tube feeds	Reduced spontaneous respiration
	No seizures	Seizures	Prolonged seizures
Outcome death or severe disability	1.5%	25%	78%

Investigations

Investigations are primarily aimed at improving prognostic information. Very few investigations are prognostic within the first six hours. Cerebral function monitoring is useful at this early stage[39,40], which is why it may be useful for targeting therapy to prevent secondary neuronal loss. The commonly performed investigations include:

- Cerebral ultrasound: shows cerebral oedema in first 24 hours.
- Resistivity index: measures cerebral blood flow velocity. Ratio < 0.55 is associated with poor outcome but only useful after first 24 hours[41].
- MRI: useful prognostic information from 7–10 days post-natal age, especially for motor disability[42].

- Electroencephalogram (EEG): useful for diagnosis of fits and provides information on background activity but can be difficult to obtain extended monitoring.
- Amplitude integrated EEG (aEEG), also known as Cerebral Function Monitor (CFM): provides continuous compressed background electrical activity with good prediction of longer term outcome within first six hours[43,44].

Management

Supportive

Management of hypoxic ischaemic encephalopathy is principally supportive and is shown in Table 14.4.

Neuroprotective treatments

The discovery that secondary neuronal injury comprises a significant portion of the total neuronal loss has led to the development of specific therapies targeted at reducing secondary neuronal loss. Many of these developments have not yet reached clinical application. Currently, the most promising therapy that has been studied in clinical trials is moderate hypothermia.

Animal studies have shown that a $3-4°C$ reduction in body temperature after a cerebral insult is associated with improved histological and behavioural outcome[45]. In order for this therapy to be effective, it must be administered within six hours of the insult and may continue to be beneficial for up to 72 hours. There are potential adverse side effects associated with hypothermia (see Table 14.5) so early identification of patients most likely to benefit is essential to avoid unnecessary treatment. A combination of evidence of intrapartum hypoxia, clinical neurological examination +/− an abnormal amplitude integrated EEG (aEEG) have been used in the published randomised controlled trials of moderate hypothermia in babies. Meta-analysis of these trials has recently been possible and appears to show reductions

Table 14.4 Examples of supportive management necessary in an infant with hypoxic ischaemic encephalopathy.

	Supportive management
Respiratory	Give oxygen therapy and/or ventilatory support to achieve normal pO_2 and pCO_2. Frequent oropharyngeal suction if poor swallow.
Cardiovascular	Arterial blood pressure monitoring with inotropic support if required.
Renal	Monitor urine output. Restrict intravenous fluids for first 48 hours and monitor urine output /electrolyte measurements and daily infant weight.
Neurology	Observe for possible signs of seizures and treat with anticonvulsants if required.
Haematology	Check clotting and platelets and treat as required with FFP, vitamin K or platelet transfusion.
Gastroenterology	Nil by mouth initially, with aspiration of gastric contents (at risk of necrotising enterocolitis). Slowly introduce nasogastric feeds. Assess suck/swallow reflex before commencing oral feeds.
Metabolic	Maintain thermoneutral environment. Commence maintenance intravenous dextrose and check regular blood sugar measurements.
Infection	Blood cultures and lumbar puncture should be sent and antibiotics started if clinically indicated.

in death and medium-term disability without significant side effects of treatment[46-48]. On this basis, some units are offering hypothermia as a treatment option. However, publication of the results of ongoing trials, more information about the safety of treatment and longer developmental follow-up data will be required before this becomes a definitive treatment for hypoxic ischaemic encephalopathy.

Prognosis

Infants with mild HIE usually have a normal neurodevelopmental outcome. Babies with

Table 14.5 Potential complications of hypothermia.

Cardiovascular	Arrhythmias
	Impaired cardiac function
Electrolyte	Hypokalaemia
Haematology	Abnormal coagulation
Infection	Increased risk sepsis

Table 14.6 Commonly used grading system for intraventricular haemorrhage.

Grade 1	Germinal matrix haemorrhage (GMH)
Grade 2	IVH without ventricular dilatation
Grade 3	IVH with acute ventricular dilatation
Grade 4	IVH with periventricular haemorrhagic infarction

severe HIE have a high mortality and survivors have cerebral palsy which may be accompanied by intellectual impairment, blindness, deafness and or epilepsy. Patients with moderate HIE have a more variable prognosis, early establishment of feeds and lack of neurological signs on discharge are encouraging signs.

Implications for practice

- Therapies to prevent secondary neuronal loss require rapid identification of infants who are most likely to have a poor outcome.
- Documenting the clinical features of the encephalopathy along with the EEG can help to identify within a few hours those infants who are most likely to have a poor outcome.
- Hypothermia shows promise as a potential treatment for hypoxic ishaemic encephalopathy but further evaluation is ongoing.

Preterm brain injury

Germinal matrix haemorrhage – intraventricular haemorrhage

The incidence of intraventricular haemorrhage (IVH) reduced through the 1980s and early 1990s and now affects about 20% of infants with a birthweight < 1500g[49,50]. It is most common in infants below 29 weeks gestation within the first 72 hours of life[51]. The origin of the haemorrhage is the germinal matrix which lies underneath the ependymal lining of the lateral ventricles. It is responsible for producing early neuronal cells which then migrate to other parts of the brain. The germinal matrix is most

prominent between 24 and 34 weeks gestation and regresses by term. During its period of rapid cell production it has a rich blood supply and is susceptible to haemorrhage, which frequently ruptures through the ependymal lining into the lateral ventricles. IVH is usually diagnosed by ultrasound and a system for recording the extent of the haemorrhage is helpful. One such grading system is shown in Table 14.6.

Clinical presentation
Occasionally, IVH occurs before birth but the majority occur within the first 72 hours. The degree of prematurity and the presence of respiratory distress syndrome are the biggest risk factors for GMH. It is hypothesised that a combination of an immature vascular anatomical structure, the natural bleeding tendency present in all newborns and poor regulation of cerebral blood flow, which is easily overloaded by swings in blood pressure, acidosis and hypoxia, make IVH more likely.

Prevention of IVH
Antenatal corticosteroids have shown a marked benefit both in reducing incidence of respiratory distress syndrome and in reducing the risk of IVH. Once the infant has been born there are factors within their post-natal neonatal care that will reduce the risk of IVH. These include:

- Early surfactant therapy
- Optimal ventilation to ensure physiological pH, pCO_2 and pO_2 and minimal exposure to barotraumas and volutrauma

- Minimal handling and suctioning
- Stable adequate blood pressure maintenance
- Treatment of coagulation disturbances

> ## Implications for practice
>
> - Antenatal steroids and early surfactant therapy reduce risk of IVH.
> - Unnecessary handling of the preterm infant should be avoided in the first few days of life.
> - Detailed physiological neonatal care reduces risk of IVH, e.g. optimisation of blood gas results, blood pressure and coagulation. ebt]

Complications of IVH

Grade I and II IVH are not associated with significant increases in cerebral palsy or mortality. The GMH gradually evolves to form a cystic lesion over 2–4 weeks, which eventually disappears.

About 30% of infants with grade III IVH go on to get post-haemorrhagic ventricular dilatation (PHVD) and there is a gradual increase in ventricular width, which may or may not be accompanied by symptoms (apnoea, seizures, irritability, feed intolerance)[52]. In half the babies the PHVD is transient and in the remainder the head circumference and ventricular size continue to increase, leading to progressive hydrocephalus. Regular monitoring of ventricular width (using ultrasound) and head circumference is required in infants with grade III hydrocephalus. Babies with rapid progressive enlargement in ventricular size, or symptoms of raised intracranial pressure should have a lumbar puncture or ventricular tap to drain cerebrospinal fluid. These babies are at risk of meningitis and fluid removed should always be sent for microscopy and culture. If the hydrocephalus persists, a ventriculo-peritoneal shunt can be placed, although this is usually delayed until the CSF protein has fallen as the risks of blockage and infection are high. About half the children with PHVD and 75% of those requiring a shunt will have a poor neurodevelopmental outcome[53]. The prognosis for neonates with grade IV IVH where there is significant haemorrhagic infarction of the periventricular white matter is poor, with 50% mortality and cerebral palsy in 85% of survivors[54]. Unilateral grade IV IVH has a significantly better prognosis than bilateral.

Periventricular leucomalacia

Periventricular leucomalacia (PVL) is the term given to damage to the periventricular white matter. This may be seen initially as persistent echodensities (flares) on ultrasound scanning. In some cases the flares become echolucent (cystic PVL), representing multiple small cavities formed as a result of necrosis and liquification of the myelinating tissue. The time from appearance of flares to development of cystic PVL is around 2–3 weeks[55].

Prenatal factors which may increase the risk of PVL are death of a co-twin, twin-twin transfusion syndrome, intrauterine infection, chorioamnionitis and inflammation[56–58]. The presence of PVL significantly increases the likelihood of a poor neurodevelopmental outcome.

Meningitis

This is covered in Chapter 16. Meningitis can occur in term and preterm infants. In the term infant the commonest cause of meningitis is that due to group B streptococcus. In the preterm infant meningitis can also occur due to GBS but these infants are also particularly vulnerable to Gram negative organisms such as E. Coli and other Gram negative species which have a devastating prognosis. The presenting symptoms and signs may include:

- Cerebral irritability
- Apnoea, bradycardia
- Poor feeding
- Seizures

It is important to have a low threshold for performing a lumbar puncture to ensure that meningitis is accurately diagnosed. Meningitis is associated with a significant mortality and neurological morbidity.

Conclusion

There are a wide variety of conditions which can affect the newborn central nervous system and many of these have associated high mortality and disability rates. However, there have been significant developments over a number of years which are changing the incidence and outcome for many of these conditions. Developments in prenatal screening and folate supplementation have seen a reduction in the incidence of some developmental neurological abnormalities. Improvements in neonatal care and a greater understanding of the underlying mechanisms for preterm intraventricular haemorrhage have led to significant reductions in the incidence of large intraventricular haemorrhage. Improvements in obstetrics have reduced the incidence of serious haemorrhage related to birth trauma.

The underlying mechanisms for some common newborn neurological conditions have been the topics of intensive research over many years. In particular, knowledge of the pathophysiology of perinatal asphyxia has led to the exciting possibility of being able to offer treatment for this devastating condition. Hypothermia has already undergone significant human trials and is on the verge of becoming an established treatment. Research in this area continues and there are a number of other potential therapeutic agents under investigation. Improvements in brain imaging and correlation of findings with neurodevelopmental outcome are another area of intensive research. Some areas of research, such as stem cell studies, are not sufficiently advanced to undergo human trials, but suggest there is potential for significant changes in outlook for some neurological conditions.

It is hoped that this chapter has given the reader an insight into the main neurological conditions affecting the newborn and will encourage an interest in further developments in this field.

References

1. Beachy P, Deacon J (1993) *Core Curriculum for Neonatal Intensive Care Nursing.* WB Saunders Company, Philadelphia.
2. Tortora GJ, Grabowski SR (1996) *Principles of Anatomy and Physiology.* John Wiley & Sons, Oxford.
3. Wong D (ed.) (1999) *Whaley and Wong's Nursing Care of Infants and Children.* Mosby, St Louis.
4. Dubowitz L, Dubowitz V, Mercuri E (eds) (1999) The neurological assessment of the preterm and full term newborn infant. In: Dubowitz L, Dubowitz V, Mercuri E (eds) *Clinics in Developmental Medicine*, 2nd edn. MacKeith Press, Cambridge.
5. Dubowitz L, Ricciw D, Mercuri E (2005) The Dubowitz neurological examination of the full-term newborn. *Ment Retard Dev Disabil Res Rev*, **11** (1), 52–60.
6. Parker S, Zuckerman B, Bauchner H, Frank D, Vinci R, Cabral H (1990) Jitteriness in full-term neonates: prevalence and correlates. *Pediatrics*, **85** (1), 17–23.
7. Casaer P, Daniels H, Devlieger H, DeCock P, Eggermont E (1982) Feeding behaviour in preterm neonates. *Early Hum Dev*, **7** (4), 331–346.
8. Amaizu N, Shulman R, Schanler R, Lau C (2008) Maturation of oral feeding skills in preterm infants. *Acta Paediatr*, **97** (1), 61–67.
9. Pillai M, James D (1990) Behavioural states in normal mature human foetuses. *Arch Dis Child*, **65** (1 Spec No.), 39–43.
10. Prechtl HF, Fargel JW, Weinmann HM, Bakker HH (1979) Postures, motility and respiration of low-risk pre-term infants. *Dev Med Child Neurol*, **21** (1), 3–27.
11. Brock DJ, Sutcliffe RG (1972) Alpha-foetoprotein in the antenatal diagnosis of anencephaly and spina bifida. *Lancet*, **2** (7770), 197–199.
12. Brock DJ, Bolton AE, Scrimgeour JB (1974) Prenatal diagnosis of spina bifida and anencephaly through maternal plasma-alpha-foetoprotein measurement. *Lancet*, **1** (7861), 767–769.
13. Botting B (2001) Trends in neural tube defects. *Health Statistics Quarterly* (www.statistics.gov.uk), 5–13.
14. Carter CO, Evans K (1973) Spina bifida and anencephalus in Greater London. *J Med Genet*, **10** (3), 209–234.

15. Gibson PJ, Britton J, Hall DM, Hill CR (1995) Lumbosacral skin markers and identification of occult spinal dysraphism in neonates. *Acta Paediatr*, **84** (2), 208–209.

16. Sparta G, Kemper MJ, Gerber AC, Goetschel P, Neuhaus TJ (2004) Latex allergy in children with urological malformation and chronic renal failure. *J Urol*, **171** (4), 1647–1649.

17. Hunt GM, Poulton A (1995) Open spina bifida: a complete cohort reviewed 25 years after closure. *Dev Med Child Neurol*, **37** (1), 19–29.

18. Hunt GM, Oakeshott P (2003) Outcome in people with open spina bifida at age 35: prospective community based cohort study. *BMJ*, **326** (7403), 1365–1366.

19. Kilani RA, Wetmore J (2006) Neonatal subgaleal hematoma: presentation and outcome –radiological findings and factors associated with mortality. *Am J Perinatol*, **23** (1), 41–48.

20. Castillo M, Fordham LA (1995) MR of neurologically symptomatic newborns after vacuum extraction delivery. *AJNR Am J Neuroradiol*, **16** (4 Suppl.), 816–818.

21. Perrin RG, Rutka JT, Drake JM, *et al.* (1997) Management and outcomes of posterior fossa subdural hematomas in neonates. Neurosurgery, **40** (6), 1190–1199, discussion 1199–2000.

22. Govaert P, Calliauw L, Vanhaesebrouck P, Martens F, Barrilari A (1990) On the management of neonatal tentorial damage. Eight case reports and a review of the literature. *Acta Neurochir (Wien)*, **106** (1–2), 52–64.

23. Govaert P, Calliauw L, Vanhaesebrouck P, Martens F, Barrilari A (1990) On the management of neonatal tentorial damage. Eight case reports and a review of the literature. *Acta Neurochir (Wien)*, **106** (1–2), 52–64.

24. Moshe SL (1993) Seizures in the developing brain. *Neurology*, **43** (11, Suppl. 5), S3–S7.

25. Estan J, Hope P (1997) Unilateral neonatal cerebral infarction in full term infants. *Arch Dis Child Foetal Neonatal Ed*, **76** (2), F88–F93.

26. Parker S, Zuckerman B, Bauchner H, Frank D, Vinci R, Cabral H (1990) Jitteriness in full-term neonates: prevalence and correlates. *Pediatrics*, **85** (1), 17–23.

27. Briggs G, Freeman R, Yaffe S (eds) (2005) *A Reference Guide to Neonatal Risk: Drugs in Pregnancy and Lactation*, 7th edn. Lippincott Williams and Wilkins, Philadelphia PA.

28. Merenstein G, Gardner S (eds) (1998) *Handbook of Neonatal Intensive Care*, 4th edn. Mosby, St Louis.

29. Edmonton A (2204) *Tobacco Basics Handbook*. Alberta Alcohol and Drug Abuse Commission, AADAC Research Services, Alberta (www.aadac.com/documents/TBH_ThirdEdition.pdf).

30. Mohammad MI, Tanveer S, Thad R (2002) Effects of commonly used Benzodiazepines on the foetus, the neonate and the nursing infant. *Psychiatric Services*, **53** (1), 39–49.

31. Hubbard M (2006) Reducing admissions to the neonatal unit: a report on how one neonatal service has responded to the ever increasing demand on neonatal cots. *Journal of Neonatal Nursing*, **12**, 172–176.

32. Volpe JJ (ed.) (2001) Teratogenic effects of drugs and passive addiction. In: *Neurology of the Newborn*. WB Saunders, Philadelphia PA.

33. Kandall SR, Gaines J, Habel L, Davidson G, Jessop D (1993) Relationship of maternal substance abuse to subsequent sudden infant death syndrome in offspring. *J Pediatr*, **123** (1), 120–126.

34. Volpe JJ (ed.) (2001) Hypoxic-ischaemic encephalopathy. In: *Neurology of the Newborn*. WB Saunders, Philadelphia PA.

35. Levene MI, Evans JV (eds) (2005) Hypoxic-ischaemic brain injury. In: Rennie J (ed.), *Roberton's Textbook of Neonatology*, 3rd edn. Churchill Livingstone, Edinburgh.

36. Levene ML, Kornberg J, Williams TH (1985) The incidence and severity of post-asphyxial encephalopathy in full-term infants. *Early Hum Dev*, **11** (1), 21–26.

37. Levene ML, Kornberg J, Williams TH (1985) The incidence and severity of post-asphyxial encephalopathy in full-term infants. *Early Hum Dev*, **11** (1), 21–26.

38. Peliowski A, Finer NN (eds) (1992) Birth asphyxia in the term infant. In: Sinclair JC, Bracken MB (eds), *Effective Care of the Newborn Infant*. Oxford University Press, Oxford. pp. 249–279.

39. Hellstrom-Westas L, Rosen I, Svenningsen NW (1995) Predictive value of early continuous amplitude integrated EEG recordings on outcome after severe birth asphyxia in full term infants. *Arch Dis Child Foetal Neonatal Ed*, **72** (1), F34–F38.

40. al Naqeeb N, Edwards AD, Cowan F, Azzopardi D (1999) Assessment of neonatal encephalopathy

by amplitude-integrated electroencephalography. *Pediatrics*, **103** (6, Pt 1), 1263–1271.

41. Archer LN, Levene MI, Evans DH (1986) Cerebral artery Doppler ultrasonography for prediction of outcome after perinatal asphyxia. *Lancet*, **2** (8516), 1116–1118.

42. Volpe JJ (ed.) (2001) Hypoxic-ischaemic encephalopathy. In: *Neurology of the Newborn*. WB Saunders, Philadelphia PA.

43. al Naqeeb N, Edwards AD, Cowan F, Azzopardi D (1999) Assessment of neonatal encephalopathy by amplitude-integrated electroencephalography. *Pediatrics*, **103** (6, Pt 1), 1263–1271.

44. Archer LN, Levene MI, Evans DH (1986) Cerebral artery Doppler ultrasonography for prediction of outcome after perinatal asphyxia. *Lancet*, **2** (8516), 1116–1118.

45. Thorensen M (ed.) (2002) Thermal influence on the asphyxiated newborn. In: Donn SM, Sinha SK, Chiswick ML (eds), *Birth Asphyxia and the Brain: Basic Science and Clinical Implications*. Blackwell, Oxford. pp. 357–368.

46. Jacobs S, Hunt R, Tarnow-Mordi W, Inder T, Davis P (2007) Cooling for newborns with hypoxic ischaemic encephalopathy. *Cochrane Database Syst Rev* (4), CD003311.

47. Shah PS, Ohlsson A, Perlman M (2007) Hypothermia to treat neonatal hypoxic ischemic encephalopathy: systematic review. *Arch Pediatr Adolesc Med*, **161** (10), 951–958.

48. Schulzke SM, Rao S, Patole SK (2007) A systematic review of cooling for neuroprotection in neonates with hypoxic ischemic encephalopathy – are we there yet? *BMC Pediatr*, 7, 30.

49. Philip AG, Allan WC, Tito AM, Wheeler LR (1989) Intraventricular hemorrhage in preterm infants: declining incidence in the 1980s. *Pediatrics*, **84** (5), 797–801.

50. Batton DG, Holtrop P, DeWitte D, Pryce C, Roberts C (1994) Current gestational age-related incidence of major intraventricular hemorrhage. *J Pediatr*, **125** (4), 623–625.

51. Linder N, Haskin O, Levit O, *et al.* (2003) Risk factors for intraventricular hemorrhage in very low birth weight premature infants: a retrospective case-control study. *Pediatrics*, **111** (5, Pt 1), e590–e595.

52. Levene MI, Starte DR (1981) A longitudinal study of post-haemorrhagic ventricular dilatation in the newborn. *Arch Dis Child*, **56** (12), 905–910.

53. Shankaran S, Koepke T, Woldt E, *et al.* (1989) Outcome after posthemorrhagic ventriculomegaly in comparison with mild hemorrhage without ventriculomegaly. *J Pediatr*, **114** (1), 109–114.

54. Guzzetta F, Shackelford GD, Volpe S, Perlman JM, Volpe JJ (1986) Periventricular intraparenchymal echodensities in the premature newborn: critical determinant of neurologic outcome. *Pediatrics*, **78** (6), 995–1006.

55. Kubota T, Okumura A, Hayakawa F, *et al.* (2001) Relation between the date of cyst formation observable on ultrasonography and the timing of injury determined by serial electroencephalography in preterm infants with periventricular leukomalacia. *Brain Dev*, **23** (6), 390–394.

56. Denbow ML, Battin MR, Cowan F, Azzopardi D, Edwards AD, Fisk NM (1998) Neonatal cranial ultrasonographic findings in preterm twins complicated by severe foetofoetal transfusion syndrome. *Am J Obstet Gynecol*, **178** (3), 479–483.

57. de Vries LS, Eken P, Groenendaal F, Rademaker KJ, Hoogervorst B, Bruinse HW (1998) Antenatal onset of haemorrhagic and/or ischaemic lesions in preterm infants: prevalence and associated obstetric variables. *Arch Dis Child Foetal Neonatal Ed*, **78** (1), F51–F56.

58. Perlman JM, Risser R, Broyles RS (1996) Bilateral cystic periventricular leukomalacia in the premature infant: associated risk factors. *Pediatrics*, **97** (6 Pt 1), 822–827.

Chapter 15

THE DYING INFANT

Zoe Wilkes and Maggie Hallsworth

Learning outcomes

After reading this chapter the reader will be expected to be able to:

- Recognise the physiological changes that characterise the terminal phase of the dying process

- Define palliative care and discuss some of the non-pharmacological and pharmacological interventions that may be required to manage the commonly observed symptoms

- Outline some of the important areas that may be affected by religious and cultural differences

- Explain the role of the coroner and give examples of cases that should be referred to the coroner

- Identify who is able to complete a death certificate

- Describe the role of the nurse in caring for the dying infant and their family

---

Introduction

The grieving process of a parent or family member following the death of a child, young person or infant is said to be 'intense, complicated and long-lasting'[1]. It is hoped that through high quality symptom management, palliative care, terminal care and bereavement support, this process could be slightly more bearable. The aim is that the child experiences a peaceful death following collaborative working amongst professionals, effective communication with the family and the empowerment of the family to make informed decisions regarding the terminal care of their child.

This chapter will expand on these areas of care for the dying infant within the following sub-headings:

- The physiology of dying
- The institution of palliative care
- Religious and cultural considerations
- Post-mortem
- Certification and registration of the infant's death
- Role of the coroner
- The clinical management of death on the neonatal unit

In neonatology there will be circumstances where parents will experience both the elation of their infant's birth and the tragedy of their death within a very short period of time[2]. Such circumstances may be where the infant is initially resuscitated only to find that it has suffered severe neurological damage, where the infant is resuscitated only to find at a later date that a malformation exists which is incompatible with life, or where the infant is born with a congenital condition for which aggressive treatment proves futile. In contrast, parents may experience a preterm birth where, following a prolonged period of neonatal intensive care, death occurs from the complications of prematurity. Each of these situations will be unique to the individual families concerned and requires a great deal of sensitivity and skill by the neonatal team, particularly the nurses, who may have developed a close professional relationship with the family.

The physiology of dying

'It is as natural to die as to be born; and to a little infant, perhaps, the one is as painful as the other.'

Sir Francis Bacon (1551–1626)

In order to discuss the end of life, it is necessary to understand the process of life, its meaning and the requirements to sustain it. There are many definitions of life and for the purpose of this chapter, the physical perspective will be considered in order that deviations from normal functioning can be detected as death nears. This perspective of life is dependent upon oxygen and food.

The following processes need to occur in order for life to be maintained:

- The neurological functioning of the brainstem in order that respiration can occur and that the lungs are able to expel carbon dioxide
- The cardiovascular system is maintained and sufficiently supplied with oxygen and blood
- Gastrointestinal functioning along with renal and liver functions are maintained and toxins are able to exit the body effectively

The physiology of dying is dependent upon infant factors which may include prematurity, size and post-natal maturity as well as a variety of factors surrounding the infant's death, such as organ damage or disease process. The dying process may also be influenced by interventions such as ventilation and medication.

As an infant enters the terminal phase of illness, many physiological changes occur, where irreversible failure of vital organs and systems within the body takes place and these include:

- Alterations in the infant's level of consciousness (becoming depressed as death becomes imminent)
- Bradycardia
- Absence of primitive reflexes
- Intermittent gasping
- Pallor

Through the ability to identify these symptoms, the needs of the infant are highlighted and appropriate interventions may then be implemented in order to ensure comfort and dignity. In some instances where the infant is ventilated, some of these processes may not occur until the ventilator is withdrawn. However, the brain will continue to become inactive, despite ventilation, where disease progression dictates this process.

As death nears, Durham and Weiss confirm that a number of occurrences take place within the body as it begins to shut down permanently[3]:

- The lungs are unable to inspire adequate levels of oxygen for gas diffusion and haemoglobin binding
- The tissues are unable to become perfused due to the heart and blood vessels being unable to maintain adequate circulation around the infant's body
- The brain becomes inactive and is no longer able to regulate vital centres required to maintain life

The effective management of this process will ensure that care is tailored to both the infant and family's individual choices and needs and that parents have been made fully aware and prepared for events following withdrawal of treatment or ventilation and the possibility that despite the withdrawal of intensive care, death may take a considerable length of time to occur[4]. Not all infants deteriorate rapidly following the cessation of intensive care.

Institution of palliative care

Palliative care can be defined in a number of ways and those definitions that convey the holistic and empowering elements of such care have been chosen and applied to this chapter in an attempt to ensure the care remains child and family focused and needs based as opposed to service based.

One such definition is:

'Palliative care includes the control of pain and other symptoms and addresses the psychological, social or spiritual problems of children (and their families) living with life-threatening or terminal conditions'[5].

Another definition that is recognised across many children's palliative care services is that stated by the Association for Children with Life-threatening or Terminal Conditions and their families (ACT)[6]:

'Palliative care is expressed as the active and total approach to care, embracing physical, emotional, social and spiritual elements. It focuses on enhancement of quality of life for the child and support for the family and includes the management of distressing symptoms, provision of respite and care through death and bereavement'[7].

The concept of palliative care is not one of simply withdrawing or ceasing treatment in a child with a life-limiting illness and equally does not imply the intent to hasten the child's death[8]. When implementing effective palliative care, some interventions may be active in nature[9], notably when undertaking symptom control in a child where pain or anxiety may be an issue. This will be discussed later in Chapter 18 where myths regarding the statement that neonates are unable to feel or experience pain are discussed and dispelled.

Wolfe fittingly states that the alleviation of a child's physical and emotional symptoms is of major importance both during the palliative and terminal phases of illness[10]. This would suggest that active interventions are required to ensure the alleviation of such symptoms and the promotion of the comfort of both the child and family.

In the very young infant this will be considerably more challenging as reactions and behaviours can be misinterpreted and appropriate treatment may be delayed as a result.

The challenge of symptom relief highlights the importance of the implementation of good quality children's palliative care where parents and relevant professionals are deemed experts in the child's care due to their knowledge and experiences of each individual infant. Such characteristics must be recognised if palliative and terminal care is to be effective and successful. In such situations, the value of the lead nurse and neonatologist become very apparent as relationships with both the infant and family have already been established and consistency and continuity of care become paramount.

When ensuring that holistic palliative care is provided, all potential symptoms need to be considered and their management planned for in advance. Such symptoms will include:

- Anorexia
- Bleeding
- Constipation
- Cough
- Dehydration
- Diarrhoea
- Dyspnoea
- Noisy breathing
- Seizures
- Gastro-oesophageal reflux
- Infections
- Muscle spasm
- Nausea and vomiting
- Pain
- Psychological issues
- Spiritual awareness

In the event that these symptoms are considered and their management planned prior to them occurring, the infant will remain in a comfortable state due to early interventions being possible. Such interventions ensure quality of life and promote a calm environment for the family.

Implications for practice

All potential symptoms must be considered and actively managed.
The individual expression of pain must be noted and actively reduced using non-pharmaceutical and pharmaceutical methods.

Religious and cultural considerations

Religious and cultural considerations are vital to consider not only following the death of the infant with regards to the funeral but also prior to death. Professionals exercising knowledge and skills around parents' individual religion and culture will encourage them to feel valued and empowered as their wishes and beliefs are heard and implemented through their infant's treatment and terminal care.

Neuberger states that through recognising the potential needs of the dying individual and their family, much comfort can be gained from the perspective of both the family and the professional through a common understanding and respect for individual beliefs and needs[11]. Such positive characteristics can be achieved through simply asking the family about obtaining religious objects or books of worship appropriate to their religion or culture or through understanding and having an awareness of the various celebrations and festivals where certain behaviours are maintained or practiced at specific times of the day.

It is recognised that there are a huge number of diverse religions and cultures and it would therefore be unacceptable to expect professionals to have a broad knowledge of all of them. However, a basic understanding of the following issues would be expected when caring for a terminally ill infant and their family:

- Beliefs in a specific God or gods
- Objects of worship
- Books of worship

- Beliefs regarding immortality of the soul/after-life beliefs
- Are last rites required?
- Who may touch the body?
- May the body be bathed?
- Times of prayer around the infant prior to and following death
- Position of infant both prior to and following death
- Beliefs regarding organ transplantation
- Period of time acceptable between death and the funeral

In many areas of practice today, spiritual and religious counsellors are in residence or are easily accessed. In some settings cultural link workers provide the above information through staff training and support sessions where they accompany the professional to the infant's bedside or home (depending on family's choice regarding place of death). Such support workers are available not only for the families but also for staff information and must be accessed and utilised in order that professional-family relationships can be maintained and enhanced as care is planned and evaluated in collaboration with the parents.

Implications for practice

- Recognise the differing beliefs and cultures of families and children where terminal care is implemented.

Post-mortem examination

Post-mortems are carried out for a number of reasons. These include the provision of vital information for both parents and clinicians and others, consisting of research and audit purposes, training and education and epidemiology. When considering the parents of a neonate following their baby's death, post-mortem

- Implications around the infant's death and funeral arrangements must be considered, noted and put into place as soon as appropriate to ensure the family and child's wishes and cultural beliefs are adhered to.

examination may answer specific questions for them regarding the circumstances around which their baby died, such as:

- Why did our baby die?
  - Was there something wrong that was not identified by the professionals caring for our baby?
  - Was there anything else either the professionals or we could have done to prevent our baby's death?
- Could this happen again if we went on to have another baby?

It is recognised, however, that approaching recently bereaved parents on the subject of a post-mortem on their baby is difficult for any professional, and a reluctance to do so is universal. When approaching such a sensitive issue, an experienced professional, who is also known to the family, is often the most appropriate individual to do so, although it is identified that regardless of experience and knowledge, such a discussion is very difficult to implement at any time and for any level of professional.

The confirmation of their infant's clinical diagnosis is very helpful for parents as their decisions around withdrawal of treatment or the withholding of various interventions becomes justified as post-mortem examination reveals findings to confirm that further treatment or intervention would have been futile, due to the progressive nature of the baby's condition. In many cases, negative findings are also very important as information can be obtained to inform future pregnancies, again to justify the difficult decisions made by parents to withhold/withdraw treatments and also to inform the future practice of professionals working in this field.

While taking into consideration the time required by the parents to spend with the body of their infant, the deceased body will begin to deteriorate rapidly if maintained at room temperature for any length of time. This in turn may result in any post-mortem findings being less reliable. Therefore, while being sensitive to the needs of the family, when post-mortem has been identified as a necessity, interventions to preserve the body need to be implemented as soon as appropriate and possible in order to preserve organ and skin cells so that future findings are accurate and concise.

In McHaffie's study, looking into the experiences of parents around treatment withdrawal from their infants, it was found that those who consented to post-mortem examination did so for the following reasons[12]:

- To obtain answers
- To help other families
- To give meaning to their baby's existence
- To confirm the right decision was made
- To provide evidence for litigation proceedings
  (McHaffie, 2001, p. 171)

It could therefore be suggested that all parents are offered the choice of post-mortem examination following the death of their infant, regardless of the conditions surrounding the baby's death. The process may go some way to helping them as they travel through the grieving trajectory in having some understanding and meaning of both the miracle of their child's birth and the tragedy of his/her death.

Implications for practice

- Ensure that the professional approaching the subject of post-mortem is experienced and qualified to do so, and is known by the family.
- Time must be given to the family to consider all the potential implications and outcomes of a post-mortem.

> • Time must be given to the family to spend with their infant following death, prior to the post-mortem.

Certification and registration of death

In the event that the infant passes away on the neonatal unit, the medic on duty will certify the death at an appropriate time. It is not necessary to document the exact moment of death and in most cases death is expected and therefore not required to be certified hastily. If the infant has been discharged into the community, or a children's hospice, either the family GP or the hospice medic will certify the infant's death.

The parents must be given as much time as they feel they need with their baby following the death. When parents have reached the point where they are able to hand over their baby to either the nurses or funeral directors (depending on place of death), the baby will be labelled in accordance with the hospital regulations or the funeral directors' protocol and taken to either the hospital mortuary or the funeral home. Parents may arrange to see their baby during the following few days if they so wish and this is usually arranged by the pathologist.

Ideally, the death certificate should be issued before parents leave the neonatal unit as it may not be easy for them to return to the hospital where their infant has just died. In order to register a death, the certificate must contain the infant's full name, date and place of death (including hospital, home or hospice address), date and place of birth, the infant's gender, the full names and occupations of both parents, along with their address or addresses (if separated) and the cause of death. Within neonatology there are two situations that can cause confusion with the certification of death and completion of documentation: These are a stillbirth and an infant born prior to 24 weeks gestation (the current gestation at which legal terminations can still be performed). In the case of an infant that is stillborn (no signs of life seen following delivery) the death certificate can be completed by the midwife attending the delivery. In the case of an infant born prior to 24 weeks gestation, if he/she is born alive then the death certificate has to be completed by a medic/doctor who saw the infant alive. In this latter case it is therefore important that even if a doctor is not attending the delivery they must be asked to briefly review the infant prior to death to enable them to legally complete the death certificate. This may be a member of the obstetric team and not necessarily a neonatologist.

The death will be registered by the registrar of births and deaths using the information on the death certificate. Each entry is registered on computer using a specific programme which the registrar is unable to override in the event of inadequate or incorrect information being provided. In such circumstances registration will be delayed, resulting in a long wait for the parents at such a stressful time. If there are any errors the parents will be asked to return to the neonatal unit for it to be completed appropriately. The infant's death is required to be registered within five days of the death unless a post-mortem or coroner's report is requested. In some cases the birth and death will be registered at the same time. There are slight differences in who can register the birth and who can register a death; a birth can be registered by:

• The mother
• The father if married to the mother at the time of birth or conception
• Rarely, a person present at the birth or guardian of the child

The death must be registered by:

• A blood relative present at death or during last illness
• Mother, father or grandparent

In the unfortunate event that there are no relatives of either stature, an individual present at the death may register as long as they have all of the information required for the process to be completed.

In the event that the baby passed away in a children's hospice, most establishments have facilities where the infant's body may be laid in a special bedroom that is cooled down to 3°C or below. Parents can then visit their baby as often as they wish to prior to the funeral. Most hospices will keep the infant until the day of the funeral and most processions will depart from the hospice itself.

Implications for practice

- Give parents time to spend with their infant following death.
- Ensure that the death certificate has been correctly completed.
- Explain thoroughly, the information they are required to take in order to register the death to prevent repetition and delays in the provision of the certificate.

The role of the coroner

The coroner is an independent officer appointed by the council to investigate any sudden or unexplained deaths. In the neonatal population this may include:

- Stillborn infants: an infant > 24 weeks gestation that has shown no signs of life following delivery
- Those that die within 24 hours of admission to the neonatal unit
- Those that die during surgery
- Those in which a medical procedure or treatment may have contributed to the death
- Where the cause of death is unknown

Once an infant death has been reported to the coroner's office, the death cannot be registered until the coroner's opinion is known. If the coroner agrees that the case needs examining the post-mortem will be a legal obligation of investigation and parents will not be able to prevent this.

Once reported to the coroner he/she may:

- Take no action: the coroner's enquiry may be able to establish that the death was due to natural causes, e.g. the stillbirth of a term infant following placental abruption. In this situation a coroner's post-mortem will not be requested although a hospital post-mortem can still be requested with consent from parents.
- Agree to investigation of the case and organisation of a coroner's post-mortem
  - If the post-mortem shows that death has occurred as a result of the disease process no inquest will be held and the death certificate can be completed to register the death
  - If the post-mortem shows that death did not occur entirely because of natural causes an inquest will be held to investigate the circumstances around the death

An inquest is a legal enquiry into the circumstances surrounding the death – it is not a trial. The doctors, and in some situations nursing staff, responsible for the infant's care will be required to be present at the inquest. Unfortunately in these situations there will be a delay of weeks or months from the infant's death to the time of the inquest but in most situations it is possible to release the infant's body for burial following the post-mortem.

Clinical management of death on the NNU

The death of every infant is a very individual and tragic experience. There are some specific situations which may be encountered on the neonatal unit which include a term infant that has experienced:

- A severe hypoxic ischaemic insult
- The diagnosis of a congenital condition for which treatment is futile

- A preterm infant with:
  - Sudden acute deterioration: for example, secondary to pulmonary haemorrhage or intraventricular haemorrhage
  - Chronic deterioration following prolonged intensive care treatment

It is not always clear when the end of life phase begins but the infant will exhibit definitive symptoms that will suggest they are entering this phase of their condition or alternatively appropriate withdrawal of life prolonging treatment may also define this phase.

The provision of care for this period of time will include:

- Symptom management
- Bereavement support for the family
- Attention to the body after death
- In some instances, preparation of the funeral

It is vital, that prior to the end of the infant's life, discussions take place in close collaboration with parents and other appropriate family members along with members of the multi-disciplinary team in order to establish decisions and plans around the infant's death. Parents and family members must be provided with informed choices and allowed to make important decisions with as much information regarding their infant as possible. This must be undertaken by a professional with experience of undertaking such a discussion and the infant's condition, and who may also be able to answer all questions and concerns honestly and promptly. The availability of a lead consultant and lead nurse in this situation is very valuable.

Who do we involve?

All family members important to the infant and parents need to be involved in any required decision making. This may include grandparents, siblings, aunts, uncles or even friends. The parents' wishes at these times for other people to be involved must be granted.

Respectful religious considerations

Discussions around the beliefs and cultures of the parents need to take place prior to this phase of the infant's condition. The family's wishes for the infant to be accepted into their own religious faith must be discussed in order that plans can be put into place promptly should this need to happen quickly.

Where should the death occur?

This decision can often be the most difficult to make and is influenced by what is felt to be in the infant's best interests, the family's wishes, the condition of the infant and the predicted time to death and the location of various appropriate venues. The venues may include:

- Home
- A children's hospice
- Intensive care room
- Quiet room on the neonatal unit
- Post-natal ward/delivery suite

Once this decision has been made, transport to this place has to be planned. This is as important when planning the transfer to a room on the neonatal unit as it is when planning a transfer to a hospice. The risk of the infant dying in transit will need to be considered and discussed with parents following this decision. An example may be the transportation of a ventilated infant through to the quiet room while bagging and then reattaching to the ventilator when in situ. It will be necessary to ensure that appropriate cribs/bedding have already been placed and prepared. The parents can then cuddle and spend time with the infant while reattached to the ventilator, rather than a professional standing over the infant while hand ventilating. Such intense discussion *will* need to take place *prior* to the commencement of this plan. Decisions around where the infant is extubated will also need to be discussed. Parents may wish to hold their infant while this is taking place, others may wish to be handed their baby following extubation.

Implications for practice

- The identification of a lead consultant and lead nurse to facilitate the dying process will provide a consistent line of communication for the family.
- It is important to prepare in detail for the place and the way in which families wish intensive care to be withdrawn or death to occur.

How is death managed on the NNU?

Following intense symptom management to ensure the infant's comfort, it may be deemed appropriate to take out many of the various lines and monitoring equipment prior to the transfer to the parents' place of choice and following discussion with the medical team, unless the infant's condition is deemed a coroner's case (such as when the infant has passed away within 24 hours of admission or surgery). A morphine infusion providing sedation may continue to be administered through a syringe driver throughout this phase. This *must* remain in situ.

Discussions may need to take place with the parents and family regarding how the infant may look, breathing changes and alterations in colour as death occurs. Some parents may not want to know this information although it is vital that they are made aware that changes will occur. It will be necessary to inform the parents that in many cases, the infant's heart rate may continue for up to two hours following what is deemed to be death. This is merely the heart's independent pump and not the act of cerebral intervention. It may also be the case when the infant appears to take the occasional gasp. This is the reaction from the primitive spinal reflex, and again not an indication of cerebral function. The infant may not be certified as dead, however, until all of this activity has ceased.

Following the infant's death, it is vitally important that *all* professionals involved (i.e. health visitor, G.P., etc.) are informed to prevent inadvertent circumstances occurring.

What to do following certification of death?

'The first rule is do not panic, do not dive in blindly'[13], listen to the parents and how they wish to move to the next phase of this very sensitive period. Some parents may wish to cuddle their infant with other family members who may not have been present at this difficult time, others may wish to spend time alone with their infant, others may wish to leave the room for a while and gather their thoughts. It is so important that their wishes are acknowledged and appreciated and that they are not judged by their behaviours at this time.

Handling of the body after death

While respecting the beliefs and culture of the family, the infant will require preparing for transportation to the mortuary or home in some cases. This will often include the removal of remaining lines and cannulas (if not a coroner's case), bathing and dressing the infant in the clothes of the parents' choice. It may be that the parents and other family members will wish to undertake this activity as they will view it as the final care they may give to their child. As professionals, we must support them through this activity and ensure dignity and privacy for its entirety. When preparing the body, the head must remain in an elevated and supported position (this can be achieved with cotton wool and various *soft* cloths) in order to prevent stasis of blood. Vaseline/moisturising cream may also be applied to the lips in order to prevent dehydration and discolouration. This needs to be undertaken on a regular basis while the body remains on the unit as discolouration can occur very quickly following death.

Memories

It is vitally important that various items are collected and kept, such as the infant's name bands/cot card, in order that parents can keep them as memories of their infant's life if they wish to do so. Many neonatal units provide memory boxes for this reason and will encourage parents to put items of the infant inside both prior to and following the infant's death. A lock of the infant's hair can also be taken by the member of staff preparing the infant. This can then be given to the family to place in the memory box.

Footprints and hand prints can also be obtained with parents' consent. This may be something the parents initially say they do not want, but often they change their minds as the grieving process progresses. Photos may also be taken both prior to and following the infant's death. Again, these may not be requested by the parents shortly after the infant's death but may be something they wish to keep in the future. (This is very dependent upon the culture of the infant and family.)

It is important that, following preparation of the infant's body, name bands are replaced if they have been removed for the parents to keep, and an identification card is placed on the wrapping *prior* to removal from the unit. Parents may wish for a particular soft toy or teddy to remain with the infant's body. This also requires labelling and placed inside with the infant.

Following the removal of the infant's body from the unit, neonatal unit staff will be able to make arrangements for the parents to see their baby in the mortuary if they wish to do so.

Implications for practice

- Helping parents to create and maintain memories is an important role for the neonatal nurse.
- Not all parents will wish to be present, discussion *must* involve the parents at all times.

Breast milk

This is one of the most overlooked activities following the death of an infant. The mother will experience many intense emotions and may also have to cope with leaking breasts where her infant should be feeding. Mothers should be given the opportunity and privacy to express their breast milk following the death of their infant and referrals may be made (following discussion with the mother) to the GP for medication to suppress lactation.

Follow-up support

Following the death of their infant, the care and support provided by the neonatal unit to the parents does not cease. Post-bereavement support will be offered by many units and referrals will be made to appropriate organisations to ensure this support meets the need of the parents, siblings and wider family and supports them through the grieving process for as long as they deem necessary.

Management of grief

It is acknowledged that everyone manages grief in various ways, all of which are individual to the person experiencing it and there are no rights or wrongs when expressing this. The previous life experiences of individuals can have major implications on the way they may express their grief and how they may deal with it. The religious and cultural beliefs of an individual can also have a huge bearing on the way their grief is portrayed.

Grief may be expressed through a number of emotions ranging from[14]:

- Shock
- Fear
- Denial
- Anger

These may become apparent at very different stages of a parent's grief after the loss of their infant and it needs to be acknowledged that both a mother and a father may express these emotions at very different times and in very different ways to one another. The role of the neonatal nurse is to support this process and to facilitate the expression of emotions as and when parents feel able. This must be provided in an environment that is comfortable for both parents.

It is acknowledged that the neonatal nurse will experience a level of grief for the loss of the infant. However, this should not be compared to that experienced by the parents, in any way. The neonatal nurse must also recognise his/her own levels of emotional involvement and obtain support through the appropriate channels and also through colleagues, to ensure their ongoing effective practice within the neonatal field of nursing and to maintain their own well-being.

It is the neonatal nurse's responsibility to recognise when their own sphere of competence has been reached. They then need to have the knowledge and networks available to them in order to ensure that an appropriate referral is then made to a more appropriate service. This will then ensure that parents may obtain continuing support appropriate to their own needs and that multi-agency working is promoted through the services. Such services may include:

- Social services – counselling service
- Neonatal unit service counsellor – outreach team
- Children's hospice community support team
- Follow-up bereavement meetings with consultant

It is acknowledged that individual localities will include services that will provide similar care and support. It is vital that the neonatal nurse is aware of these teams within his/her working locality in order that appropriate referrals can be made and a seamless service is provided to the parents.

It is also acknowledged that practice may vary from unit to unit, and services provided locally may also differ.

Conclusion

Caring for the infant and the family of an infant who is dying is very difficult for all those involved and needs to be dealt with in a sensitive manner. Where and when this takes place should be discussed with the family in order that the death may be in a place and at a pace that they are comfortable with. It is acknowledged that practice may vary from unit to unit, and services provided locally may also differ.

Helpful websites

www.suffolk.gov.uk/BirthsMarriagesAndDeaths

References

1. Rando TA (ed.) (1986) *Parental Loss of a Child*. Research Press, Champaign, Illinois.
2. Orford T (1996) Psychological support for parents whose children require neonatal intensive care. *Journal of Neonatal Nursing*, **2** (1), 11–13.
3. Durham EW, Weiss L (1997) How patients die. *American Journal of Nursing*, **97** (12), 41–46.
4. McHaffie HE (2001) *Crucial Decisions at the Beginning of Life: Parents' Experiences of Treatment Withdrawal from Infants*. Radcliffe Medical Press, Oxford.
5. Frager G (1996) Pediatric palliative care: building the model, bridging the gaps. *J Palliat Care*, **12** (3), 9–12.
6. ACT (The Association for Children with Life Threatening or Terminal Conditions and Their Families) (2003) *A Guide to the Development of Children's Palliative Care Services*, 2nd edn. ACT, Bristol. pp. 9–13 (www.act.org.uk).
7. ACT (The Association for Children with Life Threatening or Terminal Conditions and Their Families) (2003) *A Guide to the Development of Children's Palliative Care Services*, 2nd edn. ACT, Bristol. pp. 9–13 (www.act.org.uk).
8. Dyck AJ (1977) An alternative to the ethic of euthanasia. In: Reiser S, Dyck A, Curran W (eds), *Ethics in Medicine: Historical Perspectives and Contemporary Concerns*. MIT Press, Cambridge.
9. Hutchinson F, King N, Hain RDW (2002) Terminal care in paediatrics: where we are now. *Journal of Postgraduate Medicine*, **79**, 566–568.
10. Wolfe J, Holcombe Grier E, Clau N, *et al.* (2000) Symptoms and suffering at the end of life in children with cancer. *N Engl J Med*, **342** (5), 326–333.

11. Neuberger J (ed.) (2004) *Caring for Dying People of Different Faiths*, 3rd edn. Radcliffe Medical Press, Oxford.

12. McHaffie HE (2001) *Crucial Decisions at the Beginning of Life: Parents' Experiences of Treatment Withdrawal from Infants*. Radcliffe Medical Press, Oxford.

13. Jassal S (2006) *Basic Symptom Control In Paediatric Palliative Care*. The Rainbows Children's Hospice Guidelines.

14. Wyley MV, Allen J (1991) A Paradigm for parents and professionals. *Nann News (neonatal network)* (5).

Chapter 16

INFECTION IN THE TERM AND PRETERM INFANT

Alison Bedford Russell

Learning outcomes

After reading this chapter the reader will be expected to be able to:

- Describe why neonates are prone to infection

- List the common organisms to which neonates are most susceptible

- Explain what can be done to minimise the risk of infection

  ○ In the environment

  ○ In how we manage the baby

- Describe the differing ways in which neonatal infection presents

- Illustrate the principles of management when infection is suspected, including:

  ○ The investigations that should be considered

  ○ The principles of treating infection

- Describe the principles of prenatal and post-natal care for the baby of a mother with HIV infection

---

Introduction

Infection is one of the major causes of mortality and morbidity within the neonatal population. This chapter will introduce the topics of innate and acquired immunity, before discussing the common causes of early and late sepsis in neonates and the importance of strategies to prevent infection. The final section deals with congenital infections such as hepatitis B, cytomegalovirus and human immunodeficiency virus.

Development of immunity

Innate immunity

The immune system is the body's primary defence system against invasion by microbes, which include bacteria, fungi and viruses. Natural barriers to prevent invasion by these microbes, include the skin and mucous membranes. These form the first line of defence to invading organisms and are part of the 'innate' or 'non-adaptive' immune system. What follows is a brief description of the immune system; for more extensive information the reader should refer to a textbook of immunology[1].

If the skin surface is damaged (e.g. the fragile skin of a baby can easily be damaged by tape, probes or labels placed on the skin), microbes can enter the body and start to multiply. These microbes will then encounter the next component of the immune defence system; white blood cells, which engulf and ingest (phagocytose) microbes and are therefore known as 'phagocytes'. These are classified as macrophages (if present in tissues) and monocytes (if in the bloodstream) and neutrophils (recruited later on). The body also produces proteins that attract phagocytes to the sites of infection (complement components) and others that bind to invading organisms and facilitate phagocytosis (organism-specific immunoglobulins). These immunoglobulins are important in combating encapsulated organisms such as pneumococcus. Preterm babies are deficient in immunoglobulins and their phagocytic cells, especially neutrophils, may be low in number, and not function as well as in term infants. This is particularly true for those who are small for gestational age, and makes them more vulnerable to infection. Mortality and a poor outcome are much more likely when infection is associated with neutropenia (low neutrophil count) which probably reflects the consequences of a failure to mount an appropriate neutrophil response to infection.

Implications for practice

The skin and mucous membranes are an important part of the innate *immune system* and even the removal of routine ECG monitoring probes may damage the skin and increase the risk of infection.

The innate system is usually effective in destroying and removing organisms, but if it fails to clear infection rapidly, it activates the 'adaptive' or 'acquired' immune response. The two systems are connected by antigen-presenting cells and messenger molecules called 'cytokines'. Antigen presenting cells are cells that display the antigens of the foreign material on their surface in a recognisable way to the cells of the adaptive immune system. Cytokines are protein messengers produced by cells to act as signalling pathways *between* cells and *within* a cell. Some may cause inflammation, in which case they are known as 'pro-inflammatory cytokines'. Pro-inflammatory cytokines include Interleukin-6 (IL-6) and Tumor necrosis factor (TNFα) which are released at the time of infection. IL-6 stimulates the release of C-reactive protein (CRP), and CRP is often measured as a marker of infection.

Adaptive immunity

The cells of the adaptive immune system are T and B lymphocytes. The developing immune system, which is presented with thousands of bacteria and other foreign substances, called 'antigens', learns to distinguish between 'pathogenic' antigens, e.g. harmful bacteria, and harmless antigens, e.g. food antigens and non-pathogenic bacteria[2,3]. The immune system has to become immunologically reactive to harmful antigens; and to develop immunological 'tolerance' to harmless antigens, such as non-pathogenic bacteria and food antigens. The primary mechanism for distinguishing harmful from benign bacteria and antigens depends on the activation status of antigen-presenting cells (APC)[4,5].

Adaptive immune responses are complex and highly effective but may take 7–10 days to completely mobilise and the response is very specific for a particular antigen. The adaptive immune system recognises different types of bacteria and antigens by developing a huge and diverse number of 'antigen-recognition' receptors (see 1–3 in list below), whereas cells of the innate immune system (e.g. macrophages and dendritic cells) bear receptors that recognise certain pathogen-associated molecular patterns. These receptors are called 'pattern recognition receptors' and activate cells of the innate immune system before the development of adaptive immune responses.

The 'innate' or 'non-adaptive', and 'acquired' or 'adaptive' immune responses have different immunological roles, but are dependent on each other throughout the development of immune responses.

Implications for practice

The innate immune system can be considered as a system with a generalised approach (e.g. all snakes are poisonous) while the adaptive immune system has a much more specific approach (e.g. the brown snake of Australia is poisonous).

The basic differences between the two systems are summarised in Table 16.1 below.

There are several different types of antigen-recognition receptor:

(1) Antibodies (which are B-cell antigen receptors): these can be found as 'soluble' antigen-recognising molecules in the bloodstream or on the cell surface of B lymphocytes. Antibodies are also known as immunoglobulins. There are various types of immunoglobulin (G, D, A, M and E), but only immunoglobulin G (IgG), can cross the placenta.

(2) T-cell antigen receptors: these are receptors present in the membranes of T-cells. Part of the receptor is exposed to the outside of the cell, part is situated within the cell membrane and part is inside the cell.

(3) The major histocompatibility complex (MHC): the MHC genes of humans are known as human leukocyte antigen (HLA) genes and their products as HLA molecules.

Antigen receptors on each T and B-cell are unique. When a foreign antigen enters the body, it has to make contact with a lymphocyte with the matching receptor in order to bring about a response. The lymphocyte then divides up (in a process called 'clonal expansion') to produce large amounts of soluble receptor, or immunoglobulin, which specifically recognises the antigen that stimulated its production. B-cell antigen receptors (antibodies) can interact directly with antigen, if the antigen and antibody 'match'. T-cell antigen receptors only recognise antigen when it is presented to them, after being loaded into the peptide-binding groove of a specific MHC class II molecule on the surface of an antigen-presenting cell such as a monocyte. T-cells will only respond if they recognise the MHC class II molecule with the specific antigen being presented. In this way only a tiny fraction ($< 0.01\%$) of the baby's T-cell numbers are activated at any time.

An extremely important feature of the adaptive immune system is that it has 'memory' of a previous antigen. This means that the body

Table 16.1 Comparison of innate and adaptive immune systems.

	Innate	Adaptive
Characteristics	Non-specific response Response is fast (minutes) Has no memory	Very specific response Response is slow (days) Has memory
Components	Natural barriers e.g. skin Complement Neutrophils and macrophages Pattern-recognition molecules, e.g. Toll-like receptors (TLRs) and Nod proteins on dendritic and other cells	T and B lymphocytes and secreted molecules MHC-class II restricted Antigen- recognition molecules

is protected from re-infection by the same organism and is the basic mechanism by which immunisation works.

Implications for practice

The adaptive immune system can take up to 7–10 days to mount an effective response, but will then remember this response in the future when it encounters the same antigen again and mount a similar response much quicker – this is why immunisation is effective.

Superantigens

Superantigens, popularly called 'superbugs' (e.g. MRSA), are capable of triggering excessive activation of the immune system because of the way in which they bind to MHC class II molecules and to T-cell receptors, bypassing the normal procedure outlined above. The result is that up to 25% (as opposed to < 0.01%) of an individual's T-cells can be activated at one time. This results in a massive release of pro-inflammatory cytokines. Well-known examples of superantigen-producing bacteria include *Staphylococcus aureus* (not just MRSA) and *Streptococcus pyogenes*. Gram negative bacteria, mycoplasma and viruses can also produce superantigens[4]. This is why such organisms can cause such profound sepsis, with multi-organ involvement, within a very short space of time.

CD4+ and CD8+ T-cells

There are several different types of proteins which are associated with T-cell membrane surfaces and are crucial for the T-cell having specific functions. These molecules are given 'CD' numbers. CD4+ T-cells (i.e. T-cells which are 'positive' for the CD4 molecule) are known as 'T-helper cells' which differentiate into one of two helper subsets called Th1 or Th2 helper T-cells.

- Th1 T-cell subsets are generated by infection with bacteria and viruses and release IFNγ and other pro-inflammatory cytokines.

- Th2 helper T-cell subsets are generated as a result of infection with parasites, e.g. hookworm, and by allergens. Th2 helper T-cells will then release cytokines which stimulate B-cells to secrete IgE which is involved with allergic responses.

CD4 is also the cellular receptor which allows HIV to attach to T-cells and these 'T helper' cells are killed by a high HIV viral load. A low number of CD4+ cells is therefore a poor prognostic indicator for patients with HIV.

T-cells which carry CD8 have killing functions and are known as cytotoxic T lymphocytes. The number of CD8 cells tends to rise during the course of an HIV infection. The numbers of CD4 and CD8 cells as well as the ratio of CD4+ to CD8+ T-cells can be used to measure disease progression in some infections, including HIV infection.

Implications for practice

Superantigens are capable of mounting an excessive immune response that may result in multisystem failure within a short space of time.

Passive versus active immunity

The processes described above are termed 'active' immunity and describe how human beings can respond to an antigen. 'Passive' immunity is when immunity is passed from one individual to another. Passive immunity is transferred in the form of IgG across the placenta, and immune cells and immunoglobulins (antibodies) in breast milk, from mother to baby. IgG antibody transfer from mother to baby begins at 8–10 weeks' gestation, but accelerates after 32 weeks' gestation. Babies do not usually produce much immunoglobulin themselves until they are several months old. The timing of antibody transfer means that a baby who is born prematurely has less maternal antibody passively transferred than does a term infant. This contributes to the 'immune deficiency' of preterm infants.

Immunity, gastrointestinal system and feeding

The gut forms a critical part of the immune system and the infant's susceptibility to infection. This is because 80% of the cells of the immune system are present in the linings of the gut (the 'Gut-associated lymphoid system', or 'GALT') and because of the importance of bacterial colonisation of the gastrointestinal tract.

Breast milk has been shown to protect babies from necrotising enterocolitis[7]. Breast milk has also been shown to protect babies from late onset infection[8,9]. Introducing even 0.5ml/kg of 'trophic' breast milk (and only breast milk) in the first hours of life, in very immature babies, will colonise the naive gut with normal bacteria (lactobacilli and bifidobacteria)[10,11]. Such bacteria are critical for the development not only of the immune system, but also to bring about the development of mucosal barrier function, gut motility and digestive functions[12–14]. The risk of infection is greatly increased for every day a baby is not enterally fed[15,16]. This effect of early feeding is independent of the increased risk of infection with indwelling catheters (long lines, umbilical venous and arterial lines) and total parental nutrition (TPN).

The gut of a baby admitted to a neonatal unit becomes colonised with abnormal bacteria as a result of being exposed to the neonatal unit 'bacterial flora' and to antibiotics. The gut bacteria in preterm babies is dominated by Coagulase negative staphylococci (CONS or 'Staph epi' for short)[17], which is the most common organism causing late onset sepsis[18]. It is likely that bacteria from the gut 'translocate' across immature gut mucosa and lodge onto indwelling devices such as catheters and give rise to features of infection[19,20]. This is one of the reasons why it is extremely important to wear gloves when changing nappies.

Implications for practice

- In order to facilitate colonisation of the gut with healthy bacteria trophic feeds should be commenced as soon as possible with breast milk.
- Coagulase negative staphylococci dominate the colonisation of the gut in preterm infants and are the commonest cause of late onset sepsis.

Potential hazards of peripartum antibiotics

Antibiotics are increasingly prescribed in the peripartum period, for both maternal and foetal indications. Their effective use undoubtedly reduces the incidence of specific invasive infections in the newborn, such as Group B streptococcal (GBS) infection. However, the total burden of infectious neonatal disease may not be reduced, particularly if broad-spectrum agents are used, as has been shown for GBS in the USA[21]. Antibiotic prophylaxis has resulted in a reduction in the incidence of GBS infection, but there has been an accompanying increase in the incidence of infection due to antibiotic-resistant E. coli infection in low birthweight infants[22]. All antibiotics, particularly broad-spectrum antibiotics, e.g. amoxycillin/ampicillin, Augmentin, erythromycin and cephalosporins, alter the natural microflora of any living body, with possible increases in antibiotic resistance and the pathogenicity of organisms[23]. This has resulted in the well-known exponential increase in infection by bacteria such as MRSA (methicillin resistant staphylococcus aureus)[24]. Widespread use of broad spectrum antibiotics within a maternity unit will increase local persistence of resistant organisms and favour opportunistic transmission within the unit[25,26]. This is why the narrowest spectrum antibiotic should be used at all times, for treatment, rather then prophylaxis and for the shortest time possible. For this to be possible it is important to know what organisms are causing infections and what the antibiotic-sensitivity of those organisms are.

The developed world has also witnessed a substantial increase in the incidence of allergic and autoimmune disease in young children over the past three decades and this has been attributed to the 'hygiene' or 'clean child' hypothesis. The suggestion is that immune development becomes abnormal because babies are exposed to abnormal bacterial as a result of obstetric practices and inappropriate antibiotic use [27,28].

Neonatal infection: early and late onset neonatal sepsis

The highest risk group for sepsis and its sequelae are those born with birthweights of < 1500 g in whom infection is associated with prolonged ventilation and hospital stay, and increased risk of chronic lung disease of prematurity (CLD), intraventricular haemorrhage and death[29-31]. Perinatal infection has also become recognised as an important aetiological factor in the pathogenesis of cerebral cortical lesions and subsequent development of cerebral palsy in both preterm and term infants[32-36]. High concentrations of pro-inflammatory cytokines are associated with an increased risk of cardiovascular compromise, septic shock and death[37,38]. They also have effects on the developing brain during sepsis episodes, and pro-inflammatory cytokines are strongly associated with the development of brain lesions, even in the absence of meningitis[39-41].

Implications for practice

Confirmed perinatal or neonatal infection increases the risk of: neonatal death, chronic lung disease and cerebral palsy or neurodevelopmental concerns.

In the UK there is no national neonatal infection surveillance system in place. Data from 11 UK neonatal units is displayed in Table 16.2 (bacteria causing early-onset infection at < 7 days of life) and Table 16.3 (bacteria causing late

onset infection at > 7 days of life). Colonisation with organisms without signs of infection does not warrant treatment. The classic microbiological dictum summarised below remains valid:

- Never use an antibiotic unless one needs to
- Never use a broad-spectrum antibiotic when a narrow-spectrum one will do
- Treatment should be stopped as soon as there is no evidence of infection

Early onset neonatal infection

Early onset infection is less common than late onset infection and is usually caused by organisms from the maternal genital tract. Some define early-onset infection as that occurring in the first 48 hours or 72 hours of life, and others in the first seven days. Early onset infection is usually more severe than late onset and mortality is high, especially in the lower birthweight and premature baby, despite antibiotic treatment. This relates to some of these organisms being 'superantigen' producers. The organisms responsible are in order of frequency:

- Group B streptococcus ('GBS', *Streptococcus agalactiae* or Lancefield group B streptococcus);
- *Eshericia coli* (*E. coli*)
- *Listeria monocytogenes* (see Table 16.2)

Table 16.2 Positive blood cultures in the first seven days of life. Data from 11 NICUs in the UK reporting to the NEONin database (results are for 992 positive blood cultures reported for 450 patients: neonin@sgul.ac.uk).

Pathogen	Number (%)
Coagulase negative staphylococci (CONS) (Usually contaminants)	114 (11.0)
Group B streptococcus (GBS)	33 (3.3)
Mixed coagulase negative staphylococci (MCONS) (likely to be contaminants)	20 (2)
Eschericia coli	12 (1.2)
Staphylococcus aureus	7 (0.7)
Enterobacter cloacae	5 (0.5)
Bacillus	3 (0.3)
Listeria monocytogenes	3 (0.3)

Group B streptococcus (GBS)

GBS is recognised as an important cause of serious infection in neonates, infants and in immunocompromised or pregnant adults. The overall incidence of GBS infection in the UK is 0·72/1000 live births, though there are regional variations, with the highest incidence being in Northern Ireland and the lowest in Scotland [42]. These figures are based on 'culture-proven' GBS where GBS is grown in blood or cerebro-spinal fluid. Because organisms cannot always be grown even when they are present and causing infection, other studies have shown that the actual number of babies affected by GBS could be as high as 3.6/1000 [43,44].

GBS most commonly causes early onset (EO) disease which presents as sepsis or pneumonia in the first seven days of life. Late onset GBS disease (seven days to three months of life) is less common and more frequently presents as meningitis or sepsis. Risk factors for GBS infection can be identified in up to 60% of cases of early onset disease and include:

- Pre-term delivery in 37% (< 37 weeks)
- Prolonged rupture of membranes in 44% (PROM ≥ 18 hours)
- Known genital carriage of GBS during pregnancy in 4% [45]

There is also an increase risk of GBS infection in infants born to mothers with [46]:

- Pyrexia
- GBS urinary tract infection
- A previous child with GBS disease

It should, however, be noted that *GBS can cross intact membranes* and that *in 40% of cases there are no risk factors.*

Nearly 90% of neonates with early-onset GBS have signs of infection within 12 hours of delivery. The overall mortality is approximately 10%, but is significantly higher among infants born prematurely. Up to 7% of survivors of GBS infection may suffer some disability.

GBS colonisation

GBS lives in the lower gut and vagina in 10 to 25% of mothers. There are no known harmful effects of carriage or 'colonisation' itself. If a term baby is well, has a normal examination (specifically a normal respiratory rate and heart rate), and no other risk factors for infection, but is colonised with GBS, no further action need be taken. Some units monitor temperature, pulse and heart rate for a minimum of 12 hours in line with the RCOG Green-top guidelines for management of babies at risk for GBS infection [47]. A preterm baby, especially one who has delivered after spontaneous onset of labour, will warrant an infection screen and treatment with penicillin until cultures are known to be negative. This is because infection is the most common *identifiable* reason for spontaneous preterm delivery as stated above.

GBS infection

A baby may have very subtle signs of infection in the early stages. They may simply not be feeding well or possibly be excessively sleepy. Some have tachypnoea (a rapid breathing rate), and some may just stop breathing (apnoea). If infection is suspected in a baby, the baby should be carefully examined and appropriate investigations performed (see below). The baby should also be given antibiotics promptly before the results of these investigations are known. Penicillin is the antibiotic of choice for GBS.

GBS prevention

In the USA, where GBS is more common than in the UK, all mothers are screened for GBS at the end of their pregnancy and treated with penicillin if the swab is positive. Routine screening and antibiotic prophylaxis are not currently recommended in the UK [48]. There are some promising studies of GBS vaccines which may prevent GBS infection in the future, but at present there is not currently a GBS vaccine that is routinely available [49].

Implications for practice

Early group B streptococcal infection can occur when there are *no* risk factors for infection and presents as a pneumonia or overwhelming infection in 90% of infants within 12 hours of delivery.
In the preterm it can mimic idiopathic respiratory distress syndrome.

Listeria

Listeria is rare but should be suspected with any of the following:

- Maternal 'flu-like' febrile illness preceding the onset of labour, especially if there has been spontaneous premature rupture of the membranes
- An unwell baby with a rash which is usually a sparse papular eruption
- Hepatosplenomegaly
- Gram positive rods are seen in blood culture or cerebrospinal fluid (CSF)

Late onset infection

Risk factors for late onset infection

Late onset infections may be defined as those occurring after 48 hours of age or in some cases > 7 days. The risk of nosocomial sepsis is increased in:

- Low birthweight
- Extreme preterm
- Those who are not receiving enteral feeds
- Presence of indwelling catheters
- Receiving total parenteral nutrition (TPN)
- Those who have had gut surgery or gut-related problems[50,51].

Infection is more likely to occur in a baby in intensive care, and infection will prolong hospital stay and morbidity[52,53]. Breast-feeding is known to be protective for both NEC and nosocomial sepsis. This is related to colonisation of the gut with lactobacilli and bifidobacteria as well as factors present within breast milk which help 'fight' infections[54,55].

The responsible organisms are usually acquired from the post-natal environment, although the mother's genital tract is still a potential source (see Table 16.3). Infection at this stage often has an insidious onset and focal sepsis, e.g. meningitis, is more common. Sepsis should be considered as the diagnosis for any untoward event that befalls a baby until proved otherwise. Such events include:

- Bradycardia and apnoea
- Tachypnoea
- Poor feeding
- Increasing gastric aspirates
- Abdominal distension irritability
- Convulsions
- Increasing jaundice
- Unexplained increase or rapid decrease in neutrophil or platelet counts or CRP
- Signs of focal inflammation such as periumbilical cellulites or infected cannula site and for ventilated babies: unexplained increased ventilatory requirements; increased volume and 'purulence' of endotracheal secretions or increased shadowing on CXR

Table 16.3 Positive blood cultures for bacteria after the first seven days of life. Data from 11 NICUs in the UK reporting to the NEONin database (results are for 992 positive blood cultures are reported for 450 patients: neonin@sgul.ac.uk).

Pathogen	Number (%)
Coagulase negative staphylococci (CONS) (may or may not be contaminants depending on clinical situation)	459 (46.3)
Mixed coagulase negative staphylococci (MCONS) (usually are contaminants)	41 (4.0)
Enterococcus faecalis	27 (2.7)
Eschericia coli	24 (2.4)
Enterobacter cloacae	21 (2.1)
Klebsiella aerogenes	19 (1.9)
Staphylococcus aureus	18 (1.8)
Klebsiella oxytocia	14 (1.4)
Enterobacter species	10 (1.0)

Fungal infection

Systemic candidiasis is the third most common cause of late-onset sepsis in VLBW infants[56]. Recent UK data (national prospective surveillance study) showed an estimated annual incidence of invasive disease of 1.0% (0.8–1.2) amongst VLBW infants (under 1500 g) and 2.1% (1.65–2.57) in ELBW infants (under 1000g)[57]. The vast majority of cases are of late onset (i.e. > 72 hours after birth). Mortality rates range from 25–40%, which is greater than that for bacterial infection. Risk factors include:

- Birthweight < 1500 g
- TPN
- Presence of indwelling catheters
- Mechanical ventilation
- Any antibiotics, but aminoglycosides, vancomycin and cephalosporins are particularly implicated
- H-2 receptor antagonists (ranitidine)
- Peritoneal dialysis[58]

Signs and symptoms are non-specific and include:

- Temperature instability
- Respiratory distress
- Lethargy
- Apnoeas, with or without bradycardia
- Abdominal distension, bilious aspirates and blood in stools mimicking NEC, but without pneumatosis coli
- Glucose intolerance

There may be a place for prophylactic antifungal treatment in the particularly vulnerable infant.

Necrotising enterocolitis NEC
See Chapter 9.

Investigation for infection

(1) Blood culture: a minimum of 0.5 ml per blood culture bottle should be taken using a 'closed system' (the broken needle technique is not suitable)[59]. Peripheral venous samples are usually taken, but arterial samples are also suitable. Samples from a freshly sited UAC taken by the person siting the catheter, while still scrubbed up are acceptable. The first dose of antibiotics should be given before other procedures, e.g. UAC insertion is attempted in such babies; other blood tests can wait.

(2) Deep ear swab: these swabs should be taken by nursing staff using a swab passed through a sterile speculum. A deep ear swab is only useful if taken less than six hours after birth; after this time the external auditory canal will have been colonised by bacteria from the environment.

(3) Chest X-ray: a chest radiograph (X-ray) is important in the diagnosis of pneumonia and should normally be obtained as part of an infection screen. Appearances of GBS pneumonia may mimic hyaline membrane disease. Infection should always be suspected in a newborn baby who has disproportionately severe respiratory distress syndrome (RDS), especially if accompanied by a metabolic acidosis and hypotension.

(4) Lumbar puncture (LP): cerebrospinal fluid microscopy, culture and sensitivities (CSF MC & S) and CSF glucose (compared to blood glucose) and protein are required to detect meningitis. On microscopy, a raised white cell count (> 10 per high powered field in a newborn), together with a lower CSF glucose concentration than blood glucose, and a high CSF protein, indicate that a baby has meningitis. Gram staining may demonstrate the presence of organisms. In an unstable baby it is appropriate to delay an LP if it is thought this may compromise the baby. The presence and cause of meningitis can be made on a post-antibiotic CSF sample using antigen detection tests, although this is not ideal.

(5) Swabs of any focal site of inflammation: if there is pus or exudate at the site of inflammation which may be contributing to infection, this should be swabbed and sent to the laboratory for MC & S (microscopy, culture and sensitivities).

(6) FBC: white cells may be raised or low. Platelet count may be very high in the presence of

ongoing inflammation or low in the presence of acute and unresolved infection. Low platelet and white cell counts may also be a feature of intrauterine growth restriction and pregnancy-induced hypertension[60-62].

(7) Other tests may include C-reactive protein (CRP), blood glucose, bilirubin, coagulation screen and liver function tests. A CRP result is only useful if it is raised, when it can be used to monitor response to therapy. A normal CRP result does not exclude infection; it takes at least 12 hours for a CRP level to become raised, so in the acute stages, a rise may not be seen. Some babies never mount a CRP response. In the future, use of PCR techniques may lead to more rapid diagnoses[63-65].

(8) Urine: this should be obtained as part of the investigation of late onset sepsis and sent for MC & S. Urine cultures are unnecessary in the investigation of early onset sepsis. The ideal urine sample is one obtained by suprapubic aspirate. A catheter or clean catch urine is second best but should only be obtained after the genitalia have been thoroughly cleaned with sterile normal saline and sterile cotton wool. The sample must also be taken into a sterile dish or pot which has not been handled. A UTI may be associated with disseminated sepsis. All confirmed UTIs in infants need investigations as there is a high incidence of associated structural renal tract abnormalities. At minimum this will involve a renal ultrasound examination, but many will also require a micturating cystourethrogram (MCUG) and DMSA scan which are invasive and uncomfortable procedures.

(9) Maternal cultures: these may be useful in assisting with diagnosis, especially if a mother has signs of infection. Midwives or obstetricians can be asked to obtain a low vaginal swab at minimum. This will only assist if it is positive. A swab may be negative even if a potential pathogen is present, e.g. GBS.

Treatment of neonatal infection

Infections must be treated when suspected, but antibiotic use should be rationalised and treatment of colonisation or as prophylaxis should be avoided[66]. Antibiotics should be narrow spectrum with broad spectrum antibiotics being kept in reserve. They can be stopped after 48 hours if cultures are negative and there are no further signs of infection. Failure to treat infection early may result in a baby becoming extremely sick and possibly even dying.

Choice of antibiotics

Antibiotic choices for early-onset infection

The microbiologically ideal antibiotic choice for the treatment of early onset neonatal infection is the combination of benzylpenicillin with an aminoglycoside such as gentamicin. If listeria is suspected ampicillin can be given in place of penicillin although penicillin does cover 90% of listeria isolates.

Antibiotic choices for late-onset infection

As can be seen from Table 16.3, the most common nosocomial bacterial isolates are coagulase negative staphylococci (CONS). Vancomycin and teicoplanin are the antibiotics of choice for CONS, but should not be used for first-line treatment of nosocomial sepsis as this facilitates the development of vancomycin-resistant enterobacter and other Gram negative organisms[67,68]. Most units use a combination such as flucloxacillin and gentamicin as first-line nosocomial treatment and change to vancomycin or teicoplanin if clinically indicated[69]. Gentamicin treats most Gram negative infections such as E. coli. Vancomycin and gentamicin have additive toxicity and the combination should be used with caution in only the sickest babies. Vancomycin, which has good activity against CONS may be used in combination with an antibiotic such as Tazocin as second or third-line treatment of nosocomial sepsis. Once an isolate and its sensitivities have been obtained antibiotic treatment should be adapted in the light of those results[70,71].

Antibiotic safety

The bactericidal ('killing') activity of vancomycin is related to the trough concentration while the bactericidal activity of gentamicin depends on the peak gentamicin concentration. The side effects of gentamicin are partly determined genetically, but are also related to needing to have a trough level below 2 mg/l (some use a cut-off of 1 mg/l in the newborn). The goal is to achieve a high peak concentration to kill the bacterium and a low (< 2 mg/l) trough level, to avoid side effects.

Treatment of fungal infection

Liposomal amphotericin, which is a fungicidal agent (so kills fungi), is the first choice treatment used by most units. A low dose is usually commenced and the dose is increased as tolerated. Fluconazole, which is a fungistatic agent, may be used if the baby is well and all anti-inflammatory markers have settled. This is well absorbed orally so can be given in order to complete a long course of anti-fungal treatment, especially when intravenous access is compromised. Any indwelling catheters should be removed[72]. A fungal infection will not clear unless 'foreign bodies' are removed.

Where a unit has a high incidence of fungal sepsis, some evidence supports the routine use of prophylactic Fluconazole in babies < 1000g; this would not be the case for the majority of UK neonatal units[73,74].

Treatment of 'very sick septic neonates'

In addition to antibiotics, babies with infection may require an increase in intensive care support. Ventilation should be considered early and the response of blood gases carefully monitored. Other interventions may include:

- Inotropes and blood to support circulation
- Monitoring of fluid input and urine output with regular measurement of creatinine and electrolytes
- Stopping enteral feeds if there is a gastrointestinal ileus and feeds are not tolerated
- Recommencing TPN with monitoring of conjugated bilirubin, liver function tests
- Monitoring of clotting parameters and consideration to additional doses of vitamin K

Implications for practice

Infants with infection can become severely unwell and attention should be paid to:
- Ventilation
- Cardiovascular monitoring such as blood pressure
- Fluid balance including input/output and weight
- Kidney function
- Nutrition – feeds may need to be stopped and TPN recommenced

Monitoring response to therapy

Antibiotics may not necessarily clear infection. If the baby remains unwell or there are signs on investigation that the infection is not clearing (e.g. platelets remain low, raised CRP) and always if there are positive blood cultures, further sets of blood cultures should be taken 2–3 days after starting treatment. Reasons for persistent positive blood cultures include:

- Inadequate antibiotic levels or regimens
- Resistant organisms
- Colonisation of indwelling 'foreign body', e.g. long line, UAC, UVC
- Focal infection, e.g. abscess
- Osteomyelitis
- Endocarditis

Further investigation (including repeat blood cultures, checking antibiotic levels, cranial ultrasound, skeletal X-rays and echocardiogram) should be considered and therapy altered accordingly.

Length of treatment

This will depend on a number of variables such as the type of organism, antibiotic levels that have been reached and clinical response. Generally, if antibiotics are started on the possibility of infection but there is no subsequent clinical evidence of infection, and cultures are all negative, antibiotics should be stopped after 48 hours. If antibiotics are started on suspicion of infection, but cultures are negative, yet clinically it is believed that the baby was infected and responded to antibiotics, a five-day course is suggested. Likewise if there is pneumonia on a CXR, but cultures are negative, a five-day minimum course is suggested. If there are positive blood cultures, but negative CSF cultures, treatment may be appropriate for a minimum of ten days (up to three weeks for organisms such as *Staphylococcus aureus*). If a baby has positive CSF and/or blood cultures treatment may be required for up to three weeks, and for a minimum of two weeks.

Fungal infections, osteomyelitis, endocarditis and deep abscesses which are not surgically drained, may require several weeks of antibiotics. The advice of specialists will be required to manage such situations.

New developments in additional (adjuvant) treatments for infection

Antibiotic therapy alone may be insufficient to treat infection in an immune-compromised host, and long-term or recurrent use facilitates antibiotic resistance[75–77]. So far no study has demonstrated conclusively that pooled IVIG is of any definite benefit in the prophylaxis or treatment of neonatal sepsis, though there is a suggestion of benefit from using immunoglobulins in the treatment of infection[78,79]. For this reason, the 'INIS' study is investigating the potential benefit of giving pooled intravenous immunoglobulin (IVIG) to neonates with infection.

There is insufficient evidence of benefit from any of the adjuvant therapies to justify routine introduction into clinical practice, but preterm babies who have sepsis and neutropenia may benefit from treatment with rhG-CSF[80,81]. Expert advice should always be sought when considering using any such therapies.

Prebiotics and probiotics

More recently, and in recognition of the importance of the gut flora in immune development, there have been trials of prebiotics and probiotics in neonates[82].

A probiotic is defined as: a live microbial food supplement that beneficially affects the host by alteration of its intestinal microbial balance.

A prebiotic is defined as being: a non-digestible food ingredient that beneficially affects the host by stimulating the growth or activity of one or more bacterial species already present in the gut.

The benefits of these are thought to derive from normalising gut flora. Although some milk marketing companies now supply infant milks and breast milk fortifiers with added pre- or probiotics, these additives have not been subjected to rigorous scientific evaluation. There is some evidence that prophylactic use of probiotics may be associated with a reduction in NEC[83].

Prevention of infection: infection control

Every baby should always be cared for with the strictest attention to protect that baby from cross-infection and each trust will have a uniform and hygiene policy. Some general points are listed below:

- Staff and visitors should remove coats and leave bags outside the nurseries
- Arms should be naked from elbows down and freshly cleaned before touching any baby or equipment for that baby
- Bacteria live on all jewellery, particularly stones, so these should not be worn at work
- Hair and clothing should not be allowed to dangle onto a baby
- Theatre scrubs should not be worn outside the unit or theatre
- Gloves should be worn for any procedures involving bodily secretions, and discarded as soon as the procedure is completed
- Hands should have alcohol applied or be re-washed on exiting and entering a nursery from a different area, e.g. the nurses' station or staff room

- Each baby should have his/her own stethoscope, scissors, laryngoscope and any other small items of equipment
- Where equipment has to be shared, such as ultrasound machine heads and cold lights, these must always be cleaned between babies

Cohorting of babies may be necessary when a baby has particularly resistant bacteria, e.g. MRSA, or easily transmissible infection such as RSV. In this situation each baby cot should have separate pens as well as stethoscopes, scissors and other such equipment. The notes should stay outside the baby domain and not be touched by any individual on the inside of the 'baby space'. This may seem obsessive, but it is only with such attention to detail that cross-infection can be averted.

Within neonatal units, high cot-occupancy rates and high numbers of babies cared for by one nurse contribute to a greater mortality[84]. The effect of overcrowding on positive blood culture rate is less easy to discern, because bigger and busier units are likely to look after sicker babies and take more blood cultures, but the perceived wisdom is that overcrowding and high volume workload leads to greater risk of infection.

Implications for practice

Prevention of infection is better than cure. Beyond handwashing, the best way to prevent nosocomial infection in babies is to feed early with breast milk, limit antibiotic use, avoid indwelling devices, avoid overcrowding and use clean equipment. Handwashing and/or applications of alcohol between patients are critical.

Congenital infections

Congenital infection may be particularly suspected as a cause of being small for gestational age if other signs are present, e.g. microcephaly, hepatosplenomegaly, or thrombocytopenia. The management of babies with congenital infections, and their mothers, must be done in consultation with microbiologists and preferably with paediatric infectious diseases specialists.

Syphilis

Syphilis has re-emerged as a cause of congenital infection in the UK, with an antenatal seroprevalence of approximately 0.02%, and up to 0.2% in some areas. If untreated, early syphilis (defined as syphilis contracted within the past two years) will result in a 40% risk of stillbirth, spontaneous abortion or perinatal loss. The risk depends on the maternal stage of infection and how much spirochete (which is the organism causing syphilis) is in the blood. The risk of vertical transmission from a woman with late syphilis is extremely low.

Congenital syphilis in survivors may result in hydrops foetalis or preterm delivery. The clinical picture in the neonatal period may include hepatosplenomegaly, lymphadenopathy, mucocutaneous skin lesions, rash, snuffles, osteochondritis, pseudoparalysis, haemolytic anaemia and thrombocytopenia.

All women are offered testing at booking for syphilis. High risk groups (e.g. intravenous drug users, sex workers, those with contact with infectious syphilis) should also be tested towards term. Syphilis is transmitted *in utero* as well as intra-partum, so that treatment should be given as soon as syphilis is diagnosed. Treatment delayed until the third trimester must be initiated in hospital for the first 72 hours with continuous foetal monitoring as foetal distress can occur.

Cytomegalovirus (CMV)

Babies may acquire CMV trans-placentally, from breast milk or from blood products (though less so now as white blood cells are routinely removed from blood by the transfusion unit; CMV being a virus that lives inside white blood cells). CMV infection is common in mothers, with a prevalence of approximately 60% in developed countries. Two-thirds of mothers do not transmit the virus *in utero*, and the majority of neonates who are infected do not actually develop disease. The majority of neonates are therefore not affected by CMV even if their mothers do carry CMV. Symptoms and signs of intrauterine CMV infection include intra-uterine growth restriction, hepatosplenomegaly, thrombocytopenia, jaundice, microcephaly and chorioretinitis. The prognosis for such children is generally very poor, with the majority suffering from severe developmental impairment with or without hearing loss. There is evidence that babies with central nervous system (CNS) signs should be treated with the antiviral agent ganciclovir. Because of toxicity this is not offered to neonates unless they do have CNS signs[85].

Hepatitis B

Women who are carriers of the hepatitis B virus can pass this virus to their newborn baby. If a baby is not protected by immunoglobulin and/or hepatitis B vaccine at birth with follow-up vaccinations in the first year of life, there is a high risk that the baby will become infected with hepatitis from its mother. The majority of babies who become infected will have a sub-clinical infection (rather than acute hepatitis) and then become a chronic carrier for life. There is a strong association between chronic hepatitis B carriage status and the risk of development of liver cirrhosis. A minority of people go on to develop primary liver cancer in later life.

The virus is present in all body fluids such as blood, semen, vaginal secretions and saliva. It can be transmitted through unprotected sexual intercourse, intimate person to person contact, sharing infected needles, and from mother to baby, especially at birth. Some of the methods of transmission are listed below:

- Hepatitis B is transmitted *in utero* (which accounts for less than 5% of transmission as hepatitis B is a large virus and does not cross the placenta)
- In labour and delivery (most transmission is thought to occur at this point)

- Post-natally through close contact; hepatitis B antigen has been detected in breast milk, but there is no evidence that hepatitis B is transmitted through breast-feeding

Hepatitis B 'e' and 's' antigens and antibody response and how they relate to low and high risk

- Hepatatis B 's' antigen: approximately 80% of women found to have hepatitis B in pregnancy only have the 's' (or surface) antigen. They are 'low risk' carriers.
- Hepatatis B 'e' antigen positive: mothers are highly infective and are 'high risk' carriers. A baby born to an 'e' antigen positive mother has a 90% chance of becoming infected if that baby does not get both immunoglobulin ('passive' antibody) as well as vaccine soon after birth.
- Hepatitis B 's' antigen antibody: this may indicate previous hepatitis B infection or immunisation.
- Hepatitis B 'e' antigen antibody: women who have been exposed to live virus (and therefore 'e'antigen) in the past usually have 'e' antibody. This means that there is a decreased likelihood of infectivity. A person who is 'e' antigen positive is still a 'high risk' carrier even if they are 'e' antibody positive.
- Hepatitis B core antigen (HBcAg) and antibodies: this is a component of the protein envelope which encloses viral DNA and is not detectable in the blood. The presence of antibodies to HBcAg (anti-HBc Ab+) indicate present or previous hepatitis B infection.

Key for looking at laboratory results

HBV = hepatitis B virus

HBsAg+ve = surface antigen positive

HBeAg+ve = 'e' antigen positive

HBeAb+ve = 'e' antibody positive – the person is usually of low infectivity as long as the 'e' antigen is negative

Table 16.4 Interpretation of laboratory results.

	Baby should receive hepatitis B vaccine	Baby should receive hepatitis B immunoglobulin
Mother HBsAg+ve and HBeAg+ve; HBeAb-ve	+	+
Mother HBsAg+ve and HBeAg+ve; HBeAB+ve	+	+
Mother HBsAg+ve and 'e' markers not determined	+	+
Mother HBsAg+ve and HBeAg-ve; HBeAB-ve	+	+
Mother had acute hepatitis B in pregnancy	+	+
Mother HBsAg+ve and HBeAg-ve; HBeAB+ve	+	−
This will be the status of majority of mothers		

HBsAb+ve = surface antibody positive which may be induced by hepatitis B vaccine as well as natural infection.

Antibody is sometimes also written as follows:

Anti-HBe = antibody to 'e'
Anti-HBs = antibody to 's' interpreting
See Table 16.4.

If a mother has no HBsAg, she is immune and cannot infect anyone; either her baby or other contacts.

Post-natal
Hepatitis B immunoglobulin
This should be administered intramuscularly by a paediatrician within 12 hours of birth to infants that are classified as high risk. Advice should be sought from a virologist if immunoglobulin administration to a high-risk baby is delayed for 48 hours or more.

Hepatitis B vaccination
It is vital that the dose is given by *intramuscular* injection otherwise vaccine failure can result. The course of vaccine is given over one year as follows: first dose at birth; second dose at one month; third dose at two months; fourth dose at one year. *All* babies whose mothers have any antigen for hepatitis B should be given this full course of vaccine, whether the immunoglobulin is needed or not.

   (Further reading: *Drug and Therapeutics Bulletin*, 2006, **44** (6), 41–44.)

Implications for practice

Congenital infections are important causes of mortality and morbidity in the newborn infant.
- Syphilis can be treated in pregnancy.
- Treatment for neonatal CMV is only indicated in severe symptomatic cases because of the risks of gancyclovir.
- Hepatitis B can be mostly be prevented in at risk infants with strict adherence to a passive (immunoglobulin) and active immunisation protocol.

HIV (human immunodeficiency virus)

Background
HIV is now a treatable, though not curable, infectious disease. Mother-to-child transmission of HIV can be reduced to < 2% by a combination of:

- Anti-retroviral therapy (ART) to the mother and baby
- Delivering by elective caesarean section if maternal HIV viral load > 40 cp/ml
- By avoiding breast-feeding

The Department of Health advises that all women are routinely offered testing for HIV during pregnancy so that approximately 90% of mothers are tested. Some mothers are more likely to be HIV positive and these include those who have recently arrived from high prevalence countries such as those within Sub-Saharan Africa. As HIV is now treatable and the risks of mother-to-infant transmission can be significantly reduced, it is important to be alert to these risk factors. Once mothers are identified, they are best cared for by a specialised multidisciplinary team, which may include adult and paediatric HIV specialists, HIV specialist nurses, and an obstetrician, midwife, neonatologist and neonatal nurse with a special interest in HIV. A personalised birth plan of care should be developed antenatally for each mother according to her disease status as outlined in the BHIVA guidelines.

Management

Anti-retroviral therapy (ART)

The maternal HIV viral load (the amount of HIV virus circulating in the peripheral bloodstream) is critical to predicting the risk of transmission to a baby, with a higher viral load increasing the risk of transmission. Some women will already know their HIV status before pregnancy, and may be conceiving on combination anti-retroviral therapy. Other women will be newly diagnosed in pregnancy. The treatment offered to each woman is dependent on their disease status:

- Women with more advanced disease are defined as having a CD4+ count of < 200–300 or viral load >10,000 viral copies/ml. They will usually be offered triple drug therapy.
- Women with less advanced disease and a low viral load may be offered AZT alone (known as AZT monotherapy).

Some women may have reduced susceptibility to one or more anti-retroviral drugs and under such circumstances, specialist advice should be sought).

Elective pre-labour caesarian section

It is unclear whether ELCS is of any added benefit for women on ART who are delivering with an undetectable viral load. Because of the increasing success of interventions to reduce HIV viral load during pregnancy, many women with an undetectable viral load choose to deliver by normal vaginal delivery.

Emergency situations and interventions to reduce the risk of transmission

Although most deliveries will follow the prepared birth plan, some occur early or unplanned and an emergency treatment plan is required. An increased risk of HIV vertical transmission is associated with:

- Premature onset of labour before or soon after starting ART (within four weeks)
- Premature rupture of membranes and/or prolonged rupture of membranes before or soon after starting ART
- Late presentation at term on no ART, or shortly after starting ART
- Discovery of maternal HIV after delivery, where the infant is less than 72 hours old
- Poor maternal adherence to ART with risk of resistance as well as lack of viral suppression

In these situations advice should be sought from a specialised HIV team. More intensive treatment for both mother and infant may be required.

Breast-feeding

Breast-feeding approximately doubles the risk of vertical transmission and the risk continues to increase with the duration of feeding. Formula feed, bottles and steriliser may be provided by social services for asylum seeking mothers, or through local voluntary organisations for low-income families. A pre-term baby may be offered bank donor milk if available and with maternal consent.

Anti-retroviral treatment for the newborn

The drug most commonly used in the perinatal period is zidovudine (AZT). Most infants will receive AZT monotherapy for four weeks after birth. The first dose of medication must be given within six hours of delivery. Other drugs, either singularly or in combination, may also be given according to the mother's treatment regimen, viral resistance and level of perceived risk to the infant. All the medicines used are available in syrup formulation.

Premature/sick infants

The only drug with pharmacokinetic data for the premature or sick infants is AZT. As AZT is the only anti-retroviral available in an IV preparation, for premature or sick term infants unable to take oral feeds this is the only treatment possible. Once the infant is tolerating enteral feeds, further oral preparations may be administered if clinically indicated.

Laboratory diagnosis of HIV infection in non-breast fed infants

The gold standard test for HIV infection in infancy is the amplification of HIV DNA on peripheral blood lymphocytes (using the polymerase chain reaction or PCR), although some studies are now demonstrating equal or increased early sensitivity with other amplification methods for viral RNA. As most infants are infected intra-partum and blood levels of HIV may still be very low, HIV DNA is not amplified from all infected infants at birth, i.e. a negative initial HIV DNA PCR may still mean that an infant is infected. A positive HIV PCR result within 72 hours of birth is suggestive of intrauterine transmission. Within the first weeks of life the sensitivity of the test increases dramatically and by three months of age more than 95% of non-breast fed HIV infected infants will be detected. In view of the genomic diversity of HIV (viral variation between populations), a maternal sample should always be amplified with the first infant sample, to confirm that the primers used can detect the maternal virus. The BHIVA Guidelines (see below) advise that infants are tested at one day, six weeks, and twelve weeks of age. If all these tests are negative and the baby is not being breast-fed, the child is not HIV infected. Loss of maternal antibodies should subsequently be confirmed at 14–18 months of age. Neonatal ART can delay the detection of both HIV DNA and RNA in the infant. It is for this reason that further samples are collected at six and twelve weeks of age. If an infant is found to be HIV infected after perinatal ART exposure then the mother and infant should be referred to a specialist paediatrician for ongoing management.

Immunisations and clinical monitoring

Infants born to HIV infected mothers should follow the routine immunisation schedule, as the early immunisations do not contain live vaccines. However, it is vital that HIV status is known prior to the administration of live vaccines such as the BCG or MMR, due to the risk of inducing disseminated disease through inoculation with live vaccine. The hepatitis status of the HIV infected mother should be ascertained, so that hepatitis B vaccination can be carried out if necessary.

HIV remains a stigmatised disease, and those affected are often reluctant to disclose their diagnosis to others. Where possible, families should be strongly encouraged to inform primary health carers, including midwives, health visitors and family doctors about their HIV status. This will enable the local team to give appropriate support and advice, especially regarding infant feeding and where an infant or mother is unwell. It is also important that health care staff understand the importance of maintaining confidentiality and are familiar with local guidelines that support this.

Child protection

Rarely, pregnant mothers refuse treatment for their own HIV as well as interventions to reduce the risk of transmission to their unborn infant. Where the multidisciplinary team is unable to achieve a satisfactory outcome, a pre-birth planning meeting with social services should be held. Court permission should be sought at birth to treat the infant for four weeks with combination post-exposure prophylaxis and breast-feeding will be strongly discouraged. Throughout this process, staff should continue to engage with and support the mother.

Reporting and long-term follow-up

HIV services for children in the UK are organised in national networks through lead centres in London. It is the responsibility of clinicians caring for women with HIV to report women prospectively to the UK National Study of HIV in Pregnancy and the International Drug Registry antenatally, and for the neonatologist or paediatrician to report infants to the British Paediatric Surveillance Unit after birth.

The BHIVA (British HIV Association) guidelines for the management of HIV in pregnancy discuss all the issues in more detail, and can be accessed at www.bhiva.org. CHIVA (Children's HIV Association of UK and Ireland) is a subgroup of BHIVA and can be accessed on the same website. Guidelines for the management of HIV infected children can be found at the CHIVA website, along with useful resources and links to other relevant sites.

Implications for practice

The outlook for infants at risk of HIV has dramatically improved and all staff should be aware that it is possible to prevent infection in 98% of infants with the involvement of a multidisciplinary antenatal and post-natal HIV specialist team.

Respiratory viruses

These may cause serious respiratory compromise in babies with chronic lung disease. Respiratory syncytial virus (RSV), para-influenza, influenza and adenovirus are the most common isolates. RSV is most prevalent in the months of November to March each year. It causes common cold symptoms in older children and adults, and can be easily transmitted to unit babies, not only by sneezing and coughing but also from hand to object transmission. Handwashing and not touching nasal secretions is critical in the prevention of transmission of RSV.

All these viruses can be rapidly diagnosed by immunofluorescence on nasopharyngeal aspirates. A fine catheter is placed in the posterior nasopharynx and a short sharp suction applied, the resulting aspirate is flushed through into a trap with sterile saline or viral transport medium. The test requires epithelial cells stripped off by the suction and not mucous itself.

RSV-specific immunoglobulin (palivizumab, or tradename Synagis) has been developed to

Table 16.5 Childhood immunisation programme.

When to immunise	What is given	Vaccine and how it is given
Two months	Diphtheria, tetanus, acellular pertussis, killed polio and Haemophilus influenzae type B (DTaP/IPV/Hib)	One injection (Pediacel)
	Pneumococcal (PCV)	One injection (Prevenar)
Three months	Diphtheria, tetanus, acellular pertussis, killed polio and Haemophilus influenzae type B (DTaP/IPV/Hib)	One injection (Pediacel)
	Meningitis C (Men C)	One injection (Neisvac C or Meningitec)
Four months	Diphtheria, tetanus, acellular pertussis, killed polio and Haemophilus influenzae type B (DTaP/IPV/Hib)	One injection (Pediacel)
	Pneumococcal (PCV)	One injection (Prevenar)
	Meningitis C (Men C)	One injection (Neisvac C or Meningitec)
Twelve months	Haemophilus influenzae type B/ Meningitis C (Hib/ Men C)	One injection (Menitorix)
Thirteen months	Measles, mumps, rubella (MMR)	One injection (Priorix or MMR II)
	Pneumococcal (PCV)	One injection (Prevenar)
Three years, four months to five years	Diphtheria, tetanus, acellular pertussis, killed polio (dTa/IPV or DTa/IPV)	One injection (Repevax or Infanrix-IPV)
	Measles, mumps, rubella (MMR)	One injection (Priorix or MMR II)
13–18 years	Tetanus, diphtheria, killed polio (Td/IPV)	One injection (Revaxis)

prevent RSV infection and is used in those babies at highest risk of RSV, e.g. those with severe chronic lung disease[86].

Immunisations

The routine childhood immunisation programme was revised on 4 September 2006 and should be familiar to all who care for infants. Long-stay babies within neonatal units should have immunisations according to chronological and not corrected age. The schedule is summarised in Table 16.5. Further information is available from www.immunisation.nhs.uk.

Conclusion

Infection is an important cause of morbidity and mortality in the newborn, in whom the immune system is developing. The human body learns to live in harmony with normal 'colonising' bacteria, on which normal immune function depends. Recognition of which bacteria can be 'pathogenic', how infections may present, what the short and long-term consequences may be, and how best to prevent and treat infections is extremely important.

References

1. Nairn R, Helbert M (2002) *Immunology for Medical Students*. Mosby, Edinburgh.
2. Ridge JP, Fuchs EJ, Matzinger P (1996) Neonatal tolerance revisited: turning on newborn T cells with dendritic cells. *Science*, **271** (5256), 1723–1726.
3. Janeway CA Jr (1989) Approaching the asymptote? Evolution and revolution in immunology. *Cold Spring Harb Symp Quant Biol*, **54** (part 1), 1–13.
4. Ridge JP, Fuchs EJ, Matzinger P (1996) Neonatal tolerance revisited: turning on newborn T cells with dendritic cells. *Science*, **271** (5256), 1723–1726.
5. Janeway CA Jr (1989) Approaching the asymptote? Evolution and revolution in immunology. *Cold Spring Harb Symp Quant Biol*, **54** (part 1), 1–13.
6. Llwelyn M, Cohen J (2002) Superantigens: microbial agents that corrupt immunity. *The Lancet Infectious Diseases*, **2**, 156–162.
7. McGuire W, Anthony M (2003) Donor human milk versus formula for preventing necrotising enterocolitis in preterm infants: systematic review. *Arch Dis Child foetal Neonatal Ed*, **88** (1), F11–F14.
8. Hanson LA, Korotkova M, Lundin S, *et al.* (2003) The transfer of immunity from mother to child. *Ann N Y Acad Sci*, **987**, 199–206.
9. Hanson LA, Korotkova M (2002) The role of breastfeeding in prevention of neonatal infection. *Semin Neonatol*, 7, 275–281.
10. Hanson LA, Korotkova M (2002) The role of breastfeeding in prevention of neonatal infection. *Semin Neonatol*, 7, 275–281.
11. Hooper LV (2004) Bacterial contributions to mammalian gut development. *Trends in Microbiology*, **12** (3), 129–134.
12. Hooper LV, Wong MH, Thelin A, Hansson L, Falk PG, Gordon JI (2001) Molecular analysis of commensal host-microbial relationships in the intestine. *Science*, **291** (5505), 881–884.
13. Hooper LV (2004) Bacterial contributions to mammalian gut development. *Trends in Microbiology*, **12** (3), 129–134.
14. Gronlund M-M, Arvilommi H, Kero P, Lehtonen O-P, Isolauri E (2000) Importance of intestinal colonization in the maturation of humoral immunity in early infancy: a prospective follow-up study of healthy infants aged 0–6 months. *Arch Dis Child*, **83** (3), F186–F192.
15. Stoll B, Hansen N, Fanaroff A, *et al.* (2002) Late-onset sepsis in very low birth weight neonates: the experience of the NICHD Neonatal Research Network. *Pediatrics*, **110** (2), 285–291.
16. Flidel-Rimon O, Friedman S, Lev E, Juster-Reicher A, Amitay M, Shinwell ES (2004) Early enteral feeding and nosocomial sepsis in VLBW infants. *Arch Dis Child Foetal Neonatal Ed*, 89, F289–F292.
17. Gewolb IH, Schwalbe RS, Taciak VL, Harrison TS, Panigrahi P (1999) Stool microflora in extremely low birthweight infants. *Arch Dis Child Foetal Neonatal Ed*, 80 (3), F167–F173.
18. Eastick K, Leeming JP, Millar MR (1996) Reservoirs of coagulase negative staphylococci in preterm infants. *Arch Dis Child*, 74 (2), F99–F104.
19. Pierro A, van Saene HKF, Donnell SC, Hughes J, Ewan C, Nunn AJ, Lloyd DA (1996) Microbial

translocation in neonates and infants receiving long-term parenteral nutrition. *Arch Surg*, **131**, 176–179.

20. Stoll BJ, Hansen N, Fanaroff AA, *et al.* (2002) Changes in pathogens causing early-onset sepsis in very-low-birth-weight infants. *N Engl J Med*, **347** (4), 240–247.

21. Stoll BJ, Hansen N, Fanaroff AA, *et al.* (2002) Changes in pathogens causing early-onset sepsis in very-low-birth-weight infants. *N Engl J Med*, **347** (4), 240–247.

22. Stoll BJ, Hansen N, Fanaroff AA, *et al.* (2002) Changes in pathogens causing early-onset sepsis in very-low-birth-weight infants. *N Engl J Med*, **347** (4), 240–247.

23. Levy SB (1998) Multidrug resistance – a sign of the times. *New Engl J Med*, **338** (19), 1376–1378.

24. Stoll BJ, Hansen N, Fanaroff AA, *et al.* (2002) Changes in pathogens causing early-onset sepsis in very-low-birth-weight infants. *N Engl J Med*, **347** (4), 240–247.

25. Singh N, Patel KM, Leger MM, *et al.* (2002) Risk of resistant infections with enterobacteriaceae in hospitalized neonates. *Pediatr Infect Dis J*, **21** (11), 1029–1033.

26. Van Houten MA, Uiterwaal CS, Heesen GJ, Arends JP, Kimpen JL (2001) Does the empiric use of vancomycin in pediatrics increase the risk for Gram-negative bacteremia? *Pediatr Infect Dis J*, **20** (2), 171–177.

27. Bedford Russell AR, Murch SH (2006) Could peripartum antibiotics have delayed health consequences for the infant? *BJOG*, **113** (7), 758–765.

28. Montgomery SM, Wakefield AJ, Morris DL, Pounder RE, Murch SH (2000) The initial care of newborn infants and subsequent hayfever. *Allergy*, **55** (10), 916–922.

29. Stoll BJ, Gordon T, Korones SB, *et al.* (1996) Early-onset sepsis in very low birth-weight neonates: A report from the National Institute of Child Health and Human Development Neonatal research network. *J Pediatr*, **129** (1), 72–80.

30. Stoll BJ, Gordon T, Korones SB, *et al.* (1996) Late-onset neonatal sepsis in very low birth weight neonates: A report from the National Institute of Child Health and Human Development Neonatal Research Network. *J Pediatr*, **129** (1), 63–71.

31. Marshall DD, Kotelchuck M, Young TE, *et al.* (1999) Risk factors for chronic lung disease in the surfactant era: a North Carolina population-based study of very low birthweight infants. *Pediatrics*, **104** (6), 1345–1350.

32. Dammann O, Leviton A (1997) Maternal intrauterine infection, cytokines and brain damage in the preterm newborn. *Pediatr Res*, **42** (1), 1–8.

33. Murphy DJ, Sellers S, Mackenzie IZ, Yudkin PL, Johnson A (1995) Case-control study of antenatal and intrapartum risk factors for cerebral palsy in very preterm singleton babies. *Lancet*, **346** (8988), 1449–1453.

34. Grether JK, Nelson K (1997) Maternal infection and cerebral palsy infants of normal birthweight. *JAMA*, **278** (3), 207–211.

35. Jacobsson B, Hagberg G (2004) Antenatal risk factors for cerebral palsy. *Best Practice & Research Clinical Obstetrics and Gynaecology*, **18** (3), 425–436.

36. Inder TE, Volpe JJ (2000) Mechanisms of perinatal brain injury. *Semin Neonatology*, **5** (1), 3–15.

37. Roman J, Fernandez F, Velasco F, Rojas R, Roldan MR, Torres A (1993) Serum TNF levels in neonatal sepsis and shock. *Acta Pediatr*, **82** (4), 352–354.

38. Girardin EP, Berner ME, Grau GE, Suter S, Lacourt G, Paunier L (1990) Serum tumour necrosis factor in newborns at risk for infections. *Eur J Pediatr*, **149** (9), 645–647.

39. Jacobsson B, Hagberg G (2004) Antenatal risk factors for cerebral palsy. *Best Practice & Research Clinical Obstetrics and Gynaecology*, **18** (3), 425–436.

40. Inder TE, Volpe JJ (2000) Mechanisms of perinatal brain injury. *Semin Neonatology*, **5** (1), 3–15.

41. Buonocore G, Gioia D, De Filippo M, Picciolini E, Bracci R (1994) Superoxide anion release by polymorphonuclear leukocytes in whole blood of newborns and mothers during the peripartal period. *Pediatr Res*, **36** (5), 619–622.

42. Heath PT, Balfour G, Weisner AM, *et al.* (2004) PHLS Group B Streptococcus Working Group. Group B streptococcal disease in UK and Irish infants younger than 90 days. *Lancet*, **363** (9405, 24 Jan.), 292–294.

43. Luck S, Torry M, d'Agapeyeff K, *et al.* (2003) Estimated early-onset group B streptococcal neonatal disease. *Lancet*, **361** (9373, 7 June), 1953–1954.

44. Natarajan G, Johnson YR, Zhang F, Chen KM, Worsham MJ (2006) Real-time polymerase chain reaction for the rapid detection of Group B Streptococcal colonization in neonates. *Pediatrics*, **118** (1), 14–22.

45. Heath PT, Balfour G, Weisner AM, *et al.* (2004) PHLS Group B Streptococcus Working Group.

Group B streptococcal disease in UK and Irish infants younger than 90 days. *Lancet*, **363** (9405, 24 Jan.), 292–294.

46. RCOG Greentop guideline (2003) *Prevention of Early Onset Group B Streptococcal Disease*. No. 36 (http://www.rcog.org.uk/guidelines).

47. RCOG Greentop guideline (2003) *Prevention of Early Onset Group B Streptococcal Disease*. No. 36 (http://www.rcog.org.uk/guidelines).

48. RCOG Greentop guideline (2003) *Prevention of Early Onset Group B Streptococcal Disease*. No. 36 (http://www.rcog.org.uk/guidelines).

49. Heath PT, Feldman R (2005) Vaccination against group B streptococcus. *Expert Rev. Vaccines*, **4** (2), 207–218.

50. Stoll B, Hansen N, Fanaroff A, *et al.* (2002) Late-onset sepsis in very low birth weight neonates: the experience of the NICHD Neonatal Research Network. *Pediatrics*, **110** (2), 285–291.

51. Flidel-Rimon O, Friedman S, Lev E, Juster-Reicher A, Amitay M, Shinwell ES (2004) Early enteral feeding and nosocomial sepsis in VLBW infants. *Arch Dis Child Foetal Neonatal Ed*, 89, F289–F292.

52. Stoll BJ, Gordon T, Korones SB, *et al.* (1996) Late-onset neonatal sepsis in very low birth weight neonates: A report from the National Institute of Child Health and Human Development Neonatal Research Network. *J Pediatr*, **129** (1), 63–71.

53. Marshall DD, Kotelchuck M, Young TE, *et al.* (1999) Risk factors for chronic lung disease in the surfactant era: a North Carolina population-based study of very low birthweight infants. *Pediatrics*, **104** (6), 1345–1350.

54. Hanson LA, Korotkova M, Lundin S, *et al.* (2003) The transfer of immunity from mother to child. *Ann N Y Acad Sci*, **987**, 199–206.

55. Hanson LA, Korotkova M (2002) The role of breastfeeding in prevention of neonatal infection. *Semin Neonatol*, 7, 275–281.

56. Stoll B, Hansen N, Fanaroff A, *et al.* (2002) Late-onset sepsis in very low birth weight neonates: the experience of the NICHD Neonatal Research Network. *Pediatrics*, **110** (2), 285–291.

57. Clerihew L, Lamagni TL, Brocklehurst P, McGuire W (2006) Invasive fungal infection in very low birth weight infants: national prospective surveillance study. *Arch Dis Child Foetal Neonatal Ed*, **91** (3), F188–F192.

58. Clerihew L, Lamagni TL, Brocklehurst P, McGuire W (2006) Invasive fungal infection in very low birth weight infants: national prospective surveillance study. *Arch Dis Child Foetal Neonatal Ed*, **91** (3), F188–F192.

59. Isaacman DJ, Karasic RB, Reynolds EA, Kost SI (1996) Effect of number of blood cultures and volume of blood on detection of bacteremia in children. *J Pediatr*, **128** (2), 190–195.

60. Natarajan G, Johnson YR, Zhang F, Chen KM, Worsham MJ (2006) Real-time polymerase chain reaction for the rapid detection of Group B Streptococcal colonization in neonates. *Pediatrics*, **118** (1), 14–22.

61. Straka M, Cruz WD, Blackmon C, *et al.* (2004) Rapid detection of group B streptococcus and *Escherichia coli* in amniotic fluid using real-time fluorescent PCR. *Infect Dis Obst Gynecol*, **12** (3–4), 109–113.

62. Heininger A, Binder M, Schmidt S, Unertl K, Botzenhart K, Doring G (1999) PCR and blood culture for detection of *Escherichia coli* bacteremia in rats. *J.Clin.Microbiol*, **37** (8), 2479–2482.

63. Natarajan G, Johnson YR, Zhang F, Chen KM, Worsham MJ (2006) Real-time polymerase chain reaction for the rapid detection of Group B Streptococcal colonization in neonates. *Pediatrics*, **118** (1), 14–22.

64. Straka M, Cruz WD, Blackmon C, *et al.* (2004) Rapid detection of group B streptococcus and *Escherichia coli* in amniotic fluid using real-time fluorescent PCR. *Infect Dis Obst Gynecol*, **12** (3–4), 109–113.

65. Heininger A, Binder M, Schmidt S, Unertl K, Botzenhart K, Doring G (1999) PCR and blood culture for detection of *Escherichia coli* bacteremia in rats. *J.Clin.Microbiol*, **37** (8), 2479–2482.

66. Isaacs D (2000) Rationing antibiotic use in neonatal units. *Arch Dis Child Foetal Neonatal Ed*, **82**, F1–F2.

67. Singh N, Patel KM, Leger MM, *et al.* (2002) Risk of resistant infections with enterobacteriaceae in hospitalized neonates. *Pediatr Infect Dis J*, **21** (11), 1029–1033.

68. Van Houten MA, Uiterwaal CS, Heesen GJ, Arends JP, Kimpen JL (2001) Does the empiric use of vancomycin in pediatrics increase the risk for Gram-negative bacteremia? *Pediatr Infect Dis J*, **20** (2), 171–177.

69. Isaacs D (2000) Rationing antibiotic use in neonatal units. *Arch Dis Child Foetal Neonatal Ed*, **82**, F1–F2.

70. Hintz SR, Kendrick DE, Stoll BJ, *et al.* (2005) Neurodevelopmental and growth outcomes

extremely low-birthweight infants after necrotising enterocolitis. *Pediatrics*, 115 (3), 696–703.

71. de Man P, Verhoeven BAN, Verbrugh HA, Vos MC, van den Anker JN (2000) An antibiotic policy to prevent emergence of resistant bacilli. *Lancet*, 355 (9208), 973–978.

72. Karlowicz G, Hashimoto LN, Kelly Jr RE, Buescher ES (2000) Should central venous catheters be removed as soon as candidemia is detected in neonates? *Pediatrics*, 106 (5), 63.

73. McGuire W, Clerihew L, Austin N (2004) Prophylactic intravenous antifungal agents to prevent mortality and morbidity in very low birth weight infants. *The Cochrane Database of Systematic Reviews* (1), CD003850.

74. Austin NC, Darlow B (2002) Prophylactic oral antifungal agents to prevent systemic candida infection in preterm infants (protocol for a Cochrane Review). In: The Cochrane Library, 3, 2002.

75. Levy SB (1998) Multidrug resistance – a sign of the times. *New Engl J Med*, 338 (19), 1376–1378.

76. Singh N, Patel KM, Leger MM, *et al.* (2002) Risk of resistant infections with enterobacteriaceae in hospitalized neonates. *Pediatr Infect Dis J*, 21 (11), 1029–1033.

77. Van Houten MA, Uiterwaal CS, Heesen GJ, Arends JP, Kimpen JL (2001) Does the empiric use of vancomycin in pediatrics increase the risk for Gram-negative bacteremia? *Pediatr Infect Dis J*, 20 (2), 171–177.

78. Ohlsson A, Lacy JB (2006) Intravenous immunoglobulins for preventing infection in preterm and/or low birthweight infants. *Cochrane Database of Systematic Reviews* (3).

79. Ohlsson A, Lacy JB (2006) Intravenous immunoglobulins for treatment of suspected or subsequently proven infection in neonates. *Cochrane Database of Systematic Reviews* (3).

80. Bedford Russell AR, Emmerson A, Wilkinson N, *et al.* (2001) A trial of recombinant human granulocyte colony stimulating factor for the treatment of very low birth weight infants with presumed sepsis and neutropenia. *Arch Dis Child*, 84 (3), F172–F176.

81. Bernstein HM, Pollock BH, Calhoun DA, Christensen RD (2001) Administration of recombinant granulocyte colony-stimulating factor to neonates with septicemia: a meta-analysis. *J Pediatr*, 138 (6, June):917-20

82. Murch SH (2001) Toll of allergy reduced by probiotics. *Lancet*, 357 (9262), 1057–1059.

83. Schanler RJ (2006) Probiotics and necrotizing enterocolitis in premature infants. *Arch Dis Child Foetal Neonatal Ed*, 91 (6), F395–F397.

84. The UK Neonatal Staffing study group (2002) Patient volume, staffing, and work-load adjusted outcomes in a random stratified sample of UK neonatal intensive care units: a prospective evaluation. *Lancet*, 359 (9301), 99–107.

85. Griffiths PD (2001) Cytomegalovirus infection in pregnancy. Chapter 18 in: Maclean AB, Regan L, Carrington D (eds) *Infection and Pregnancy*. RCOG Press, London.

86. Sharland M, Bedford Russell AR (2001) Preventing respiratory syncytial virus bronchiolitis. *BMJ*, 322 (7278), 62–63.

Chapter 17

HAEMATOLOGY IN THE TERM AND PRETERM NEONATE

Tim Watts, Karissa Jowaheer and Ping Corcoran

Learning outcomes

After reading this chapter the reader will be expected to be able to:

- Describe the common pathophysiological problems of the haematological system in the context of the foetus and newborn

- Explain the causes and contributing factors in each of the haematological conditions described within this chapter

- Identify and interpret the clinical signs and symptoms associated with the common haematological conditions described within this chapter

- Contribute confidently to the effective care and management of this group of neonates

- Provide the parents and families of the neonates with accurate information on each of the haematological conditions described

- Discuss the support needed by the parents of neonates with haematological complications and the relevance of social, psychological and cultural context of care provision

---

Introduction

This chapter focuses on haematology and will provide a current perspective on common haematological issues relating to the neonatal period, with particular emphasis placed on the implications for nursing practice. An overview of blood and a brief outline of blood cell production, particularly that of red blood cells (erythropoiesis), and how it develops during foetal life will be included to help clarify matters for the reader. (For detailed physiology, please refer to a standard anatomy and physiology textbook.) The aim is to discuss the role of the nurse in the management of the neonates and their family with the following haematological problems:

- Anaemia
- Jaundice
- Polycythaemia
- Coagulation problems

Haematology is the study of blood and the blood forming tissues, i.e. the formation of blood vessels, the appearance of blood and its composition, the volume of blood, the production of different types of blood cells and their functions. Blood is a tissue and the only fluid tissue in the body; Marieb describes it as the river of life that flows within us transporting almost everything that must be carried from one part of the body to another[1].

Disturbances of the haematology of newborn, particularly preterm, babies are very common. This is due to many factors, with the relative immaturity of their blood cell production and the stress that newborn illnesses place on this system being the common underlying themes. For example, red blood cell production falls immediately after birth at a time when sick newborn babies may have significant blood loss from phlebotomy during neonatal intensive care[2]. It is not surprising, then, that this often leads to anaemia. In addition, the small size and therefore low volumes of blood in the newborn baby increases this risk. Neonatal blood volume per kg decreases as the neonate approaches term[3]. A term neonate has a blood volume of about 82–85 mls/kg while a preterm neonate has approximately 100 mls/kg. This will equate to as little as 100 ml total blood volume in a 1 kg 28-week gestation baby.

Implications for practice

Newborn babies are vulnerable to haematological problems due to their:
• Immature blood-producing systems
• Small size

Components of blood

Blood is slightly alkaline and has a pH of 7.35–7.45. Its appearance as a homogeneous liquid is deceptive; blood is a bionetwork made up of living blood cells suspended in plasma, the non-living medium (see Figure 17.1)[4]. A brief overview is outlined below; a full description of every component in the blood can be obtained from other relevant resources.

The two distinct parts of the blood are plasma and the living blood cells which are elaborated on below.

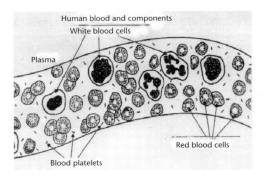

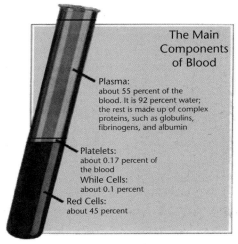

Figure 17.1 The main components of blood.

Plasma (the non-living medium of the blood)

This straw-coloured, sticky fluid makes up 55% of the blood volume (see Figure 17.1). It is 92% water, with a variety of other substances including dissolved complex proteins (globulins, fibrinogens and albumin), nutrients, electrolytes, hormones and metabolic wastes, held in suspension[5]. The plasma composition is kept fairly constant; the liver is responsible for the blood protein levels, the kidneys and respiratory systems maintain the blood pH, while the pancreas controls the blood glucose.

Laboratory analysis of plasma can provide useful information of the state of health/condition of the infant. For example, babies undergoing care on the neonatal unit will have regular measuring of plasma levels of a variety of plasma constituents to monitor kidney function (urea and creatinine) and blood salts (for example, sodium and potassium) to ensure normal function and enable appropriate intervention to be taken to correct problems.

Formed elements (the living blood cells)

Platelets

Platelets are anucleate (no nucleus), small cell fragments with a short life span of about ten days. They make up about 0.17% of the blood and their formation is regulated by a hormone called thrombopoietin. They have a vital role in the clotting process and are sometimes referred to as thrombocytes (*thromb* means clot)[6]. Platelets help to initiate the clotting process by releasing chemical enzymes to orchestrate a series of events that lead to blood clot formation. They also temporarily seal the ruptured area in the blood vessel by forming a plug to arrest the bleeding. Low platelet number (thrombocytopenia) is quite common in the newborn baby and may increase the chance of bleeding complications (see below)[7].

White cells

The white blood cells (WBCs) or leucocytes (*leuko* means white) are the only complete cells in the blood with nuclei and the usual organelles. They make up 0.1% of the blood and there are about 4000 to 11,000 WBCs in each cubic millilitre of blood. They are the body's mobile army and have a vital role in protecting the body from invading organisms. Leucocytosis refers to an increase in the white cell count (WCC) of > 11,000 cells per cubic millilitre of blood and occurs in response to infection, as long as the infant is well enough to mount this response. A suppressed WCC is a serious concern.

The white cells can slip in and out of capillary vessels through a process called 'diapedesis' and when out of the bloodstream, they move through the tissues by amoeboid motion. Their capacity to engulf and destroy (phagocytosis) foreign bodies or dead cells is critical to the body's ability to fight and eliminate infection[8].

This ability of the body to respond to infection by increasing leucocyte numbers and sending them to areas of need within the body is another that is relatively reduced in the newborn baby due to the immaturity of the haematological system[9]. This is one of the reasons that severe infection is such a common problem in the first weeks of life (see Chapter 16)[10].

Implications for practice

Reasons why newborn babies are at increased risk of infection include that, compared to infants and children, they have a:
- Reduced ability to increase white cell count
- Reduced white cell function

Red cells

Mature red blood cells (RBCs) or erythrocytes are anucleate, flexible biconcave-shaped discs. Their major role is the transportation of oxygen to all the tissues in the body to meet their metabolic needs and the partial removal of the by-product carbon dioxide ($\simeq 20\%$). Their structure, constituents and regulation all reflect this central role. For example, they are smaller than leucocytes and are remarkably flexible, which allows them to change shape when passing through the smallest capillaries without rupturing, thereby preserving blood and oxygen delivery[11].

They make up 45% of the blood volume and each cubic millilitre of blood should have about 5,000,000 of RBCs. The number of RBCs varies with age (a newborn baby has more than an adult), sex (males have more than females) and environment (the altitude at which a person lives affects the number of RBCs present in his or her system). This variation with environment is another example of the body's attempt to maintain adequate oxygenation through regulation of red cells. At high altitude, where the oxygen concentration in the air is lower, RBC production increases leading to an increase in red cell number and therefore oxygen carrying capacity. A RBC has a normal life span of about 120 days, whereas the RBC of a preterm infant has only approximately an 80-day life span. (This reduction in life span of newborn babies' red cells can contribute to the development of both jaundice and anaemia in the newborn period.)

The volume of RBCs, the relative amount of space that the RBCs occupy within the blood, is measured as the packed cell volume (PCV) or haematocrit. If whole blood (the cellular portion together with the plasma) is placed in a capillary tube and then 'spun down' in a centrifuge, the heavier formed elements will quickly settle to the bottom of the tube (see Figure 17.2). During the haematocrit procedure, the RBCs are forced to the bottom of the tube first because they are the heaviest element in the blood. The white blood cells and platelets then settle out in a layer called the *buffy coat*. Above the buffy coat is the plasma. From the capillary tube, one can approximate the percentage of space that the RBCs occupy in the total sample using the haematocrit device. At sea level, the haematocrit of a normal adult male averages about 47 (which means that 47% of the blood volume is RBCs), while that of a normal adult female is 42.

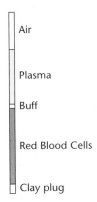

Figure 17.2 Measuring PCV: a capillary tube is centrifuged so that the high density red blood cells are forced to the bottom of the tube and the low density plasma sits on the top. The buffy coat is made up of the white blood cells and platelets and separates the other two parts.

The number of RBCs determines the blood viscosity. If the number of RBCs exceeds the normal range, the blood viscosity increases and the blood flows more slowly. Likewise, if the number of RBCs is below the normal range, the blood is thinner; therefore the blood flows faster. A newborn baby usually has a haematocrit of 50–60, which gives the blood a higher viscosity than adults. In some babies at birth, this can be higher, up to 70 or more (polycythaemia), which can begin to impair blood flow and oxygen delivery to tissues and may have clinical implications (see later in chapter)[12].

Implications for practice

The foetus compensates for being in a low oxygen environment by having:
- More red cells and a higher haematocrit
- Foetal haemoglobin (HbF), which holds on to oxygen with higher affinity than adult haemoglobin.

The oxygen-carrying component of the red blood cell (RBC) is known as the haemoglobin. It is made up of the protein 'globin' bound to the red 'heme' pigment (the iron component). The globin is a complex structure made up of four polypeptide chains, its synthesis is genetically controlled and it changes as the foetus grows. The globin chain determines the type of haemoglobin[13]. Foetal haemoglobin (HbF) is made up mainly of alpha (α) and gamma (γ) chains. As the foetus matures, the γ-chain is replaced by the beta (β) chain in preparation of the foetus for an *ex utero* existence. Adult haemoglobin (HbA) is made up of two α-chains and two β-chains.

The synthesis of haemoglobin occurs in the RBCs and heme production takes place in the mitochondria[14]. Each globin chain encircles round the heme and the iron atom is set in the centre of the heme. As each iron atom can combine reversibly with one molecule of oxygen, haemoglobin with its four polypeptide chains and four iron atoms can transfer four molecules of oxygen[15]. A RBC is 97% haemoglobin, each containing 250 million haemoglobin molecules; therefore each RBC can transport 1 billion oxygen molecules[16,17].

One of the physiological changes that needs to occur in late foetal and early neonatal life is the conversion of the foetal haemoglobin (HbF) to adult haemoglobin (HbA). The structure of HbF means that the oxygen molecules are more strongly held to the haem component. This allows the foetus to maintain oxygen delivery to its tissues in the relatively low-oxygen (hypoxic) environment of *in utero* life.

The normal haemoglobin values are:

Adult (male) → 13–18 g/100 mls blood
Adult (female) → 12–16 g/100 mls blood
Infant → 14–20 g/100 mls blood

Blood cell production (haemopoiesis)

In common with all of the cells that make up the body, blood cells (red cells, white cells and platelets) are produced from stem cells[18]. These are special cells that are capable of developing into many different types of cells, such as skin cells, brain cells (neurons) and blood cells. A single type of haemopoietic stem cell is capable of developing into all types of blood cells by a process called differentiation[19,20]. In adults, haemopoiesis from stem cells to functioning blood cells occurs in the bone marrow. In the embryo and foetus, there are different sites of blood cell production depending on the stage of foetal development[21,22].

Figure 17.3 shows the process of haemopoiesis. Under the influence of a variety of naturally

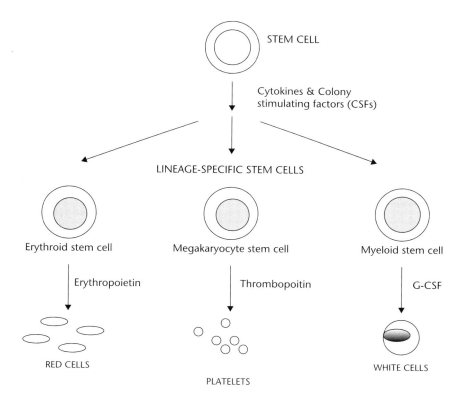

Figure 17.3 The process of haemopoiesis.

occurring substances called cytokines, stem cells are stimulated either to divide to form more stem cells or to differentiate. At a certain point they become committed to becoming a certain type of blood cell, such as a red cell, and are said to be differentiating down the red cell lineage. Erythropoietin is the cytokine that stimulates erythropoiesis.

The term *erythropoiesis* (*erythro* means red and *poiesis* means 'to make') is used to describe the process of RBC formation. The amount of RBCs in the circulatory system is regulated within very narrow limits so that an adequate number of red cells are always available to provide sufficient tissue oxygenation. The bone marrow of essentially all bones produces RBCs from birth to about five years of age. Above age 20 most RBCs are produced primarily in the marrow of the vertebrae, the sternum, the ribs and the pelvis. Our body produces RBCs every day to replace the old RBCs. (The old RBCs are 'eaten' by the spleen and the liver and most of the leftover components are recycled to form new RBCs.)

The body can use the regulation of red cell production to increase production in response to special needs, such as after blood loss or living in high altitude. The organ responsible for 'turning on the faucet' of RBC production is the *kidney*. The kidney responds to low levels of oxygen by stimulating the release of erythropoietin which, in turn, acts on the bone marrow to increase the rate of RBC production. At this point, the number of RBCs increases (and so does the haematocrit), thereby increasing the oxygen-carrying capacity of the blood. When the oxygen level in the blood is sufficient, the kidneys suppress the erythropoietin activity until the next need arises[23,24].

The ontogeny of erythropoiesis

Primitive blood cell production starts as early as 19 days' gestation in the *yolk sac* of the embryo. Subsequently, this process ceases and haemopoiesis starts in the embryo itself, and the main site for this is the foetal liver from about 6–8 weeks' gestation. Although bone marrow blood production starts at about 11 weeks' gestation, the liver is the main organ of haemopoiesis until the third trimester of pregnancy, when the bone marrow takes over[25,26].

Production of red cells, white cells and platelets is well established during the second trimester of pregnancy. However, it is likely that the large changes that occur in the processes and site of haemopoiesis are in part responsible for how vulnerable newborn, particularly preterm newborn, babies are to haematological problems after birth.

Implications for practice

Changes in the process of haemopoiesis during foetal life are still occurring in the third trimester of pregnancy, which makes premature babies more susceptible to haematological problems such as anaemia and thrombocytopenia.

Blood group

Red cells have a variety of antigenic molecules expressed on their cell surface that are used to classify blood into *blood groups*. A copy of each antigen can be inherited from either parent (e.g. a newborn may have the A antigen from the mother and the B antigen from the father and has blood group AB). Associated with these blood group antigens are related antibodies (e.g. anti-A and anti-B) and it is the reaction between mismatched antigens and antibodies in these systems that cause problems such as blood transfusion reactions, graft rejection in organ transplantation and haemolytic disease of the newborn (HDN, see below). Antibodies to specific blood group antigens can occur spontaneously or in response to a sensitisation event, such as a blood transfusion or foeto-maternal haemorrhage during pregnancy. There are many blood group systems (e.g. ABO, Rhesus, Kell, Duffy) but the commonest blood groups to cause immunological reactions are the ABO and the Rhesus systems[27].

ABO blood group

Red cells can either express A antigen, B antigen or O antigen. Due to the O antigen being functionally silent, this results in a person being classified as:

- Blood group A (either homozygous AA or heterozygous AO)
- Blood group B (homozygous BB or heterozygous BO)
- Blood group AB (heterozygous for A and B)
- Blood group O (homozygous OO) (see Table 17.1)

The ABO blood group antigens are also present on the surface of other types of cells. Antibodies are produced to A and B antigens, but not to O. They occur naturally and develop, after the newborn period, to the antigen(s) not present on the innate red cells[28,29].

Rhesus blood group

There are a number of Rhesus antigens (including D, c and E), although the commonest disease-causing antigen-antibody reaction is from Rhesus D (RhD). Red cells will either inherit D antigen or not, resulting in a person being either:

- RhD positive (homozygous or heterozygous for RhD)
- RhD negative (homozygous for the gene on this allele that does not code for RhD)

Unlike with the ABO blood group, antibodies for RhD only occur after sensitisation. Because RhD is highly immunogenic, when exposure of an RhD negative person occurs (for example, an RhD negative mother to an RhD positive baby), antibodies will occur rapidly and in relatively high titre, making a significant reaction very likely at the next exposure (for example, in a subsequent pregnancy).

Blood group incompatibility between mother and baby is the source of significant morbidity, and in the past mortality, in the newborn period through the development of haemolytic disease of the foetus and newborn with resulting jaundice, with or without anaemia (see below)[30,31].

Implications for practice

It is crucial to assess the baby's risk of developing haemolytic disease in the newborn period. Points in the history to note are:
- Maternal blood group.
- Previous neonates with significant jaundice.
- Antenatal evidence of circulating antibodies against other blood group antigens.
- Post-natal evidence of circulating antibodies (Coombs test).

Anaemia

Anaemia is a disorder characterised by a decrease in haemoglobin in the blood to levels below the normal range. The causes are due to:

- Decreased red cell production
- Increased red cell destruction
- Blood loss[32,33]

A neonate with a haemoglobin value of less than 12 g/dl in the first week or less than 10 g/dl later in

Table 17.1 The ABO blood group – different phenotypes, genotypes, antigens expressed on red cells and associated antibodies.

Blood group	A	B	AB	O
Genotype inherited	AA or AO	BB or BO	AB	OO
Antigen(s) expressed on red cells	A or A and O	B or B and O	A and B	O
Antibodies in serum	anti-B	anti-A	None	anti-A and anti-B

infancy is anaemic[34]. Symptoms and signs of anaemia relate to the fall in oxygen carrying capacity due to the low Hb and, in the acute setting, to the loss of circulating blood volume. This may cause an anaemic baby to present with organ dysfunction due to reduced oxygen delivery, which includes:

- Respiratory symptoms
  - Increasing oxygen requirement
  - Apnoea
- Cardiovascular symptoms
  - Hypotension
  - Bradycardia
  - Poor perfusion
- Non-specific symptoms: poor feeding and lethargy

Acute anaemia is far more likely to present with symptoms than chronic anaemia and it demands immediate intervention. Sudden and severe blood loss can be life threatening. Failure to arrest or control bleeding will result in cardiovascular collapse followed closely by respiratory failure [35]. However, probably the most common presentation of anaemia on NNU is a low Hb in a premature neonate with no apparent symptoms.

Implications for practice

Acute anaemia is a medical emergency. However, babies with chronic anaemia of prematurity can tolerate Hb as low as 7–8 g/dl.

Causes of anaemia

The causes of anaemia can be considered as antenatal, perinatal and post-natal and these are listed below[36.]

Antenatal[37–39]
- Intrauterine twin-to-twin transfusion, where the larger twin is plethoric and the smaller twin is anaemic
- Rhesus haemolytic disease

- Foeto-placental haemorrhage from abnormal placental site or injury
- Foetal internal haemorrhage (e.g. intraventricular haemorrhage)
- Impaired red cell production (α-thalassaemia)
- Foetal congenital infection (especially parvovirus)

Perinatal[40,41]
- Placenta praevia, vasa praevia, placental abruption
- Laceration of placenta at caesarean section
- Bleeding from the umbilical cord (velamentous insertion of cord, inadequately clamped umbilical cord), rupture of anomalous vessels

Postnatal[42,43]
- Acute anaemia
  - Internal bleeding: intraventricular haemorrhage, trauma, deficiency in clotting factors
  - Mechanical: losing blood from defective or poorly connected umbilical catheters
  - Acute red blood cell destruction: infection
- Chronic anaemia
  - Repeated blood sampling
  - Chronic haemolysis and marrow suppression in small sick infants
- Physiological anaemia
  - Erythropoietin (EPO) is a significant cause. The production of EPO switches off after birth and increases only very slowly in the neonatal period[44,45]. Premature babies have a slower erythropoietin recovery.
  - Folic acid deficiency can be corrected through supplementation. Common practice is to prescribe folic acid supplements for babies with a history of haemolytical disorders, e.g. haemolytic disease of the newborn, spherocytosis, etc.

Principles of management in anaemia

Management of foetal and/or neonatal anaemia depends on a number of important principles, regardless of cause[46–48]. However, there will be variation depending on the time of presentation (especially with antenatal causes) and whether the presentation is acute or chronic.

(1) Preparation and communication
  (a) Acknowledge parental concerns and ensure that the parents are kept fully informed and understand the situation
  (b) Ensure excellent communication between staff, e.g. inform NNU if baby found to be compromised on labour ward
  (c) Ensure presence of adequate staff of appropriate seniority
  (d) Know where to access the neonatal emergency blood – this will depend on local protocols, but there should be access to immediate O negative blood for acute emergencies
  (e) Arrange for a medical member of staff to speak to parents as soon as possible

Implications for practice

Babies may be born unexpectedly severely anaemic. This may require transfusion with emergency uncrossmatched O Rh negative blood in the labour ward or soon after admission to NICU.

(2) Prevention is better than treatment
  (a) Prevent further blood loss if possible
  (b) Careful attention to reducing phlebotomy losses has been shown to reduce the need for blood transfusion in the newborn period
  (c) Appropriate supplementation of iron, vitamins and folic acid depending on clinical circumstances (e.g. prematurity, evidence of haemolysis) and local protocols

Implications for practice

A careful policy aimed at reducing blood sampling in preterm babies can significantly lower the number of transfusions these babies receive, which in turn reduces their blood donor exposure and risk of complications.

(3) Clinical assessment
  (a) Perform an immediate general assessment of the infant's condition and need for resuscitation, i.e. airway, breathing, circulation (ABC)
  (b) Ensure you have baseline assessment of the vital signs (temperature, pulse, respiration and blood pressure)
  (c) Ensure the baby is kept warm
  (d) Assist in the establishment of respiratory support and gaining venous assess
  (e) Monitor fluid intake and output

(4) Transfuse if benefit of transfusion outweighs risk
  (a) Infant may require just volume expander initially to improve circulatory output
  (b) Blood transfusion should be given only if necessary
  (c) Refer to hospital policy for blood transfusion
  (d) Prompt blood transfusion, if there is clear compromise or blood loss is severe, can be life-saving
  (e) Infant with haemolytic disease of the newborn may require exchange transfusion

There will be particular considerations in babies who have been diagnosed as anaemic antenatally. This will include referral to an appropriate counsellor, allowing parents to visit the neonatal unit and a careful multidisciplinary approach to planning of the optimal time to deliver the baby. Liaison with the blood transfusion department in advance will ensure rapid access to appropriate blood products (including blood for exchange transfusion) to expedite management at birth.

Blood transfusion

Blood transfusion is a frequent procedure on the NNU, particularly for preterm babies, as the frequency of anaemia is high[49]. However, there has been increasing recognition over the last 10–15 years that neonatal practice has not always carefully balanced the risks of blood transfusion with the proven benefits[50,51]. Transfusion is usually of paediatric packs of packed red cells, although exchange transfusions will require greater volume and may have a lower haematocrit than standard packed red cells.

Risks of blood transfusion[52,53]

It should be remembered that these risks pertain to all blood products, which includes fresh frozen plasma and 4.5% (or 20%) albumin.

(1) Immune reactions
(2) Infection
    (a) Bacterial infection due to bacterial contamination of blood and blood products
    (b) Viral infections, e.g. HIV, hepatitis, etc.
    (c) Other, e.g. new variant CJD
(3) Infusion-related, e.g. tissued cannula, scarring, etc.
(4) Suppression of innate erythropoiesis

Benefits of blood transfusion

In a baby who is symptomatic of anaemia, the benefits of transfusion to restore oxygen delivery to the tissues and support the circulation are clear. However, particularly in sick premature babies with respiratory problems, it is not always straightforward to decide when symptoms or signs of anaemia are present and the evidence base for the benefit of blood transfusion in this circumstance is not strong. In addition, there is a developing body of evidence that supports the safety of transfusion at lower Hb values than have traditionally been used[54,55]. In all cases the decision to transfuse should be based on an assessment of risk versus benefit.

Indications for blood transfusion in newborn

A decision to transfuse a baby in the newborn period will depend on the post-natal age (lower transfusion thresholds will be tolerated in older babies), the rapidity with which the anaemia has occurred (acute onset is more likely to require intervention) and the presence of clinical signs and symptoms (particularly respiratory and cardiovascular compromise). Each NNU should have guidelines for local practice[56].

Implications for practice

Appropriate care should be taken when deciding whether a baby requires transfusion, to weigh up the potential risks and benefits. There is increasing recognition that carefully reducing the number of transfusions that premature babies receive does not lead to harm.

Jaundice

Jaundice is the yellow discolouration to the skin and sclera that is produced when there is a build-up of bilirubin in the blood and tissues (hyperbilirubinaemia). It is extremely common, occurring in approximately two-thirds of all newborn babies, is most often benign and usually does not require treatment. However, hyperbilirubinaemia can be significant for the following reasons:

• Very high jaundice levels, particularly in the first days of life, can be toxic to the brain and lead to death or long-term disability (kernicterus)
• Persistent jaundice, particularly beyond two weeks of life, can be an indication of underlying pathology requiring investigation, such as liver disease[57]

Bilirubin metabolism

Bilirubin is produced after the metabolism of heme released from haemoglobin after red cell breakdown. Red cells are broken down under normal circumstances as they reach the end of their life span, but may also be broken down (haemolysed) prematurely by pathological processes as outlined below. Normal newborn babies are likely to develop jaundice due to a combination of factors including:

- Large red cell load (higher haematocrit as previously mentioned)
- Shorter red cell life span
- Reduced bilirubin clearance by and from the neonatal liver[58]

Causes of excess haemolysis in newborn babies [59–61]

- Immune haemolysis: most commonly blood group incompatibility (see below)
- Red cell membrane abnormalities, e.g. hereditary spherocytosis
- Red cell enzyme abnormalities, e.g. glucose-6-phosphate dehydrogenase deficiency
- Haemoglobinopathies (rarely present in the newborn period)
- Sepsis

Haemolytic disease of the newborn secondary to blood group incompatibility

Immune haemolytic disease in the foetus and newborn is most commonly due to either Rhesus or ABO incompatibility. The spectrum of presentation and the management of this condition have changed markedly since the introduction of routine post-natal prophylactic anti-D immunoglobulin for RhD negative women led to a massive reduction in the number of babies being born with significant haemolysis, leading to severe anaemia and jaundice requiring exchange transfusion[62,63]. The predominant presentations of haemolysis in the neonatal period now are:

- Antenatally diagnosed haemolysis, with rising maternal anti-D antibody titres, with or without anaemia
- Rapidly developing or severe jaundice not predicted by antenatal antibody screening

RhD negative women may begin to produce anti-D antibodies if they become pregnant with an RhD positive foetus (sensitisation). In these circumstances, an RhD positive foetus will have inherited an RhD antigen from the father. For sensitisation to occur there must have been a previous pregnancy or an event in the current pregnancy that causes transfer of red cells from the foetus to the blood of the mother. This most often occurs during normal birth, but may also occur following a miscarriage, amniocentesis or antepartum haemorrhage. If the woman subsequently becomes pregnant with another RhD positive foetus, the antibodies may cross the placenta causing haemolysis. However, provision of anti-D to RhD negative mothers post-natally (and also now at 28–32 weeks' gestation) has been found to stop endogenous antibody production in response to exposure to their RhD positive baby.

During pregnancy RhD negative women are monitored to look for rising antibody levels and ultrasound is used to recognise signs of foetal anaemia secondary to haemolysis. Signs of anaemia, such as changes in cerebral blood flow on Doppler ultrasound, may require intervention with foetal blood sampling to measure foetal haemoglobin and possibly intrauterine foetal blood transfusion. Alternatively, the baby may require early delivery to manage the increasing haemolysis.

Implications for practice

Haemolysis due to Rhesus incompatibility can be avoided in most circumstances by careful management of pregnancies in Rh negative women. However, babies are still being born with anaemia and/or severe jaundice due to failure of anti-D prophylaxis.

Babies with ABO incompatibility will usually present either with jaundice diagnosed in the first 24 hours of life or often after referral from the community, with severe jaundice noted after discharge from post-natal ward on day three to five. This condition occurs almost exclusively in babies of women of blood group O and most commonly with babies who are blood group A. Approximately 15–25% of maternal/foetal pairs are ABO-incompatible, but only in about 1% of these will significant HDN occur, as only in these circumstances is there a sufficiently high titre of IgG antibody produced by the mother to cross the placenta and cause disease[64]. The complications of significant jaundice include:

- Mild to moderate neurological damage affecting cognitive development
- Sensory hearing loss in premature babies
- Abnormal functioning of the acoustic nerve in jaundiced but otherwise healthy infants
- Neurological handicap (cerebral palsy)[65]

Implications for practice

Most causes of severe neonatal jaundice not caused by Rhesus incompatibility cannot be predicted antenatally. Babies need to be assessed for jaundice regularly in the first days of life, whether they are still in hospital or have been transferred to the community.

Management of jaundice

Phototherapy

Phototherapy is the use of light to alter the composition of the bilirubin to allow it to be excreted more easily. An example of this is the conversion of bilirubin (structural isomerisation) into a water soluble substance known as lumirubin which can be effectively excreted by the kidneys. The most effective light spectrum for converting the yellow bilirubin pigment to the photoisomer lumirubin is blue light and the wavelength of blue light is in the 425–475 nm range. Two other reactions also occur as a result of the bilirubin absorbing a photon of light[56]:

- Photo-oxidation: a slow process that may not contribute significantly to elimination of bilirubin
- Configurational isomerisation: a rapid conversion process but the excretion of the isomer is slow.

- A rapid conversion process but excretion of the isomer is slow

The factors that influence the effectiveness of phototherapy are:

- Total dose of light delivered
- Energy output of light source
- Number of light sources
- Distance from infant
- Maximum skin surface area exposed to those lights

Phototherapy can be delivered in a variety of ways which include:

- Overhead unit
- Bilirubin blankets
- 360 unit: this is the most effective, but reduces the ability to perform nursing observations as the infant is surrounded by phototherapy units and so care must be taken when utilising

Exchange transfusion

Whereas this procedure was once common due to the high incidence of Rhesus incompatibility, even busy neonatal units may only be required to perform them a handful of times in a year. Even babies presenting with very high bilirubin levels or evidence of significant haemolysis may often be effectively treated with phototherapy (with or without intravenous immunoglobulin, see below)[67]. Therefore, exchange transfusion should be restricted to those babies with haemolysis and either:

- Severe anaemia, or
- Severe or rapidly increasing hyperbilirubinaemia unresponsive to phototherapy

Other treatment strategies

- Supportive care: as with other neonatal illnesses, appropriate emphasis on cardiorespiratory stability, fluid balance and general care is extremely important in the jaundiced baby. In addition, jaundice can be worsened by dehydration and the neurological effects can be exacerbated by concurrent problems such as prematurity, acidosis and sepsis which all need to be managed accordingly.

- Evidence is accumulating that giving babies with HDN intravenous immunoglobulin may reduce the likelihood of needing an exchange transfusion[68]. However, this has not become a standard of care at this time.

Implications for practice

- Neonatal jaundice is very common and usually resolves without treatment.
- It is important to be vigilant to identify and aggressively treat potentially dangerous jaundice which is mainly caused by haemolysis and infection.
- Jaundice presenting within 24 hours of birth is pathological until proved otherwise.

Polycythaemia

Polycythaemia, refers to an increase in the PCV above the normal range, which is generally held to be up to 65%[69]. This is relatively common, occurring in about 5% of newborn babies. Its clinical significance lies in the accompanying increase in blood viscosity, as it is this that may lead to impaired blood flow and tissue ischaemia. The increase in blood viscosity that occurs as a direct consequence of polycythaemia is not routinely measured in the newborn, but it has been shown to increase markedly above 65%[70].

Implications for practice

Polycythaemia produces its effects due to the increase in the viscosity of the blood, leading to reduced blood flow and oxygen delivery to the tissues.

Neonatal polycythaemia is more likely to be seen in the following circumstances[71,72]:

- Placental insufficiency/intra-uterine hypoxia
  - IUGR and maternal pre-eclampsia
  - Maternal diabetics
  - Maternal smoking
- Increased blood volume: twin-to-twin transfusion (recipient)
- Foetal abnormalities: trisomy 21 (Down's syndrome)

Most babies with polycythaemia will be asymptomatic. However, symptoms and signs of polycythaemia can affect all systems[73], such as:

- Nervous system
  - Lethargy, jitteriness, poor feeding
  - Polycythaemia has been shown to cause reduced cerebral blood flow[74]; however, although this is probably the most concerning aspect of polycythaemia, it is not clear whether polycythaemia alone can also cause seizures and/or lead to long-term neurodevelopmental problems, particularly in the absence of significant symptoms
- Metabolic: jaundice (due to increased red cell load), hypoglycaemia
- Cardiorespiratory: respiratory distress, cyanosis
- Gastro-intestinal: may predispose to necrotising enterocolitis (NEC)

Treatment of polycythaemia

Protocols for the treatment of neonatal polycythaemia vary. It is generally agreed that overtly symptomatic babies should be treated regardless of the PCV. However, as the presentation is often non-specific and mimics other neonatal conditions (e.g. respiratory distress), uncertainty as to when to treat may still remain. In addition, even babies with very high haematocrits may remain asymptomatic and the evidence for treating these babies is slight[75].

- Supportive care
  - As with other neonatal conditions, close attention to respiratory and cardiovascular support is crucial.

○ Monitoring of fluid balance, hypoglycaemia, jaundice, etc.
○ Attention to feeding, monitoring for NEC, particularly in the preterm and/or IUGR infant
• Dilutional exchange transfusion: this is the mainstay of treatment once the decision to reduce the PCV is made. This involves the careful removal of a calculated volume of the baby's blood (depending on the degree of polycythaemia) and replacement with a diluting agent (in modern practice, usually a crystalloid solution such as normal saline).

Coagulation problems

Blood clotting is achieved by the complex interaction between blood vessels, platelets and substances (factors) that enhance or inhibit clot formation (the 'clotting cascade'). An understanding of coagulation problems is important in the newborn baby because there are a number of significant disorders of coagulation that can present in the newborn period and the consequences of bleeding can be catastrophic[76].

The normal process of clot formation and regulation is as follows:

• Endothelial injury precipitates platelet adhesion and release of tissue factor
• Platelets are activated to change shape and release substances, which leads to platelet aggregation and the start of a clot
• A cascade of clotting factors are released and activated (initiated by tissue factor), which leads to formation of thrombin from prothrombin and fibrin from fibrinogen and the growth and maturation of the clot
• Simultaneously, mechanisms to control and inhibit clot formation are stimulated, particularly via the activation of plasmin

As with many other systems, the coagulation system in a newborn baby is in a state of development[77]. The liver is responsible for production of many of the clotting factors and their levels can be low at birth. Although in normal circumstances the baby's coagulation control is adequate, adverse clinical situations may lead to rapid and severe haemorrhage as the system is overwhelmed[78]. Premature babies may be particularly vulnerable to bleeding in this way, which may result in intraventricular, pulmonary or gastrointestinal haemorrhage.

The causes of coagulation problems in the newborn period can be grouped as follows:

• Platelet problems – usually thrombocytopenia
• Clotting factor deficiencies, e.g. vitamin K deficient bleeding, haemophilia

Thrombocytopenia

Thrombocytopenia (low platelet count $< 150 \times 10^9/l$) is the commonest coagulation problem in the newborn. It is present in 1–5% of all newborns and in up to 50% of sick preterm babies on NICU[79,80]. Thrombocytopenia is usually the result of reduced platelet production or increased platelet destruction or a combination of both.

The two commonest presentations of thrombocytopenia in the foetus and newborn are described below[81,82].

Signs of haemorrhage in an otherwise healthy term baby
This baby presents with purpura or petechiae, but may present with severe haemorrhage (e.g. intracranial). This may be picked up in a foetus antenatally or early in the newborn period. Specific causes of this presentation are:

(1) Neonatal alloimmune thrombocytopenia: this is caused by a similar mechanism to haemolytic disease of the newborn. The antibodies that cross the placenta from the mother are against antigens on the baby's platelets that have been inherited from the father, which means that the mother has a normal platelet count. This baby can have

very severe thrombocytopenia ($< 10 \times 10^9$/l) and is at high risk of bleeding. Urgent treatment is required by transfusion with specific platelets that will not react with the mother's antibody.

(2) Neonatal autoimmune thrombocytopenia: this is also caused by antibodies, but they are antibodies to maternal platelets when the mother has idiopathic (immune-mediated) thrombocytopenic purpura (ITP) and therefore the mother will also be thrombocytopenic. The baby is less at risk of bleeding and will often not require treatment. If the platelet count is very low, treatment with infusion of immunoglobulin is generally recommended.

(3) Congenital or inherited thrombocytopenias: there are many of these and they are all very rare e.g. Wiskott-Aldrich syndrome, Fanconi's anaemia[83].

Implications for practice

With neonatal alloimmune thrombocytopenia:
- The baby may present only with an incidental finding of petechiae.
- The risk of haemorrhage is high and prompt treatment may prevent severe sequelae such as intracranial haemorrhage.

Thrombocytopenia in a baby requiring neonatal intensive care

This is the most common presentation of neonatal thrombocytopenia and occurs mainly in preterm babies. It can be thought of as occurring as 'early' and 'late' presentations:

(1) Early thrombocytopenia: this presents in the first few days of life. It is generally agreed that there is a degree of reduced platelet production underlying this and it is commonly seen in babies who are extremely premature (< 28 weeks gestation) or in babies with IUGR, asphyxia or infection.

(2) Late thrombocytopenia: this presents usually after 72 hours and is most commonly due to septicaemia or necrotising enterocolitis. It may be severe and require platelet transfusion.

These sick premature babies are particularly at risk of bleeding and severe bleeding may lead to death and significant morbidity[84,85]. It is for this reason that this group of babies are quite commonly transfused with platelets, although there is not general agreement as to the best time to do this and at what platelet level it should be done.

Clotting factor deficiencies

The diagnosis of a bleeding problem due to abnormal clotting factors is based on the measurement of a 'coagulation profile'. The tests performed in a coagulation profile will vary between haematology laboratories, but will usually include the Prothrombin Time (or ratio) (PT) and the Activated Partial Thromboplastin Time (or ratio) (APTT). The results of these tests will give some idea of the cause, but more complicated and/or specific tests are also available to help with diagnosis (for example, blood levels of specific clotting factors)[86].

Vitamin K deficient bleeding (VKDB)

Although there are a number of causes of abnormal coagulation (other than thrombocytopenia) in the newborn period, VKDB is particularly important as it is almost entirely preventable with appropriate vitamin K provision after birth[87]. The underlying problem in this condition is a deficiency of vitamin K in the newborn baby coupled with the low amount of vitamin K found in breast milk. It may present in a variety of ways from minor bleeding from the umbilical stump or circumcision site to catastrophic intracranial haemorrhage[88].

There are many factors in the clotting cascade (traditionally numbered I to XIII). Four of them, II (prothrombin), VII, IX and X, need vitamin K for their production by the liver and for their function.

The foetus has relatively low stores of vitamin K and without provision of vitamin K babies are at risk of severe bleeding in the newborn period[89]. Some babies are at particular risk of VKDB:

- Babies who have inadequate vitamin K intake after birth: this is most commonly babies who are exclusively breast-fed and is due to the levels of vitamin K in breast milk being insufficient to supply the liver with adequate vitamin K for clotting factor production
- Babies with liver disease (e.g. biliary atresia) that are unable to produce adequate vitamin K-dependent factors

Babies with VKDB are divided into:

(1) Early (< 24 hours of life): this may be due to abnormal maternal vitamin K metabolism (and therefore very low neonatal vitamin K levels), for example if the mother is taking anti-convulsant medication
(2) 'Classic' VKDB (in the first week of life): this occurs predominantly in babies who have not been given vitamin K at birth and who are exclusively breast-fed
(3) Late VKDB (1–8 weeks post-natally): babies presenting at this time will either have the same risk factors as the 'classic' form or may have underlying liver disease

VKDB can be almost completely prevented by vitamin K prophylaxis given at birth. The best way of providing this has been extensively debated and varies within and between countries. It can be given either as:

- Single dose intramuscularly at birth: this will prevent more or less all cases of VKDB and is the recommended route in the current UK National Institute of Health and Clinical Excellence (NICE) guidelines, or
- Multiple doses orally: if given in adequate doses at the correct times this will also prevent VKDB; however, it has been associated with more failures from problems with compliance

Formula milk is supplemented with vitamin K and therefore formula fed infants are also protected. VKDB occasionally occurs due to parental refusal for any vitamin K prophylaxis[90].

Implications for practice

Adequate hospital protocols to ensure adequate newborn vitamin K prophylaxis are crucial to prevent VKDB (previously known as hemorrhagic disease of the newborn).

Haemophilia

Haemophilia A and Haemophilia B are caused by specific inherited deficiencies of Factor VIII and IX respectively. Haemophilia B is the most common and has an X-linked inheritance (although at least 30% of cases occur spontaneously and therefore will not have a family history).

Haemophilia most commonly presents with oozing from an umbilicus or circumcision site. However, it should be suspected in any baby presenting with bleeding of unknown cause and may present with intracranial haemorrhage. The diagnosis rests on measuring blood levels of the appropriate clotting factor and treatment involves replacement therapy with synthetically produced (recombinant) clotting factor[91].

Disseminated intravascular coagulation (DIC)

DIC is caused by the uncontrolled activation of the clotting cascade, which causes consumption of platelets (leading to thrombocytopenia) and clotting factors (leading to their depletion and derangement of coagulation profiles).

The exact incidence of DIC is unknown in the newborn. Until recently, many episodes of thrombocytopenia in sick newborns were thought to be due to DIC, although platelet consumption frequently occurs in the absence of significant clotting factor consumption. However, prolonged coagulation times are common in newborn, particularly preterm, babies due to normal low factor levels and reduced liver production; thereby introducing diagnostic uncertainty.

DIC is most commonly caused by either hypoxia-ischaemia (usually presents as early thrombocytopenia) or sepsis (usually presents as late thrombocytopenia)[92].

Conclusion

Newborn babies have a variety of haematological problems. Like problems affecting other body systems, they are often the result of their developing physiology coming under pressure from external forces, such as premature delivery, infection or maternal influences. Additionally, foetal and newborn haematological abnormalities can be the result of genetic defects.

Knowledge of the causes and safe management of the common haematological conditions is crucial to a good outcome for the newborn infant.

References

1. Marieb E (2004) *Human Anatomy and Physiology*, 6th edn. Pearson International Edition, London.
2. Widness JA (2000) Pathophysiology, diagnosis and prevention of neonatal anemia. *NeoReviews*, 1 (4), e61–e67.
3. Shaw N (1998) Assessment and Management of Hematologic Dysfunction. In: Kenner C, Lott JW, Flandermeyer AA (eds) *Comprehensive Neonatal Nursing – a Physiologic Perspective*, 2nd edn. WB Saunders, Philadelphia.
4. Widness JA (2000) Pathophysiology, diagnosis and prevention of neonatal anemia. *NeoReviews*, 1 (4), e61–e67.
5. Marieb E (2004) *Human Anatomy and Physiology*, 6th edn. Pearson International Edition, London.
6. Marieb E (2004) *Human Anatomy and Physiology*, 6th edn. Pearson International Edition, London.
7. Castle V, Andrew M, Kelton J, Giron D, Johnston M, Carter C (1986) Frequency and mechanism of neonatal thrombocytopenia. *J Pediatr*, 108 (5, part I), 749–755.
8. Marieb E (2004) *Human Anatomy and Physiology*, 6th edn. Pearson International Edition, London.
9. Cairo MS (1989) Neonatal neutrophil host defence. *American Journal of Diseases in Childhood*, 143, 40–46.
10. Stoll BJ, Gordon T, Korones S, *et al.* (1996) Late-onset neonatal sepsis in very low birth weight neonates: a report from the National Institute of Child Health and Human Development Neonatal Research Network. *J Pediatr*, 129, 63–71.
11. Oski FA (1993) The erythrocyte and its disorders. In: Nathan A, Oski FA (eds) *Hematology of Infancy and Childhood*. WB Saunders, Philadelphia. pp. 18–43.
12. Werner EJ (1995) Neonatal polycythemia and hyperviscosity. *Clinic Perinatol*, 22 (3), 693–710.
13. Bell SG (1999) An Introduction to Hemoglobin Physiology. *Neonatal Network*, 18 (2), 9–15.
14. Bell SG (1999) An Introduction to Hemoglobin Physiology. *Neonatal Network*, 18 (2), 9–15.
15. Marieb E (2004) *Human Anatomy and Physiology*, 6th edn. Pearson International Edition, London.
16. Marieb E (2004) *Human Anatomy and Physiology*, 6th edn. Pearson International Edition, London.
17. Oski FA (1993) The erythrocyte and its disorders. In: Nathan A, Oski FA (eds) *Hematology of Infancy and Childhood*. WB Saunders, Philadelphia. pp.18–43.
18. Emerson SG (1991) The stem cell model of hematopoiesis. In: Hoffman R, Benz E, Shattil SJ (eds), *Hematology: Basic Principles and Practice*. Churchill Livingstone, New York. pp. 72–81.
19. Ogawa M (1993) Differentiation and proliferation of hemopoietic stem cells. *Blood*, 81, 2844–2853.
20. Roberts IAG, Murray NM (2005) Haematology. In: Rennie JM (ed.), *Roberton's Textbook of Neonatology*. Elsevier, Philadelphia. pp. 739–772.
21. Forestier F, Daffos F, Catherine N, Renard M, Andreux JP (1991) Developmental hematopoiesis in normal human foetal blood. *Blood*, 77 (11), 2360–2363.
22. Tavian M, Cortes F, Charbord P, Labastie MC, Peault B (1999) Haematopoietic stem cell emergence and development in the human embryo and foetus: perspectives for blood cell therapies *in utero*. *Semin Neonatol*, 4, 55–66.
23. Oski FA (1993) The erythrocyte and its disorders. In: Nathan A, Oski FA (eds) *Hematology of Infancy and Childhood*. WB Saunders, Philadelphia. pp.18–43.
24. Emerson SG (1991) The stem cell model of hematopoiesis. In: Hoffman R, Benz E, Shattil SJ

(eds), *Hematology: Basic Principles and Practice.* Churchill Livingstone, New York. pp. 72–81.

25. Forestier F, Daffos F, Catherine N, Renard M, Andreux JP (1991) Developmental hematopoiesis in normal human foetal blood. *Blood*, **77** (11), 2360–2363.

26. Tavian M, Cortes F, Charbord P, Labastie MC, Peault B (1999) Haematopoietic stem cell emergence and development in the human embryo and foetus: perspectives for blood cell therapies *in utero*. *Semin Neonatol*, **4**, 55–66.

27. Oski FA (1993) The erythrocyte and its disorders. In: Nathan A, Oski FA (eds) *Hematology of Infancy and Childhood*. WB Saunders, Philadelphia. pp.18–43.

28. Oski FA (1993) The erythrocyte and its disorders. In: Nathan A, Oski FA (eds) *Hematology of Infancy and Childhood*. WB Saunders, Philadelphia. pp.18–43.

29. Murray NA, Roberts IAG (2007) Haemolytic disease of the newborn. *Foetal Neonatal Ed*, **92**, F83–F88.

30. Oski FA (1993) The erythrocyte and its disorders. In: Nathan A, Oski FA (eds) *Hematology of Infancy and Childhood*. WB Saunders, Philadelphia. pp.18–43.

31. Murray NA, Roberts IAG (2007) Haemolytic disease of the newborn. *Arch Dis Child Foetal Neonatal Ed*, **92** (2), F83–F88.

32. Anderson KN, Anderson LE (1995) *Mosby's Pocket Dictionary of Nursing*. Medicine and Professions Allied to Medicine, UK Edition, England.

33. Widness JA (2000) Pathophysiology, diagnosis and prevention of neonatal anemia. *NeoReviews*, **1** (4), e61–e67.

34. Rennie JM, Roberton NRC (2002) *Neonatal Intensive Care*, 4th edn. Arnold, London.

35. Stephenson T, Grant J, Marlow N, Watkin S (2000) *Pocket Neonatology*. Elsevier, Amsterdam.

36. Widness JA (2000) Pathophysiology, diagnosis and prevention of neonatal anemia. *NeoReviews*, **1** (4), e61–e67.

37. Shaw N (1998) Assessment and Management of Hematologic Dysfunction. In: Kenner C, Lott JW, Flandermeyer AA (eds) *Comprehensive Neonatal Nursing – a Physiologic Perspective*, 2nd edn. WB Saunders, Philadelphia.

38. Rennie JM, Roberton NRC (2002) *Neonatal Intensive Care*, 4th edn. Arnold, London.

39. Stephenson T, Grant J, Marlow N, Watkin S (2000) *Pocket Neonatology*. Elsevier, Amsterdam.

40. Shaw N (1998) Assessment and Management of Hematologic Dysfunction. In: Kenner C, Lott JW,

Flandermeyer AA (eds) *Comprehensive Neonatal Nursing – a Physiologic Perspective*, 2nd edn. WB Saunders, Philadelphia.

41. Stephenson T, Grant J, Marlow N, Watkin S (2000) *Pocket Neonatology*. Elsevier, Amsterdam.

42. Shaw N (1998) Assessment and Management of Hematologic Dysfunction. In: Kenner C, Lott JW, Flandermeyer AA (eds) *Comprehensive Neonatal Nursing – a Physiologic Perspective*, 2nd edn. WB Saunders, Philadelphia.

43. Werner EJ (1995) Neonatal polycythemia and hyperviscosity. *Clinic Perinatol*, **22** (3), 693–710.

44. Rennie JM, Roberton NRC (2002) *Neonatal Intensive Care*, 4th edn. Arnold, London.

45. Widness JA (2000) Pathophysiology, diagnosis and prevention of neonatal anemia. *NeoReviews*, **1** (4), e61–e67.

46. Ramasethu J, Luban NLC (1999) Red blood cell transfusions in the newborn. *Semin Neonatol*, **4**, 5–16.

47. Murray NA, Roberts IAG (2004) Neonatal transfusion practice. *Arch Dis Child Foetal Neonatal Ed*, **89** (2), F101–F107.

48. British Committee for Standards in Haematology (2004) Transfusion guidelines for neonates and older children. *British Journal of Haematology*, **124**, 433–453.

49. Widness JA (2000) Pathophysiology, diagnosis and prevention of neonatal anemia. *NeoReviews*, **1** (4), e61–e67.

50. Ramasethu J, Luban NLC (1999) Red blood cell transfusions in the newborn. *Semin Neonatol*, **4**, 5–16.

51. Murray NA, Roberts IAG (2004) Neonatal transfusion practice. *Arch Dis Child Foetal Neonatal Ed*, **89** (2), F101–F107.

52. Galel SA, Fontaine MJ (2006) Hazards of neonatal blood transfusion. *NeoReviews*, **7** (2), e69–e74.

53. Busch MP, Kleinman SH, Nemo GJ (2003) Current and emerging infectious risks of blood transfusions. *JAMA*, **289** (8), 959–962.

54. Widness JA, Seward VJ, Kromer IJ, Burmeister LF, Bell EF, Strauss RG (1996) Changing patterns of red blood cell transfusion in very low birth weight infants. *J Pediatr*, **129** (5), 680–687.

55. Kirpalani HK, Whyte RK, Andersen C, *et al.* (2006) The Premature Infants in Need of Transfusion (PINT) study: a randomized, controlled trial of a resprictive (low) versus liberal (high) transfusion threshold for extremely low birth weight infants. *J Pediatr*, 149, 301–307.

56. British Committee for Standards in Haematology (2004) Transfusion guidelines for neonates and older children. *British Journal of Haematology*, **124**, 433–453.

57. Ives NK (2005) Gastroenterology: neonatal jaundice. In: Rennie JM (ed.) *Roberton's Textbook of Neonatology*, 4th edn. Elsevier, Philadelphia. pp. 661–678.

58. Ives NK (2005) Gastroenterology: neonatal jaundice. In: Rennie JM (ed.) *Roberton's Textbook of Neonatology*, 4th edn. Elsevier, Philadelphia. pp. 661–678.

59. Oski FA (1993) The erythrocyte and its disorders. In: Nathan A, Oski FA (eds) *Hematology of Infancy and Childhood*. WB Saunders, Philadelphia. pp.18–43.

60. Roberts IAG, Murray NM (2005) Haematology. In: Rennie JM (ed.), *Roberton's Textbook of Neonatology*. Elsevier, Philadelphia. pp. 739–772.

61. Murray NA, Roberts IAG (2007) Haemolytic disease of the newborn. *Arch Dis Child Foetal Neonatal Ed*, **92** (2), F83–F88.

62. Murray NA, Roberts IAG (2007) Haemolytic disease of the newborn. *Foetal Neonatal Ed*, **92** (2), F83–F88.

63. Ives NK (2005) Gastroenterology: neonatal jaundice. In: Rennie JM (ed.) *Roberton's Textbook of Neonatology*, 4th edn. Elsevier, Philadelphia. pp. 661–678.

64. Murray NA, Roberts IAG (2007) Haemolytic disease of the newborn. *Foetal Neonatal Ed*, **92** (2), F83–F88.

65. Connoly AM, Volpe JJ (1990) Clinical features of bilirubin encephalopathy. *Clin Perinatol*, **17** (2), 371–379.

66. Ennever JF (1992) Phototherapy for neonatal jaundice. In: Polin RA, Fox WW (eds) *Foetal and Neonatal Physiology*. WB Saunders, Philadelphia. pp.1165–1173.

67. Murray NA, Roberts IAG (2007) Haemolytic disease of the newborn. *Foetal Neonatal Ed*, **92** (2), F83–F88.

68. Gottstein R, Cooke RWI (2003) Systematic review of intravenous immunoglobulin in haemolytic disease of the newborn. *Arch Dis Child Foetal Neonatal Ed*, **88** (1), F6–F10.

69. Watts T, Roberts A (1999) Haematological abnormalities in the growth-restricted infant. *Semin Neonatol*, **4**, 41–54.

70. Werner EJ (1995) Neonatal polycythemia and hyperviscosity. *Clinic Perinatol*, **22** (3), 693–710.

71. Watts T, Roberts A (1999) Haematological abnormalities in the growth-restricted infant. *Semin Neonatol*, **4**, 41–54.

72. Werner EJ (1995) Neonatal polycythemia and hyperviscosity. *Clinic Perinatol*, **22** (3), 693–710.

73. Werner EJ (1995) Neonatal polycythemia and hyperviscosity. *Clinic Perinatol*, **22** (3), 693–710.

74. Swetman SM, Yabek SM, Alverson DC (1987) Hemodynamic consequences or neonatal polycythemia. *J Pediatr*, **110**, 443–447.

75. Watts T, Roberts A (1999) Haematological abnormalities in the growth-restricted infant. *Semin Neonatol*, **4**, 41–54.

76. Manco-Johnson M, Nuss R (2000) Hemostasis in the neonate. *NeoReviews*, **1** (10), e191–e195.

77. Andrew M (1997) The relevance of developmental hemostasis to hemorrhagic disorders of newborns. *Semin Perinatol*, **21** (1), 70–85.

78. Manco-Johnson M, Nuss R (2000) Hemostasis in the neonate. *NeoReviews*, **1** (10), e191–e195.

79. Castle V, Andrew M, Kelton J, Giron D, Johnston M, Carter C (1986) Frequency and mechanism of neonatal thrombocytopenia. *J Pediatr*, **108** (5, part I), 749–755.

80. Roberts I, Murray N (2003) Neonatal thrombocytopenia: causes and management. *Arch Dis Child Foetal Neonatal Ed*, **88** (5), F359–F363.

81. Roberts I, Murray N (2003) Neonatal thrombocytopenia: causes and management. *Arch Dis Child Foetal Neonatal Ed*, **88** (5), F359–F363.

82. Murray NA (1999) New concepts in the aetiology and management of neonatal thrombocytopenia. *Semin Neonatol*, **4**, 27–40.

83. Clarke P, Shearer M (2007) Vitamin K deficiency bleeding: the readiness is all. *Arch Dis Child*, **92** (9), 741–743.

84. Castle V, Andrew M, Kelton J, Giron D, Johnston M, Carter C (1986) Frequency and mechanism of neonatal thrombocytopenia. *J Pediatr*, **108** (5, part I), 749–755.

85. Roberts I, Murray N (2003) Neonatal thrombocytopenia: causes and management. *Arch Dis Child Foetal Neonatal Ed*, **88** (5), F359–F363.

86. Manco-Johnson M, Nuss R (2000) Hemostasis in the neonate. *NeoReviews*, **1** (10), e191–e195.

87. Hey E (2003) Vitamin K – what, why and when. *Arch Dis Child Foetal Neonatal Ed*, **88** (2), F80–F83.

88. Roberts I, Murray N (2003) Neonatal thrombocytopenia: causes and management. *Arch Dis Child Foetal Neonatal Ed*, **88** (5), F359–F363.

89. Hey E (2003) Vitamin K – what, why and when. *Arch Dis Child Foetal Neonatal Ed*, **88** (2), F80–F83.

90. McNinch A, Busfield A, Tripp J (2007) Vitamin K deficiency bleeding in Great Britain and Ireland: British Paediatric Surveillance Unit surveys, 1993–1994 and 2001–2002. *Arch Dis Child*, **92** (9), 759–766.

91. Manco-Johnson M, Nuss R (2000) Hemostasis in the neonate. *NeoReviews*, **1** (10), e191–e195.

92. Roberts I, Murray N (2003) Neonatal thrombocytopenia: causes and management. *Arch Dis Child Foetal Neonatal Ed*, **88** (5), F359–F363.

Chapter 18

DEVELOPMENTAL CARE

Inga Warren

Learning outcomes

After reading this chapter the reader will be expected to be able to:

- Compare and contrast the conceptual models of developmental care

- Define NIDCAP and summarise the benefits to the individual and family

- Discuss the developmental influences on the preterm brain

- Explain some of the strategies that can be employed within the neonatal unit to support development of the preterm brain

- Describe ways in which an infant communicates with its surroundings

- Explain the principles of support for a preterm infant's posture and comfort

---

Introduction

Developmental care covers a range of interventions that intend to improve the developmental outcomes of preterm infants, and other infants with perinatal problems needing treatment in hospital, usually in neonatal units. It is also perceived as a way to combat stress and pain, and as such should be a basic standard of humane care in the neonatal unit. It complements conventional medical and nursing care with strategies drawn from biological, social and psychological sciences.

Models of developmental care

Developmental care can be summarised in five overlapping conceptual frameworks (see Figure 18.1).

Ethical developmental care

A compelling argument for developmental care is that it is a kinder, more humane way to care for babies, supporting the rights of mother and baby to be together, the right to be protected from unnecessary pain and distress, and the right to breast-feed.

Although 24-hour parent access to infants is reported to be the norm in Northern Europe there continue to be barriers to this in neonatal units in the UK. These include lack of comfortable seating beside the baby, lack of overnight facilities and the exclusion of parents from nurseries during ward rounds and handovers. It seems that paediatric wards are expected to accommodate parents but that neonatal units are not, in spite of the distress that separation so soon after birth obviously generates. While staff may feel that they do not have enough

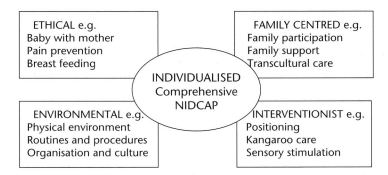

Figure 18.1 Frameworks of developmental care.

time to support parents it is interesting that in a European survey the most negative views about parents' presence were expressed by units who actually had least contact with them[1].

Recent studies demonstrating changes in cortical haemodynamics in response to painful stimuli have strengthened the view that the preterm infant is capable of experiencing pain[2,3]. There is also growing concern about the short and long-term developmental consequences of painful experience during critical early phases of neuromaturation[4]. Nevertheless few neonatal services have reported comprehensive approaches to assessing and managing acute or chronic pain and there are many unresolved issues around pain in the neonatal unit, particularly around the value of analgesia[5,6]. It does appear that there is widespread agreement about the benefits of non-pharmacological (environmental and behavioural) strategies and developmental care has become a front-line defence in the management of stress and pain. Studies of procedures such as venepuncture, heel prick, eye exams, and nappy change show that such strategies reduce signs of pain and distress[7].

The World Health Organisation promotes breast-feeding worldwide for well established health and development benefits. The majority of preterm babies can have expressed breast milk, and can become successful breast-feeders provided that appropriate parent information, with support for mother and baby, is available. Developmental care can make more successful breast-feeding on the neonatal unit a reality[8].

There is a considerable overlap between the philosophy of developmental care and the main points outlined in Levin's manifesto for humane neonatal care[9]. Alderson and colleagues draw on models of developmental care to illustrate the relevance of the United Nations Charter for Children's Rights to infants in neonatal units[10]. Many centres that have integrated developmental care into their philosophy and practice now feel that it is unethical to withhold it, on the basis of both experience and research.

Implication for practice

Developmental care supports the rights of mothers and infants to be together, protected from pain and distress, and the right to be supported in breast-feeding.

Family centred developmental care

Family centred care acknowledges the baby as part of a family unit, and values this unit as the most constant developmental force in the infant's world. The health and well-being of the family are important for the future of the child.

Early attachment relationships are believed to be the foundation of emotional development, and influence the relationships we form throughout our lives. Infant attachment is the sense of trust in the primary caregiver that gives the infant the security and confidence to explore, to play and learn. Attachment is a two-way process. Attached parents are fiercely protective of their children and are constantly looking out for them, which can be challenging for staff on the neonatal unit. Preterm infants are more likely than those born at term to suffer from disorganised attachment, particularly if they have a disability, and also are more likely to have emotional problems later in life and to find it more difficult to relate to their peers[11]. The fostering of strong bonds between the infant and parents as early as possible after birth is therefore a positive investment in development.

A family centred philosophy encourages parents to provide comfort for their baby, to be active partners in their daily care and in decision making, and to be advocates for their baby. Professional psychological support should be provided to enable parents to deal with the emotional roller coaster of having a baby in neonatal intensive care. Every baby changes relationships within the family, often in ways that are not anticipated, but the arrival of a preterm baby can generate shock waves that may radiate throughout the whole circle of family and friends.

The influence of paediatricians, psychoanalysts and psychologists such as T Berry Brazelton, Daniel Sterne and Heidelise Als have raised awareness of the communication skills of preterm/newborn infants and the developmental significance of attunement between parent and infant. Studies have shown that the mother's sensitivity to her infant's behavioural cues influences development[12,13]. Several intervention programmes that have helped parents with the art of reading their baby have had positive outcomes[14–16].

Implication for practice

A family centred philosophy of care facilitates the development of early attachment.

Environmental developmental care

There is growing awareness of how the physical environment affects the well-being and development of infants. Guidelines for the physical and developmental environment have been generated by a consensus group that meets biannually in the USA to agree evidence based standards for the physical and developmental environment of neonatal nurseries[17]. These make recommendations for environments that protect the baby from harm and facilitate developmentally appropriate experience, and will be referred to later.

The impact of bright light, loud noise and noxious smells on preterm infant behaviour can be demonstrated, but controlling for a single factor in an otherwise chaotic environment is unlikely to have an impact on health and development. Studies that have claimed to find effects from controlling light exposure have failed to take into account the impact of the experimental measures on staff behaviour and the way infants were cared for. Temporary adjustments to create a benign hiatus, for example 'quiet hours', are unlikely to make an impact on a brain that is developmentally susceptible for 24 hours a day. Adaptations to the physical environment to make it less stressful and more developmentally appropriate are just one step in the complex process of reaching a successful level of developmental care.

Temporal and social organisation in the nursery is part of the environment. Routines reduce effort, and can be particularly helpful for novices as they learn to cope with the demanding complexities of neonatal care; therefore the shift to baby focused developmental care is challenging; it means that caregiving becomes centred on the baby, blending with the baby's sleep-wake patterns and creating opportunities for family participation. Organisational structures within institutions and neonatal services also influence the way developmental care is implemented, and how change in practice is achieved. It can take years for a nursery to reach a standard of developmental care that could be expected to make a difference to outcomes. Lack of cost effectiveness studies makes it difficult for hesitant organisations to make the commitment to allocate resources for this.

Developmental interventions

Developmental interventions involve doing something to the baby with the expectation of improving outcomes. Within this category are activities such as positioning, kangaroo care and sensory stimulation programmes, including massage.

As a biomechanical intervention, positioning is often recommended to improve physiological functions or motor development. Studies mainly compare prone with supine positions using an array of outcomes including respiration, circulation, digestion, heat loss and energy expenditure, head shape, postural development, sleep and risk of cot death. Although the results are variable and sometimes inconsistent these studies have certainly influenced caregiving in neonatal units, with proliferation of positioning protocols that focus more on the bedding than the baby. Positioning that improves comfort and enhances self-regulatory behaviours is built into the comprehensive, individualised model of developmental care. The merits of infants sleeping on their backs at home to reduce the risk of cot death make this an imperative, particularly for preterm infants as they prepare for discharge from hospital.

The practice of the mother holding her baby upright against her chest for skin-to-skin or kangaroo care was born out of necessity in Colombia and has spread across the developing world as a way to improve mortality and morbidity in communities that have limited access to high tech neonatal care [18]. In developed countries kangaroo care is a way to humanise the technical environment and culture of neonatal units, encouraging closeness between parent and baby, and successful breast-feeding. There is some evidence that kangaroo care can enhance physiological stability, improve breast-feeding uptake and also make the mother feel more confident. However, kangaroo care is an example of an intervention that, without quality control, can be a good or bad experience for parent and baby. As Charpak tells us nurses need to be properly trained to do this sensitively and safely, and each nursery needs its own guidelines [19–20].

Sensory stimulation programmes in which babies are subjected to controlled stimulation in one or more modalities were particularly popular in the early days of neonatal intensive care when preterm babies were larger and were thought to suffer from sensory deprivation. This was followed by a phase in which, as babies began to survive at earlier and earlier ages, the neonatal unit was perceived as being too stimulating and the idea of reducing stimulation through 'minimal handling' was born. Minimal handling is not likely to reduce the number of medical procedures a baby has, but it does discourage loving contact between baby and parents, and nursing care that is responsive to the infant's behavioural cues [21], and is thus inconsistent with current thinking about the importance of care being orientated around the baby's expressed needs. Minimal handling encourages clustering of procedures and cares, which may sometimes be sensible but is often overwhelming, particularly with smaller babies [22].

There is little evidence that sensory stimulation programmes generalised for all babies in the nursery are effective; some infants may respond positively to these interventions while others may have a negative reaction, and so the sensory stimulation paradigm has shifted from the quantitative to the qualitative, with stimulation for the infant guided by knowledge about foetal and newborn developmental expectations, and an understanding of the baby's behavioural repertoire.

Massage is a controversial intervention on the NICU. In spite of a large body of research indicating that nurturing touch is not harmful, massage on the neonatal unit needs to be considered carefully and cautiously due to the vulnerability of small fragile infants to handling [23, 24]. The idea that nurses should massage other people's babies or that babies should experience prescribed doses of massage using specific techniques is not compatible with the philosophy of the International

Infant Massage Association, or with family centred or individualised developmental care. Cherry Bond's 'Positive Touch' programme, which emphasises the dialogue of touch between infant and parent is an example of how a potentially overwhelming intervention can be adapted to meet the most sensitive baby's needs, with parents as the natural medium for loving touch[25].

Implications for practice

Low light and noise levels with opportunities for 'skin to skin' care contribute to an environment that suits the developmental needs of preterm infants.

Individualised developmental care: NIDCAP

The Newborn Individualised Developmental Care and Assessment Programme (NIDCAP), developed by Heidelise Als and colleagues at Harvard Medical School and the Children's Hospital Boston in the 1980s, has had wide-reaching influence on developmental care. NIDCAP is a complex, inclusive, dynamic programme that is individualised to suit the changing needs of each baby and family. The baby's needs are assessed through detailed observation and analysis of behavioural interactions with the caregiving environment. NIDCAP is unique in that it is quality controlled through rigorous, formal training and quality assurance policies governed by an international board (NIDCAP Federation International).

The synactive theory underpinning NIDCAP describes the continuous interaction between the baby's autonomic, motor and state subsystems of functioning, and between the baby and the environment[26,27]. The baby reveals competence and vulnerability in each subsystem, with behaviours that indicate approach or avoidance. Approach behaviours signify that the baby is coping with challenges and is comfortable, while avoidance behaviours show that the baby is feeling uncomfortable or overwhelmed. Approach behaviours

typically included flexed and groping movements, while avoidance behaviours are typically extended, defensive, or withdrawing. If stimulation and caregiving are pitched right the baby will stay in balance, move forwards, relax or pay attention; if not the baby will pull away, shut down or become disorganised. The baby's ability to self-regulate and stay in balance has to be matched by the caregiver's co-regulatory role. The caregiver permits developmentally appropriate challenges while offering the baby enough support to meet these challenges successfully without crossing stress thresholds.

Regular and frequent NIDCAP reporting for all babies is unlikely to be practical in most nurseries but a NIDCAP trained leader is able to help everyone in the NICU team to appreciate the subtle, individual and changing needs of each baby, raising awareness of their capabilities and furnishing examples of ways to act as co-regulators of the baby's own efforts to cope and move on[28]. NIDCAP strategies can be incorporated into all aspects of neonatal care. Surveys of staff working on units that practice NIDCAP show decidedly positive support for NIDCAP, with few reservations[29,30].

It has been extremely difficult to carry out large randomised control trials with NIDCAP due to the complexity of the interventions, the small number of babies available for single site studies, and insufficient numbers of staff trained to the required standard to ensure quality control. Six randomised controlled trials (RCTs) have been completed and published to date and are included in the Cochrane Review[31]. An additional study in Canada is awaiting publication. These RCTs show that NIDCAP is safe and has benefits for health (e.g. lower incidence of chronic lung disease, less need for intensive care) and developmental outcomes, re-confirming NIDCAP as the leading and most promising model of developmental care. Another recent meta-analysis confirmed a statistically significant developmental advantage for NIDCAP babies compared to controls on developmental testing at 9 months: 1 year corrected age[32]. Longer term outcomes are awaited.

Implication for practice

NIDCAP advocates detailed observation to assess the infant and proposes individualised caregiving strategies.

Why does developmental care make sense? Influences on preterm/newborn development

During the last trimester of pregnancy the brain undergoes the most rapid and significant period of brain development in the human lifespan. For babies who are born prematurely and are discharged from the expected eco-niche of the healthy uterus the neonatal team are in fact the guardians of those brains at a particularly vulnerable period. While much of this growth and development is genetically driven and has its own momentum the preterm baby's experience is also important at this time[33]. We should therefore consider how to provide the best possible climate for preterm brain development. Two studies have examined the impact of developmental care on brain structure and/or function (both of them are NIDCAP studies) and both show more mature brain development in the NIDCAP intervention cohort[34,35]. The influences on brain development that are susceptible to intervention are outlined below.

Implications for practice

Key elements of the NIDCAP are expert observation skills and the art of narrative writing to tell the baby's story, portraying the baby as a competent individual with goals. Recommendations reinforce strategies that appear helpful to the baby and suggest ideas for caregivers to consider. NIDCAP encourages reflective practice and clinical reasoning, moving us away from a task and protocol based outlook to one that is dynamic and interactive. Parents are a key part of this process.

Physiological stability

The developing preterm brain requires a stable physiological climate. This includes factors such as well-regulated temperature, blood circulation, hormonal balance and appropriate supply of oxygen and nutrients. Physiological stability is influenced by physical, social and temporal aspects of the environment: light and noise, positioning and handling, pain and comfort, the timing and pacing of caregiving and procedures. These can all be adjusted to make a positive difference, for example helping the baby breathe more easily, thus reducing the need for ventilation and associated developmental risks. Similar strategies can conserve energy for growth, and improve digestion so that nutrition is more effective, and as the baby prepares to go home, environmental strategies promote successful feeding, state regulation and ability to pay attention and interact socially.

Stress and pain

Stress and pain are not good for the brain. High levels of stress hormones may be damaging and repeated painful experiences in infants have been shown to interfere with later pain perception and the ability to mount an adequate stress response[36]. Preterm infants endure many painful and stressful events in the course of treatment and the use of analgesia and sedation is being questioned. Even apparently non-painful events such as nappy change and weighing generate considerable signs of distress[37]. Developmental care offers non-pharmacological strategies that can be tailored to fit the baby and the task in hand.

Sleep

Sleep, both quiet and active, has been cited as an important influence on brain development[38]. Growth hormone release takes place during quiet sleep and neuronal organisation is particularly dependent on active (REM) sleep. It is difficult to imagine what would be the normal sleep pattern of a preterm infant in the neonatal unit, for the infant is without the moderating influence of the mother's circadian rhythms and sleep is constantly disrupted by alarming sounds and unexpected handling. Developmental care has been shown to increase sleep time in one study by Bertelle *et al.*[39].

Sensory stimulation

During the last trimester of pregnancy when the vast majority of neurones have already migrated to predetermined locations in the cortex the process of sculpting useful pathways of communication within the brain is in progress. The generation of synapses to pass information between cells is a somewhat promiscuous process. Not all of these connections will be used or needed and the pruning of surplus connections, refining the pathways to make the brain more efficient, begins before term. Many synaptic connections are activated by sensory stimulation occurring at critical periods when the brain expects them. Evidence from animal studies shows how interference with expected sensory inputs at critical phases can permanently alter brain structure and function[40]. Not so much is yet known about critical periods in foetal and preterm brain development but it is speculated that inappropriate and out of phase sensory inputs contribute to the cognitive and perceptual problems often seen in children born prematurely. The job of developmental care is to provide appropriate sensory experience in all modalities, keeping pace with the infant's developmental trajectory.

Parenting

The relationship between infant and parent has a crucial determining influence on development. Through close bodily contact parents provide the physiological climate for well-being, and the sensory experience the newborn infant normally needs. Touch and smell have particular influence

on the chemistry of attachment, the strong emotional bond that grows mutually between parent and child. Healthy attachment ensures that the child is kept safe and well, and contributes to the developing sense of self-worth that enables children to play, explore and learn. Concerns about the separation endured by parents and infants as a result of admission to the neonatal unit and the possible effect this may have on later development has been heightened by evidence that children born preterm are more likely to suffer abuse[41].

A child's development is influenced by the mother's sensitivity to her infant's behavioural cues. The children of mothers who can read their babies' cues do better developmentally[42,43]. The process of learning to parent a premature baby is complicated, not just by separation, the emotional impact of giving birth prematurely and anxiety about the baby, but also because the behaviour of preterm babies is more difficult to read. Positive Touch Parent Infant Transaction Programmes[44–47] and NIDCAP are all examples of developmental care programmes that enhance early parent-infant communication.

Implications for practice

Developmental care plans will be influenced by the baby's gestational age as well as medical condition.

Strategies for developmental care

It appears from the evidence currently available that complex, multidimensional interventions are more likely to be effective than single strategies. The evidence also supports an individualised approach[48]. Making universal recommendations for all babies can be harmful. Examples of this are insisting that all babies are kept in complete darkness at all times regardless of developmental stage or need to be observed, or playing background music on the grounds that this is therapeutic for all babies. Strategies like quiet hours, while providing welcome respite from the hullabaloo of intensive care are unlikely to enhance development as the baby's brain is susceptible to the environment for 24 hours of the day and a calm, quiet atmosphere is something to aim for all day and all night. These points may seem common sense, but in a complex, high-risk, protocol driven setting such as the modern neonatal unit, task orientated care based on rules and routines tends to dominate.

Implication for practice

Perhaps the most important rule in developmental care is that everything we do should involve dialogue with the baby.

The strategies outlined below should be combined in a comprehensive approach. Clinical governance issues can be addressed by ensuring staff have the knowledge to engage in problem solving around the individual needs of babies in the context within which care will be implemented. The needs of a ventilated 24-week gestation infant will obviously be different to those of a healthy 35 week gestation infant; in both cases strategies will need to reflect the infant's and parents' individual characteristics as well as current health and development status. Opportunities for implementing some strategies will be influenced by staffing levels and the structural properties of the building; nevertheless many strategies can be implemented anywhere, with some imagination and reorganisation.

Create a comfortable environment for babies, parents and staff

Sound

Sound levels recommended by the Florida consensus group are an average of not more than 45 decibels (dB) per hour for background noise levels, and peak noises of no more than 65 dB[49].

Noise levels are influenced by building design and materials, locations and equipment, but the greatest impact on sound levels is likely to be staff behaviour. In practice most sounds over 55 dB can be modified or eliminated. Preterm infants have well developed hearing but lack the ability to habituate to meaningless stimuli or to distinguish between background and foreground noise. So while staff may get so used to the sounds of alarms, taps, packaging, bin lids and cupboard doors slamming, loud talking and laughing, and hardly notice them, the very preterm may be unsettled by every sound. In the face of this cacophony the baby may 'shut down' and be unable to arouse for social interaction or to feed. (See Care Example 18.1.)

Staff who wish to have music playing while they work should bear in mind that, apart from the

---

Care Example 18.1

Maryam gave birth to Ali unexpectedly when she and her family were visiting London. She lives in Dubai. Her husband and other two children have already gone home and she is desperate to join them with Ali. Today the doctors have told her that he will be able to leave hospital as soon as he can manage all his feeds. Because Maryam needs medication that is contraindicated for breast-feeding Ali is bottle-fed with formula. The nurses tell her that he took all his bottles in the night. She is sitting in the special care nursery with Ali on her lap, his bottle feed half finished. His arms dangle by his sides, he is asleep, his mouth drooping open. The small nursery is crowded; a doctor is doing tests and all the lights are on; a baby is crying; a monitor alarm is ringing; people are walking backwards and forwards past Maryam and Ali; parents and nurses are talking. There is a smaller room next door and we suggest that Maryam takes Ali in there. The curtains are drawn and the lights switched off. It is quiet and shady. As soon as they are settled in this room Ali opens his eyes. He opens and closes his mouth. Maryam offers him the bottle again and he sucks readily, grasping her hand, finishing his feed.

Copyright I. Warren

fact that music can have undesirable physiological effects, from the baby's perspective music added to other sounds in the room amounts to more noise, noise that makes it difficult to pick out the familiar mother's voice, difficult to sleep properly, difficult to feed and pay attention. It is not only babies who are affected; noise is not good for parents or staff either[50]. Tolerance to sounds (including music) varies from person to person but working in a noisy place impairs work performance, increases the risk of errors and interferes with communication.

Light

Preterm infants are not adapted to cope with bright light and the developmental expectation is for darkness. Eyelids are thin and pupil constriction does not begin until 30–32 weeks gestation so the very preterm infant has weak defences against bright light. If babies are not individually protected with incubator covers and canopies, constant moderate background lighting will be better than abrupt changes from dim to bright as lights are switched on and off for procedures. Term babies need enough light to see shapes and forms clearly in order for vision to develop normally.

In the absence of clear evidence about light and circadian rhythms in preterm infants, two options can be considered. The first is to adjust lighting to fit the baby's behaviour and developmental stage, taking into account foetal expectation for darkness and sensitivity to light. The second approach, recommended by the Vermont Oxford Potential best practice project is to break constant low level of light with a two-hour period of moderate lighting during the day from 32 weeks gestation onwards[51]. Moderate lighting of 200–300 lux during the day is sufficient to entrain circadian patterns, and also for staff to perform most caregiving tasks and procedures safely.

Lowering the light seems to have a calming effect on everyone in the nursery, reducing noise and the pace of activity, but working in low-level lighting is a concern for some people who fear this will affect their own well-being, and

safe working. Lighting affects staff performance and alertness[52]. Preparation for a demanding task that requires high visual performance must include lighting that is sufficient for safe performance *and* light protection for the baby.

Visual array

The range of equipment in intensive care presents an intimidating barrier to parents and whenever possible equipment should be fitted discretely using wall mountings or attachments to the distal end of the incubator so that parents have direct access and a view of their baby on entering the nursery. Colour and organisation of space may also affect relaxation and mood. There should be soft colours, open spaces and mild nursery motifs suggesting gentle, baby-centred care, in contrast to bright colours and walls busily covered in pictures, notices and murals, which can create a distracting, disconcerting atmosphere. The bold, bright patterns that are marketed as developmental accessories for newborn babies are likely to be overwhelming when placed at close range. (See Care Example 18.2.)

Care Example 18.2

Gus was dangling a black and white disc in front of Shanika's face. At first Shanika stared at it with a panicky expression, and then she turned her head away, poking out her tongue. She got hiccups and shut her eyes. Her arms dangled by her side. Gus put the toy away, pulled the blanket more closely around Shanika and sat quietly gazing at his daughter. After a few minutes Shanika wriggled, and opened her eyes looking towards her father. She shut her eyes again. Gus moved his face a little further away and this time when Shanika opened her eyes she looked towards him, her face softening. Gus smiled. 'I think she knows me,' he whispered.

Copyright I. Warren

Smell and taste

Smell and taste are important, underrated, moderators of behaviour. Preterm infants are affected by irritants and unpleasant odours and may react negatively to chemicals such as cleaning fluids and perfume. Conversely, they react positively to familiar maternal odours[53]. The ability of infants to recognise the characteristic maternal odours of amniotic fluid and breast milk may play a part in attachment, breast-feeding and reducing stress; therefore opportunities for close physical proximity, e.g. kangaroo care, are important and efforts should be made to avoid masking maternal odour with perfume or other chemicals.

Parent participation and support

In a NICU that supports developmental care parents will be wholeheartedly welcomed to be present and involved in their baby's care as much as possible. Comfortable seating that is suitable for kangaroo care will be provided; there will be adjacent facilities for parents to relax, eat and make hot drinks, welcome family and friends; rooms for sleeping over night will be available; ward rounds will be organised away from the bedside or will be conducted discretely in small groups so that parents are not required to leave the room.

An important role for parents is to comfort their baby. The Positive Touch programme developed by Cherry Bond, works on the principle of a four-step dialogue to guide parents to give their baby comfort (see Box 18.1). This

Box 18.1 The dialogue of Positive Touch: a guide for parents

Step 1 *Preparation*: set the scene with a quiet calm, softly lit background. Prepare yourself with comfortable seating, warm hands, relaxed breathing.
Step 2 *Permission*: let your baby know you are there. Watch for a reaction and adjustment before touching your baby. Be prepared in case your baby's response tells you that he/she is not ready just now. Tell your baby what is going to happen next. At the first touch wait for your baby to relax before moving on.

Step 3 *Pacing*: as you proceed, watch carefully for signs that your baby is becoming wary, upset or tired, then pause and help your baby to settle.
Step 4 *Parting*: let your baby know you are leaving. Make your baby comfortable in the bed, say goodbye and gradually withdraw your hands.
Adapted from Bond C, 2002. Copyright C Bond (2002) Positive Touch and massage in the neonatal unit: a British approach. Semin *Neonatol*, **7** (6), 477–486.

leads parents towards an understanding of how their baby communicates, how individual temperament and characteristic will shape the way they will develop as a parent – baby dyad.

Addressing parents' concerns will help to create an atmosphere in which parents will feel more confident about engaging in their baby's care. High on the list is the appearance of the baby. Positioning of the baby, bedding, clothing and personal items in the bed can all contribute to the baby's comfort, softening the impact of the many lines, tapes and tubes required for intensive care and emphasising the much appreciated personal touch. Privacy is another issue and being able to show love for your baby in the way you want can be very difficult in full view and hearing distance of doctors, nurses and other parents. The way we share information and decisions also makes a difference to parenting confidence.

Gentle procedures and cares

Strategies that support the baby's comfort and stability during difficult procedures are those that facilitate behaviours such as grasping and hand clasping, foot bracing or clasping, arms and legs folded towards body, hands on face or to mouth, sucking. (See Care Example 18.3.)

Care Example 18.3

When Claire came back from her coffee break the new doctor had already started to take a blood sample from Amy. He was preparing a second attempt on her right foot. Amy lay on her back, the spot light full on her, her bedclothes in a tangle. She was thrusting her arms in the air, fussing and grimacing, alternately pulling her knees up and then stiffly stretching her legs out. She was breathing more quickly than usual and looked dusky around the chin and eyes. Claire got some sucrose from the fridge. She directed the spotlight away from Amy's face and talked quietly to her, telling her what was happening as she turned her to her side and made her comfortable. She kept talking to Amy, one hand resting on her shoulder, and telling her what was going to happen. The doctor placed a drop of sucrose in Amy's mouth. Claire found the little dummy that Amy's mother had agreed she could use for comfort, and offered it to Amy who hesitated before accepting it and then sucked rhythmically. Claire folded a blanket into a strip, laid it over Amy's shoulder and tucked it firmly in under the mattress. Amy brought her hands together and clasped them under her chin. She lay quietly, eyes closed, her feet resting on a rolled blanket at the bottom of her bed. Claire cupped Amy's head with one hand, shading her eyes. Amy tensed briefly as the doctor pricked her foot and then relaxed, appearing to sleep. After a few moments she stretched her legs a little as he squeezed her foot harder and then relaxed again. Claire asked the doctor to tell Amy when he had finished. He looked a little puzzled but did as he was asked, saying 'Well done Amy'. Claire slowly removed her hands and watched Amy for a few minutes. Amy lay quietly sleeping, she breathed more gently and began to look pinker.

Copyright I. Warren

A step-by-step approach to managing procedures effectively with the minimum of distress to the baby begins with careful preparation, choosing an advantageous time for the baby, setting the scene with a calm atmosphere, having everything ready so the baby receives the caregiver's full attention. If additional support will help the baby this may be planned with parents or a colleague. The baby is approached in a gradual way to help achieve a smooth transition and the activity is paced to keep within the infant's

stress thresholds, pausing for recovery time as necessary. Opportunities to grasp, brace and suck are offered and bedding or hands provide gentle support to keep the baby calm and comfortable. At the end of the procedure the baby is made comfortable and held gently to allow him/her to settle. These measures are likely to make it easier to complete procedures successfully, and babies will be more settled and less demanding afterwards.

Developmental care strategies that help to alleviate chronic pain and distress may also make it easier to regulate the use of medication[54,55]. Systematic attention to details, such as posture that encourages self-regulation, containment of tiring movement, management of stressors in the environment, and energy conservation should be part of routine observations.

Many procedures that are not thought of as painful can also cause distress and disorganisation[56]. Effective developmental care is integrated into all aspects of neonatal care and many ways can be found to adapt potentially stressful procedures to increase infant comfort. The following are some examples (each task can be adapted in other ways):

(1) *Weighing* is more easily accomplished with two people and can often be smoothly integrated with other activities such as bedding change or kangaroo care. Parents keenly awaiting the news of progress towards homecoming will eagerly assist. The baby can be undressed and gently transferred to the scales wearing a nappy and wrapped in a sheet, both of which have already been weighed. The baby can then be transferred directly to the parent's chest for skin-to-skin kangaroo care.

(2) *Nasogastric tube insertion* usually goes more smoothly if the baby is laid on the side and given a dummy to suck while the tube is inserted. The narrower the tube the less it will irritate the baby. Like many other procedures this can often be done while the baby is held by a parent.

(3) *Nappy change* can also be done in the side lying position, discouraging caregivers from distressing the baby by lifting legs in the air. The arms and shoulders can be wrapped to keep hands close together and to help the baby stay settled. Sucking can also be encouraged if the baby has a dummy. The caregiver rests one hand on the baby, hooking the upper knee in his/her thumb to flex the leg, making access to the genital area easy for cleaning with the other hand. The baby is gently rolled over, with both of the caregiver's hands supporting the body, to allow the nappy to be fastened on the underside.

(4) *Bathing* should be reserved for parents. The first bath is a special occasion and fathers often like to be present. There is no need for nurses to bath babies. Parents may have their own ideas of how a baby should be bathed, which can be discussed. The process is rehearsed with dolls so parents can anticipate what they will do. During the first bath it is easier if the baby is wrapped in a cloth. The baby is slowly lowered into a bath of deep, warm water, feet first, pausing with any sign of tension to allow the baby to adjust. Once in the water the baby is placed with feet in bracing range of the wall of the bath while the sheet is gradually unwrapped.

Timing events to suit the baby is another challenge on a busy unit and nurses have an important coordinating role, negotiating rest for the baby, responding when the baby needs help, adjusting the day to fit round parents and essential tasks such as feeding, changing nappies, or medical tests, taking vital signs, arranging kangaroo care. Anecdotal evidence suggests that individualised developmental care does not take more time, because babies are more settled.

Support for functional posture and organised movements

Until close to the end of pregnancy the foetus is very active in the womb, twisting and turning, stretching and grasping, sucking fingers and toes, and acquiring a considerable amount of experience in the process. The work of Heinz Prechtl and colleagues shows that in spite of the disadvantage of gravity, preterm infants in the period equivalent to the last two months of pregnancy produce waves of spontaneous, varied and fluent movements involving the whole body and including rotations. In light of this knowledge positioning has to be a dynamic rather than a static intervention.

Postural support is a careful balance between facilitating development of natural movement patterns that the baby uses for self-regulation, exploration or exercise, and containing or limiting disorganised movements that lead to instability. It also involves support for the sleeping, medicated or exhausted baby to prevent long periods in static positions that lead to muscle shortening and postural patterns that will slow later development, e.g. retracted shoulders (preventing bringing hands together and to mouth), torticollis (leading to asymmetrical orientation) and tightness of hip extensors and abductors (leading to frog-leg posture, delayed sitting and 'Charlie Chaplin' walk).

Positioning is much more complex than the 'flexion with midline orientation' paradigm that dominates positioning protocols. The baby's own goals may include being able to stretch and wriggle when he/she needs to get his/her breathing going again, to be able to put his/her hands over his/her eyes or ears to fend off light and noise, to be able to steady him/herself by bracing or clasping his/her feet, by grasping and holding on to his/her own hands, or anything else that is handy, by being able to stretch out if he/she is too hot, and perhaps anchor his/her hands under his/her head or chin to stay quietly asleep. These are not, of course, conscious choices but belong to a repertoire of innate behaviours that human beings use to survive. The creative use of bedding arranged *around the baby* to provide support where and when it is needed, whether the baby is on the front, back or side, is an art that is based on an understanding of what the baby is striving towards. The degree of support necessary will depend on how the baby is managing in all the domains outlined in the synactive model, i.e. autonomic, motor and state.

Side lying, the least researched position, is often recommended in developmental care because this position reduces the need to work against gravity and thus maximises the baby's competence, and active efforts to settle (self-regulate). Although prone positioning is often recommended for stabilising the chest wall to improve ventilation, to increase sleep and improve energy conservation, babies can often be made equally comfortable on their side. The baby will indicate when a position change is needed. (See Care Example 18.4).

Care Example 18.4

Martin was 35 weeks gestation when he was born. On arrival at the NICU he was breathing with difficulty, his chest wall recessing. His nurse put him on his front to help with his breathing. Martin cried and struggled, lifting his head and moving it from side to side. His nurse turned him over, placing him on his side. He lay quietly, eyes open, scanning his surroundings, still breathing with great effort. After ten minutes he began to fuss again and his nurse turned him back on to his tummy. Martin immediately went to sleep.

Copyright I. Warren

Perhaps the most obvious position for any baby is to be attached to his mother in the skin-to-skin kangaroo care style. Charpak emphasises correct positioning and binding of the baby to the mother and suggests a minimum of two hours to get the full benefit[57]; the baby will let it be known when he/she has had enough. Kangaroo care may be suggested for ventilated babies; several people will be needed to manage the transfers safely as this is the riskiest and most destabilising phase of kangaroo care. Other guidelines have suggested that kangaroo care should not be offered with extremely preterm babies in the first week, to give the skin a chance to mature and to reduce the risk of temperature instability. As several authors point

out it is important that each neonatal unit has well thought out guidelines for kangaroo care[58] (see Care Examples 18. 5 and 18.6).

Care Example 18.5

The nurse placed a rolled sheet in an oval shape on the mattress in the incubator and covered it with a blanket to make a 'nest' for Jamil. She placed him on his tummy with a small roll under his hips, in the middle of the ring. Jamil stretched out his legs, looking for something to press his feet on and extended them over the rim of the nest. He continued to wriggle, twisting his head round, arching his back, pressing up on his hands, and stretching out his legs. Half an hour later he was lying half in and half out of the blanket ring, the roll had shifted and now lay under his abdomen. He looked limp, breathed quickly and was dipping his oxygen levels every few minutes.

The shift changed and Pam, his new nurse, greeted Jamil and gently lifted him back into the dip in the nest, removing the roll under him and turning him onto his side. She deconstructed the old nest and rolled up a towel which she placed to support his back. She rolled another into a firm fat roll and placed it where his feet touched it as he stretched out his legs. She folded a small soft blanket and placed it so that he could wrap his arms around it. Around this construction she arranged a rolled sheet to hold everything together and laid a soft blanket over his body and legs. Jamil put one hand near his mouth, resting the other on the blanket before him. He pushed his feet against the roll at the bottom of his bed, relaxed and drifted off to sleep. He settled his breathing and stabilised his oxygen saturation level.

Copyright I. Warren

Care Example 18.6

Maria is in the SCBU because she has difficulty keeping herself warm. Maria's nurse told Carlos and Delia that they could bring some personal things for Maria and they have arrived with a soft cotton wrap and a little hat and jacket. Maria is just waking and is squinting in the light coming in from the window above her. There are several other mothers and fathers in the room. Delia speaks softly to her daughter and strokes her face. Maria's feed is due and the nurse asks Delia if she would like to breast-feed Maria. Delia is keen and settles down in the chair with Maria, who is wearing a thick cardigan over her baby suit. Delia loosens her blouse and bra and puts Maria close to her breast. Maria opens her mouth and moves her head from side to side brushing against her cardigan and her mother's clothing. She starts to get upset. The nurse brings a screen to give them some privacy so that Delia feels comfortable exposing more of her breast for Maria. The nurse suggests that they take off the bulky cardigan, wrap Maria in her new blanket and put on her new hat to keep her warm. She also adjusts the blinds to shut out the sunlight. After a couple of attempts Maria latches on to the breast and takes three sucks. Her first successful breast feed!

Copyright I. Warren

Sensitive feeding

Feeding is an important part of the emotional, nurturing relationship between mother and baby. Feeding is about communication as well as nutrition, whether it is by tube, breast or bottle. Breast-feeding is undoubtedly the method for which the baby is developmentally adapted, and is possible for almost every baby in the NICU. The developmental approach to feeding is an individualised approach emphasising observation, pacing, comfort and dialogue with the baby. Feeding and nutrition will be addressed in detail elsewhere in this book. The following examples are given to illustrate how developmental care supports successful feeding.

(1) *Tube feeding*: while a baby is tube fed the caregiver can rest a hand on the baby to feel the baby's reactions, anticipate discomfort and respond by slowing or pausing the flow of milk according to the baby's behavioural signs. If the baby is awake the tube feed can be done with the baby lying chest to chest, preferably against the parent's skin where

the advantages of oxytocin release can have a beneficial effect on digestion. The size of the feeding tube may make a difference to the baby's comfort and the smallest possible diameter tube is recommended (size 4 preferable to size 6 for example).

(2) *Breast-feeding*: this is the normal developmental progression and can be the standard for neonatal units provided staff are able to provide the right information and support for the mother and baby, including helpful scene setting (see Care example 18.6). Breast-feeding has the advantage of being inevitably baby led as the baby has control of when and how much he/she can manage. Breast-feeding can be introduced as early as the baby shows interest in licking or nuzzling the breast.

(3) *Bottle feeding*: this is occasionally necessary. Insensitive bottle feeding can be an ordeal for any baby and can result in aversive feeding disorders so it is particularly important that the baby is carefully observed and approached, and avoidance signs are noted. Successful feeding very much depends on well regulated breathing and it is particularly important to help the baby to pace suck/swallow bursts with breathing. Bottle feeding can be introduced in a position that more closely simulates breast-feeding with the baby lying on the side, head higher than feet, chin slightly raised, with the back supported. In this position the baby is able to move away from the teat when he/she wants to, and if more milk is taken into the mouth than can be swallowed it will leak out rather than forcing the baby to gulp. Back support in this position keeps the head and trunk comfortably aligned for efficient breathing, stomach emptying and release of wind.

Conclusion

The evidence we have to date is enough to reassure the enthusiasts that a comprehensive, individualised approach to developmental care, most clearly conceptualised in the Newborn Individualised Developmental Care and Assessment Program (NIDCAP), is the right thing to do, but not yet enough to convert the sceptics who would like large good quality randomised controlled trials with long-term outcomes, which will probably never be possible for such a complex intervention. Deconstructing developmental care to single elements may look an attractive research proposition but is theoretically implausible and results are likely to be drowned by interfering variables. Many leaders in neonatology are coming to the conclusion that, regardless of the evidence on long-term developmental outcomes, this is a better, kinder way to care for babies. The real debate now hinges on whether or not one needs knowledge and skills to make it work.

Like any other form of treatment one should expect developmental care to depend on careful observation of signs, evidence based recommendations for treatment and evaluation of results. Thus, the caregiver needs to be skilled at observing and interpreting preterm and newborn behaviour, and knowledgeable about foetal, preterm and newborn development, about mothers and fathers, families and cultural influences. Developmental leaders need to be rigorous in their critical evaluation of research, old and new, in order to draw on evidence regardless of whether or not they think that developmental care is common sense; in this field, as in others, accepted truths have been turned on their head. Like any other innovation, developmental care needs to be evaluated, whether this is for safety or cost effectiveness, parent or staff satisfaction, infant comfort or medical and developmental benefits. When it is perceived to be effective it will be accepted. To be effective it requires knowledge and skill.

To practice developmental care is not merely a question of knowledge and skill, or even approval: it requires organisational change. The biggest challenges are relationships and systems within the neonatal service. For developmental care to be truly effective it needs to be part of the NICU culture rather than a personal choice. Becoming proficient in developmental care is a process, and while each member of the team can be expected to be at a different stage in that process, whether or not the team moves forwards as a whole will depend on the vision and support of its leaders

A developmental care ethos extends to staff as well as parents and babies. Individualised, family centred care encourages us to focus on the baby and family, shifting the emphasis from tasks to relationships. This makes us more conscious of our feelings about what we are doing. Managing these emotions can be difficult and opportunities for reflective supervision are important to help staff deal with the complexities of relationship based practice.

As Cohen points out, in order for us to keep the baby and family in mind we need to keep each other in mind[59]. Developmental care is part of a nurturing, supportive culture for everyone within the neonatal nursery. At the heart of this is the baby. The dialogue between each baby and his/her special caregivers is the essence of developmental care.

Acknowledgements

I would like to thank Cherry Bond for her contributions to this chapter, and Beryl King for her suggestions in the finishing stages. The care examples are based on true stories but names and personal details have been changed.

NIDCAP training

More information is available at: www.nidcap.org

Positive touch

More information from: www.cherrybond.com

Recommended reading

1. Charpak N (2006) *Kangaroo Babies*. Souvenir Press, London.
2. Cohen M (2003) *Sent Before My Time*. Karnac Books (The Tavistock Clinic Series), London.
3. Kenner C, McGrath JM (eds) (2004) *Developmental Care of Newborns and Infants: a Guide for Health Professionals*. National Association of Neonatal Nurses. Mosby, St Louis.
4. Philbin MK, Graven SN, Robertson A (2000) The influence of auditory experience on the foetus, newborn, and preterm infant: report of the Sound Study Group of the National Resource Centre: the Physical and Developmental Environment of the High Risk Infant. *Journal of Perinatology*, **20** (8), part 2.
5. Sizun J, Browne JV (2005) *Research on Early Developmental Care for Preterm Neonates*. John Libbey Eurotext, Paris.
6. Vergara ER, Bigsby R (2004) *Developmental and Therapeutic Intervention in the NICU*. Paul Brookes Publishing Co., Baltimore.
7. White D (ed.) (2004) The sensory environment of the NICU: scientific and design related aspects. *Clinics in Perinatology*, **31** (2), 199–388.

Video series from VIDA Health Communications Inc.: www.vida-health.Com

Focus on the brain. Part 1: The science of preterm infant development

Focus on the brain. Part 2: Clinical practices for special care nurseries

For parents: No matter how small.

References

1. Cuttini M, Chiandotto V, Barba BD, Cavazzuti GB, Zanini R, Reid M (2000) Visiting policies in neonatal intensive care units: staff and parents' views. *Arch Dis Child Foetal Neonatal Ed*, **82** (2), F172.
2. Slater R, Boyd S, Meek J, Fitzgerald M (2006) Cortical pain responses in the infant brain. *Pain*, **123** (3), 332, author reply 332–334.
3. Bartocci M., Bergqvist LL, Lagercrantz H, Anand KJ (2006) Pain activates cortical areas in the preterm newborn brain. *Pain*, **122** (1–2), 109–117.
4. Grunau RE, Holsti L, Peters JW (2006) Long-term consequences of pain in human neonates. *Semin Foetal Neonatal Med*, **11** (4), 268–275.
5. Redshaw M (2005) Infants in a neonatal intensive care unit: parental response. *Arch Dis Child Foetal Neonatal Ed*, **90** (2), F96.
6. Anand KJ, Aranda JV, Berde CB, *et al.* (2006) Summary proceedings from the neonatal pain-control group. *Pediatrics*, **117** (3, Pt 2), S9–S22.
7. Leslie A, Marlow N (2006) Non-pharmacological pain relief. *Semin Foetal Neonatal Med*, **11** (4), 246–250.
8. Warren I, Tan GC, Dixon P, Ghaus K (2000) Breast feeding success and early discharge for preterm infants. Results of a dedicated breast feeding programme. *Journal of Neonatal Nursing*, **6** (2), 43–48.
9. Levin A (1999) Humane Neonatal Care Initiative. *Acta Paediatr*, **88** (4), 353–355.
10. Alderson PH, Hawthorne J, Killen M (2005) The participation rights of premature babies. *International Journal of Children's Rights*, **13**, 31–50.
11. Wolke D (1998) Psychological development of prematurely born children. *Arch Dis Child*, **78** (6), 567–570.
12. Meins E, Fernyhough C, Fradley E, Tuckey M (2001) Rethinking maternal sensitivity: mothers' comments on infants' mental processes predict security of attachment at 12 months. *J Child Psychol Psychiatry*, **42** (5), 637–648.
13. Smith KE, Landry SH, Swank PR (2006) The role of early maternal responsiveness in supporting school-aged cognitive development for children who vary in birth status. *Pediatrics*, **117** (5), 1608–1617.
14. Resnick MB, Eyler FD, Nelson RM, Eitzman DV, Bucciarielli RL (1987) Developmental intervention for low birth weight infants: improved early development outcome. *Pediatrics*, **80** (1), 68–74.
15. Rauh VA, Nurcombe B, Achenbach T, Howell C (1990) The Mother-Infant Transaction Program. The content and implications of an intervention for the mothers of low-birthweight infants. *Clin Perinatol*, **17** (1), 31–45.
16. Melnyk BM, Feinstein NF, Alpert-Gillis L, *et al.* (2006) Reducing premature infants' length of stay and improving parents' mental health outcomes with the Creating Opportunities for Parent Empowerment (COPE) neonatal intensive care unit program: a randomized, controlled trial. *Pediatrics*, **118** (5), e1414–e1427.
17. White RD (2007) Recommended standards for the newborn ICU. *J Perinatol*, **27** (Suppl. 2), S4–S19.

18. Charpak N, Ruiz-Pelaez JG (2006) Resistance to implementing kangaroo mother care in developing countries, and proposed solutions. *Acta Paediatr*, **95** (5), 529–534.

19. Charpak N, Ruiz-Pelaez JG (2006) Resistance to implementing kangaroo mother care in developing countries, and proposed solutions. *Acta Paediatr*, **95** (5), 529–534.

20. Black K (2005) Kangaroo care and the ventilated neonate. Infant, **1** (1), 14–18.

21. Werner NP, Conway AE (1990) Caregiver contacts experienced by premature infants in the neonatal intensive care unit. *Maternal Child Nursing Journal*, **19** (1), 21–43.

22. Holsti L, Grunau RE, Whifield MF, Oberlander TF, Lindh V (2006) Behavioral responses to pain are heightened after clustered care in preterm infants born between 30 and 32 weeks gestational age. *Clin J Pain*, **22** (9), 757–764.

23. Field T (2002) Preterm infant massage therapy studies: an American approach. *Semin Neonatol*, **7** (6), 487–494.

24. Browne JV (2000) Considerations for touch and massage in the neonatal intensive care unit. *Neonatal Netw*, **19** (1), 61–64.

25. Bond C (2002) Positive Touch and massage in the neonatal unit: a British approach. Semin *Neonatol*, 7 (6), 477–486.

26. Als H (1997) The neurobehavioral development of the preterm infant. In: Fanaroff AA, Martin RJ (eds), *Neonatal-Perinatal Medicine*. Mosby, St Louis. pp. 964–989.

27. Als H (1999) Reading the preterm infant. Nurturing the premature infant. In: Goldson E (ed.), *Developmental Interventions in Newborn Intensive Care*. OUP, London.

28. Browne JV, VandenBerg K, Ross E S, Elmore AM (1999) The newborn developmental specialist: definition, qualifications and preparation for an emerging role in the neonatal intensive care unit. *Infants and Young Children*, **11** (4), 53–64.

29. Sell E (1997) Views of physicians/ANNPs in USA NIDCAP training centres on NIDCAP and philosophy of family centred care. In: *NIDCAP Trainers Meeting*. McCall, Idaho.

30. Westrup B, Stjernqvist K, Kleberg A, Hellstrom-Westas L, Lagercrantz H (2002) Neonatal individualized care in practice: a Swedish experience. *Semin Neonatol*, 7 (6), 447–457.

31. Symington A, Pinelli J (2006) Developmental care for promoting development and preventing morbidity in preterm infants. *Cochrane Database Syst Rev* (2), CD001814.

32. Ohlsson AJ (2006) *Newborn Individualized Care and Assessment Program (NIDCAP): A Systematic Review.* Society of Pediatric Research, San Francisco. Poster session.

33. Gressens P, Rogido M, Paindaveine B, Sola A (2002) The impact of neonatal intensive care practices on the developing brain. *J Pediatr*, **140** (6), 646–653.

34. Buehler DM, Als H, Duffy FH, McAnulty GB, Liederman J (1995) Effectiveness of individualized developmental care for low-risk preterm infants: behavioral and electrophysiologic evidence. *Pediatrics*, **96** (5 Pt 1), 923–932.

35. Als H (2004) *Program Guide: Newborn Individualized Developmental Care and Assessment Program (NIDCAP)*. National NIDCAP Training Center, Harvard Medical School, Children's Hospital, Boston MA. www.nidcap.org

36. Grunau RE, Holsti L, Peters JW (2006) Long-term consequences of pain in human neonates. *Semin Foetal Neonatal Med*, **11** (4), 268–275.

37. Evans JC, Vogelpohl DG, Bourguignon CM, Morcott CS (1997) Pain behaviors in LBW infants accompany some 'nonpainful' caregiving procedures. *Neonatal Netw*, **16** (3), 33–40.

38. Simunek VZS (2005) Sleep in preterm neonates; organisation, development and deprivation. In: Sizun J (ed.), *Research on Early Developmental Care for Preterm Neonates*. John Libbey, Paris.

39. Bertelle V, Mabin D, Adrien J, Sizun J (2005) Sleep of preterm neonates under developmental care or regular environmental conditions. *Early Hum Dev*, **81** (7), 595–600.

40. Lickliter R (2000) Atypical perinatal sensory stimulation and early perceptual development: insights from developmental psychobiology. *J Perinatol*, 20 (8, Pt 2), S45–S54.

41. Spencer N, Wallace A, Sundrum R, Bacchus C, Logan S (2006) Child abuse registration, foetal growth, and preterm birth: a population based study. *J Epidemiol Community Health*, **60** (4), 337–340.

42. Meins E, Fernyhough C, Fradley E, Tuckey M (2001) Rethinking maternal sensitivity: mothers' comments on infants' mental processes predict security of attachment at 12 months. *J Child Psychol Psychiatry*, **42** (5), 637–648.

43. Smith KE, Landry SH, Swank PR (2006) The role of early maternal responsiveness in supporting school-aged cognitive development for children

who vary in birth status. *Pediatrics*, **117** (5), 1608–1617.

44. Cuttini M, Chiandotto V, Barba BD, Cavazzuti GB, Zanini R, Reid M (2000) Visiting policies in neonatal intensive care units: staff and parents' views. *Arch Dis Child Foetal Neonatal Ed*, **82** (2), F172.

45. Rauh VA, Nurcombe B, Achenbach T, Howell C (1990) The Mother-Infant Transaction Program. The content and implications of an intervention for the mothers of low-birthweight infants. *Clin Perinatol*, **17** (1), 31–45.

46. Melnyk BM, Feinstein NF, Alpert-Gillis L, *et al.* (2006) Reducing premature infants' length of stay and improving parents' mental health outcomes with the Creating Opportunities for Parent Empowerment (COPE) neonatal intensive care unit program: a randomized, controlled trial. *Pediatrics*, **118** (5), e1414–e1427.

47. White RD (2007) Recommended standards for the newborn ICU. *J Perinatol*, **27** (Suppl. 2), S4–S19.

48. Symington A, Pinelli J (2006) Developmental care for promoting development and preventing morbidity in preterm infants. *Cochrane Database Syst Rev* (2), CD001814.

49. Charpak N, Ruiz-Pelaez JG (2006) Resistance to implementing kangaroo mother care in developing countries, and proposed solutions. *Acta Paediatr*, **95** (5), 529–534.

50. Thomas KA, Martin PA (2000) NICU sound environment and the potential problems for caregivers. *J Perinatol*, **20** (8, Pt 2), S94–S99.

51. Liu WF, Laudert S, Perkins B, MacMillian-York E, Martin S, Graven S (2007) The development of potentially better practices to support the neurodevelopment of infants in the NICU. *J Perinatol*, **27** (Suppl. 2), S48–S74.

52. Rea M (2004) Lighting for caregivers in the neonatal intensive care unit. *Clin Perinatol*, **31** (2), 229–242, vi.

53. Schaal B, Hummel T, Soussignan R (2004) Olfaction in the foetal and premature infant: functional status and clinical implications. *Clin Perinatol*, **31** (2), 261–85, vi–vii.

54. Heller C, Constantinou JC, VandenBerg K, Benitz W, Fleisher BE (1997) Sedation administered to very low birth weight premature infants. *J Perinatol*, **17** (2), 107–112.

55. Godambe SW (2007) Managing neonatal pain while rationalising the use of morphine – a retrospective observational study. At: Pediatric Academic Societies' Annual Meeting, 5–8 May, Toronto.

56. Evans JC, Vogelpohl DG, Bourguignon CM, Morcott CS (1997) Pain behaviors in LBW infants accompany some 'nonpainful' caregiving procedures. *Neonatal Netw*, **16** (3), 33–40.

57. Charpak N, Ruiz-Pelaez JG (2006) Resistance to implementing kangaroo mother care in developing countries, and proposed solutions. *Acta Paediatr*, **95** (5), 529–534.

58. Black K (2005) Kangaroo care and the ventilated neonate. *Infant*, **1** (1), 14–18.

59. Cohen M (2003) *Sent Before My Time*. Karnac Books (The Tavistock Clinic Series), London.

Chapter 19

NEONATAL ETHICS

John Wyatt

Learning outcomes

After reading this chapter the reader will be expected to be able to:

- Summarise and explain the three core ethical principles

- Compare and contrast these principles with those highlighted by the United Nations

- Explain the term 'informed consent'

- Describe an example of a situation where intensive care has been replaced by palliative care; examine the ethical principles behind the decision

- Recognise the importance of religious and cultural differences

---

Introduction

Neonatal care is an area of increasing ethical debate both amongst health professionals and the public. A number of high profile cases have received extensive coverage in the media. Several harrowing legal cases, involving apparently irreconcilable conflicts between parents and doctors about whether intensive care should be continued or withdrawn, have received prime time coverage. As the technical possibilities of neonatal care continue to develop, ethical debates and problems are likely to become more widespread. It is essential, therefore, that all staff caring for newborn babies understand the fundamental ethical and legal principles which should govern their actions.

Fundamental ethical principles

There are some core or fundamental terms that are often used when medical ethics are discussed and it is useful to begin with some definitions of these terms before discussing them in more depth in relation to specific situations.

Autonomy

This refers to the respect that should be shown for an individual's capacity for self-determination and their own personal goals.

Beneficence and non-maleficence

These terms refer to the duty of providing benefit (beneficence) and not inflicting harm (non-maleficence), which are central to the medical and nursing professions.

Justice

This encompasses several other principles, which include non-discrimination and protecting the vulnerable, the latter of which is particularly relevant to the care of infants.

When considering the area of neonatology these terms contribute to the philosophy of acting in the best interests of the child.

Acting in the best interests of the child

The over-riding ethical principle, derived from more than two thousand years of medical and nursing practice, is that as health care professionals we have a duty of care to act in our patients' best interests. In other words, we are here to do the best for each individual baby in our care. The principle of always acting in the best interests of the patient is particularly important in neonatal care, because babies are uniquely vulnerable and dependent on others for all aspects of their care. It has always been a foundational value of neonatology that every baby deserves the very best medical treatment and care that can realistically be provided and that every effort should be made to protect them from harm or abuse. Behind this is the belief that every baby, however small or sick, has intrinsic value as a unique human person.

This perspective is also enshrined in the United Nations Convention on the Rights of the Child[1]. The Convention spells out the basic human rights that children everywhere have:

- The right to life
- The right to survival and development
- To protection from harmful influences, abuse and exploitation
- To participate fully in family, cultural and social life

The four core principles of the Convention are:

- Non-discrimination
- Devotion to the best interests of the child

- The right to life, survival and development
- Respect for the views of the child

It is clear, legally and morally, that every baby possesses these impressive rights from the moment of birth. As health professionals, we have a duty to put our patients' interests and well-being before our own interests, before the interests of the hospital or health service, and before the interests of anyone else.

But what about the baby's parents and family? Should we not take their interests into account? Whose interests come first? In the vast majority of cases, the interests of both the baby and the parents coincide. The interests of a baby are inextricably intertwined with those of the parents and wider family.

Health professionals should therefore start with the presumption that, in nearly all cases, the actions and decisions of parents will be for their baby's best interests. So an essential part of all good neonatal practice will be to involve parents as much as possible in the care of their baby and to enable them to share in important decisions about the welfare of their baby. We have a primary responsibility to communicate as fully as possible with parents and involve them in all aspects of their baby's care. In particular, when there are questions about whether intensive treatment should be continued or withdrawn, we have a legal and professional duty to inform and involve parents in these difficult decisions. But the basis on which such decisions are made must always be what is best for the individual baby.

Implications for practice

The importance of professional empathic communication and the involvement of parents in decisions about their child cannot be overemphasised.

Informed consent

It is a foundational principle of medical ethics that medical treatment should only be given with the informed consent of the patient, or of the parent in the case of a child. In the case of a newborn baby we have a responsibility soon after birth to ensure that parents are fully informed about the medical condition their child suffers from, and of the various treatment options, and that we request the parents' consent for the treatment we wish to give. In the case of an acute emergency health staff may act in good faith in order to save life, without obtaining explicit consent, but at the first opportunity the parents must be informed and their agreement confirmed. It is therefore good practice, as soon as a baby is admitted to a neonatal intensive care unit, to ensure that parents are informed about the procedures and treatments which are routinely used, and to ensure their agreement. Failure to request consent threatens the relationship of trust which is essential between health staff and parents. Some parents may react in a negative and even hostile manner if they discover that procedures such as lumbar puncture or cranial ultrasound scanning have been performed without their knowledge or agreement.

Implications for practice

On the admission of an infant to the neonatal unit it is good practice to inform parents about the procedures and treatment that are likely to be used and to ensure their agreement or consent.

In legal terms, only a person with 'parental responsibility' is able to give legally valid consent to treatment. People with parental responsibility include:

- The mother of the baby
- The father of the baby if the parents are married at the time of birth
- The father of the baby if he is named on the birth certificate
- A person (such as a social worker) who has been designated as having parental responsibility by the legal authorities

In addition, the person with parental responsibility must have legal capacity to give informed consent. This means that they must be able to *understand* and *retain* the information given, *weigh up* the information in order to come to a decision and then be able to *communicate* this decision to others. It is important that health care staff should seek legal advice if they are uncertain about the capacity of the parents to give valid consent. In an emergency the staff must act in what they perceive to be the best interests of the baby, but further advice must be sought as soon as the acute emergency has passed. The Department of Health and the medical defence organisations provide detailed guidance in this area[2].

Making treatment decisions in partnership with parents

The aim of all treatment decisions is to act for the baby's good, to protect and enhance his or her welfare. However, in some of the agonising clinical decisions concerning babies born at the limits of viability, or those with profoundly disabling congenital malformations or severe brain injury, it may not be at all clear which course of action is genuinely in the baby's best interests.

In this situation it is important that there is open communication and discussion, first between the different professionals directly involved in the care of the baby, and then subsequently between the senior doctor in charge of the baby's care and the parents. The nursing staff have an important contribution to make to these discussions and their perspective is often complementary to that of the medical team:

- First, experienced neonatal nurses can provide first-hand observations of the baby's moment-to-moment behaviour and responses to intensive care procedures. It is particularly important in these situations to assess how much distress a baby is suffering, their unique responses to different forms of stimulation, and the effectiveness of pain relieving and other medication.

- Second, the nursing staff can provide unique insights into the involvement and attitudes of the parents and wider family and the interactions between the parents and their baby.
- Finally, nursing staff can play a vital role in facilitating communication between the medical team and the parents in discussions about the care of their baby.

Parents may find personal discussions with a consultant or senior doctor intimidating and difficult. This may be particularly likely if the parents come from a minority cultural or ethnic background. Parents may feel that they are not in possession of sufficient knowledge or expertise to participate in discussion about treatment options. They may also feel that doctors should make these decisions by themselves and that it is impossible for parents to take this responsibility. On the other hand, some parents may feel that they alone should decide what is best for their babies and that the professional staff should not play a role. It is important that health care staff are sensitive to differing attitudes and perspectives of parents to the care of their baby, and that they spend time exploring and discussing these issues in an open and unthreatening manner.

Implications for practice

Neonatal nurses have an important role to play in difficult ethical decisions and should be proactive in facilitating communication between the medical team and the parents.

The 'expert-expert' relationships

It is helpful to think of the partnership relationship between health care staff and parents as an 'expert-expert' relationship. The health care staff have special expertise in the diagnosis, prognosis and treatment of neonatal conditions and will be able to share their experience of treatment options and likely outcomes. In addition to technical expertise, health professionals should also demonstrate a commitment to professional and ethical values, including integrity, truthfulness,

compassion and humanity. However, parents also have their own 'expertise' – in their family background, their history, their shared beliefs and values, and their concerns for their child.

Expert-expert relationships are effective when they are based on mutual respect. As health care professionals we need to demonstrate that we recognise the expertise of the parents, and in turn we ask parents to recognise our expertise. The aim is for professionals and parents to come to a consensus through a process of open and honest explanation and discussion. These discussions are often emotionally charged, time-consuming and difficult, but with patience and persistence a consensus can usually be reached. However, it may take several meetings for a consensus to be achieved and wherever possible the same professionals should be involved in discussions with parents from day to day. Unfortunately, this is becoming increasingly difficult with modern working practices and shift patterns, and loss of continuity of care is an important cause of misunderstanding and conflict between parents and health staff.

On occasion there may be a major disagreement between professionals and parents on the best course of action. It may be that some form of compromise can be reached which all parties can agree to. A second opinion from an independent specialist may be valuable, and the involvement of religious leaders or emotional support from a counsellor is often helpful. In some hospitals a clinical ethics committee may be available to provide independent review and consideration when there is a dispute about the best course of action. However in the UK, clinical ethics committees can only provide advice and support, and the legal responsibility for clinical decisions remains with the medical team and ultimately with the consultant who is responsible for the care of the baby.

From a legal standpoint, the UK courts have consistently judged that they do not wish to become involved in medical decisions about starting or withholding intensive care, provided that the parents are fully informed about the decision and that there is agreement on the best course of action between the medical team and the parents about the decision.

On the rare occasions that there is complete disagreement between the medical team and the parents, it may be necessary to involve the courts for a legal adjudication. However, the involvement of the courts should only be seen as a last resort, as it has many unfortunate consequences. Because of the adversarial nature of our legal system, lawyers and expert witnesses are instructed to act for the different parties. This tends to exacerbate and highlight the conflict between the parents and the health care staff caring for their baby. Both parents and staff may find the long-drawn-out and intensive process of making statements and writing reports, extremely distressing, and even psychologically damaging. Although in the past, court cases involving the care of children have nearly always been held in private, with strict confidentiality, there is now an increasing tendency for judges to lift reporting restrictions. This means that these painful and difficult cases are sometimes held in the full glare of publicity, with extensive media interest.

The involvement of the courts also implies that a decision which is of enormous personal and emotional significance to the parents will be finally settled by legal professionals who are effectively strangers to the parents and baby. Hence, recourse to the courts has to be seen as a last resort. The recently published report on neonatal care from the Nuffield Council for Bioethics recommended that the involvement of professional mediators might be considered, prior to referral to the courts. However, there is little experience with this approach so far in the UK.

When parents do not act in their child's best interests

We always start from the basic assumption that parents will act in the best interests of their child. But of course we also recognise that there are uncommon cases where the actions of the parents may not be genuinely for the good of their baby. There are situations where parents are at risk of harming their babies, because of psychiatric illness or substance abuse, for instance. There are also situations where the particular religious convictions of the parents cause them to act in ways which seem to go against the interests of the child. For example, parents who are convinced members of the Jehovah's Witnesses Church may not wish their baby to receive a blood transfusion, even if there is evidence of life-threatening haemorrhage. In other cases parents may threaten to take their sick baby away from the hospital. In some cases honest discussion and gentle persuasion may enable a suitable conclusion, with parents agreeing to essential treatment. However, if no agreement can be reached and if there is any serious concern that the actions and decisions of parents or families are not in the baby's best interests, it is our duty as health professionals to put the baby's interests first. In an emergency, life-saving treatment can be provided against the parents' wishes. The indications for emergency treatment must be carefully documented. Subsequently, it will be necessary to seek urgent legal advice and where necessary a court order should be obtained to confirm the legality of continued treatment.

Implications for practice

Both patience and persistence are necessary with difficult ethical decisions. Although it is often sensible to seek legal advice, involvement of the courts should be avoided if at all possible.

Implications for practice

In rare cases where the decisions of the parents are not thought to be in the child's best interests, the role of the professional is to act for the child. In these cases clear communication and documentation are essential and legal advice is often sought.

Withholding or withdrawing life-sustaining treatment

Our fundamental duty as health professionals is to act to protect and preserve health and to minimise suffering and harm to our patients. We start with a primary orientation towards the protection and the preservation of life. However, we recognise that there are situations in which the consequences of disease or developmental abnormality are so severe, that medical treatment can bring no benefit to that individual. In these circumstances it is appropriate to withhold or withdraw life-sustaining treatment with the knowledge that death is likely to follow. The report of the Royal College of Paediatrics and Child Health provided a number of clinical situations in which it might be appropriate to withhold life-sustaining treatment[3]. Of these, three in particular are relevant to the care of newborn babies, the 'no chance' situation, the 'no purpose' situation, and the 'unbearable' situation.

The 'no chance' situation refers to terminal illness where death is imminent and inevitable and where the effect of medical treatment is to delay death without alleviating suffering.

The 'no purpose' situation refers to a condition in which although the patient may survive with treatment, 'the physical and mental impairment will be so great that it is unreasonable to expect them to bear it'. This idea has also been expressed in the concept of 'intolerability', when the prolongation of life imposes an intolerable burden upon the child.

The 'unbearable' situation refers to progressive and irreversible illness where treatment is causing pain and suffering which cannot be controlled.

It is this second concept of the 'intolerable life' or the 'life which has no purpose' which causes the most controversy and difficulty for health staff and for parents. Is it ever possible or appropriate for one person to decide that another person's life is 'intolerable' or has 'no purpose'? The judgements involved are subjective and personal, and it is easy to see how this concept might be used to support discrimination against individuals with chronic disabling conditions.

Balancing the burdens and benefits of treatment

An alternative way of thinking about withholding or withdrawing life-sustaining treatment is in terms of the balance between burdens and benefits. It is a fundamental principle of health care that we should only provide a medical treatment if the benefits of the treatment outweigh the burdens and risks of the treatment.

So in deciding whether or not to commence or withdraw intensive life support treatment, we have to balance the likely benefits of that treatment with its burdens and risks. If the benefits exceed the burdens we should give the treatment, but if the burdens exceed the benefits then we should stop. Indeed, to continue to give intensive treatment when its burdens exceed its likely benefits could be regarded as abusive and immoral.

This balancing process is complex – it involves judgement about the future probability of certain events, such as the likelihood that the child will have such severe brain injury that they will be unable to communicate. It also involves balancing burdens in the present against likely benefits in the future. And we can't ask the baby what their own wishes would be. We have to act on their behalf and in what we judge to be their best interests. But the principle is clear – we should only give invasive medical treatment if the benefits we can expect exceed the burdens we will inflict on the baby.

With most babies admitted to a neonatal intensive care unit, it is clear that the benefits of days or weeks of intensive care outweigh the burdens and risks. But we must give special attention to those cases where intensive care has either very *limited benefits* or *excessive burdens*.

Limited benefits of intensive treatment

Cases in which the benefits are very limited include, first, the baby in whom death is inevitable. This is the clinical situation where there is a progressive and untreatable decline in respiratory, cardiac and metabolic function. In this case intensive treatment can only prolong the dying process, and the burdens clearly outweigh the benefits. It is very important that medical and nursing staff are able to recognise the point at which death becomes inevitable so that needless and burdensome treatment is not prolonged. On rare occasions it may be justified to continue intensive support for a short period – if, for example, the parents are in another hospital and have not yet arrived to see their baby. However, we should always ensure that appropriate pain relief and symptom control is given and intensive treatment should be stopped as soon as possible.

Second, there are cases where life expectancy is limited, such as major chromosomal disorders like trisomy 13 or 18, severe pulmonary hypoplasia, or rare disseminated malignancies. Third, there are infants born at the limits of viability in whom the chances of survival are minimal and there are very high risks of brain injury. The recent report of the Nuffield Council on Bioethics has recommended that intensive care should not normally be provided below 23 weeks of gestation[4], unless in exceptional circumstances and as part of a formal research protocol, and that treatment at 23 weeks should only be given with the clear and informed agreement of the parents. Although these general guidelines based on gestational age are helpful, it is important that benefits and risks are assessed in each individual baby and that treatment decisions are individualised rather than decided on the basis of inflexible rules.

Finally, there are the most difficult cases in which very severe and permanent brain injury has occurred, and even if the child survives to discharge there is little or no chance that he or she will be able to develop the ability to communicate or interact with others. In these cases health care staff and parents may come to an agreement that it is not fair to submit the child to many weeks or months of intensive care when the benefit it can bring is so limited. It is often

said in such circumstances that the future quality of life is so poor that treatment should be stopped. However, I (and others) have concerns about this way of expressing our conclusion. It implies that we as health care professionals are able to make a final judgement about the value or worth of another individual's life. In my view we are not able to judge whether a *life* is worth living – what we can and must do is decide whether a *treatment* is worth giving.

Techniques such as ultrasound scanning or magnetic resonance imaging of the brain can give vital information about the presence of brain injury in the critical first hours and days after delivery. Although it will never be possible to foresee the long-term outlook with complete reliability, it is increasingly possible to use brain scans to give a moderately accurate prediction of the likely long-term development for an individual baby. Of course brain scans allow the extent of brain injury to be assessed but do not solve the painful ethical dilemmas concerning the appropriateness of intensive care for a malformed or critically sick newborn. However, scans and other diagnostic tests provide objective information which can be discussed in detail with the parents and with other concerned individuals, and on which ethical decisions about intensive care can be based. In this way respect for the dignity and worth of the individual baby, and concern for their best interests, can be translated into practical decisions about medical care.

Implications for practice

We are not able to judge whether a *life* is worth living – what we can and must do is decide whether a *treatment* is worth giving.

Excessive burdens of intensive treatment

In most cases babies undergoing intensive care should not suffer severe distress provided that appropriate pain relief and sedation is provided. But there are rare clinical circumstances in which intensive care procedures may cause excessive suffering and distress. This may be seen, for instance, in the most severe forms of epidermolysis bullosa, the rare skin condition in which the epidermis is abraided and injured even by the lightest contact. This can cause extreme pain and distress which is resistant to maximal pain relief and symptom control. There are other rare circumstances where repeated painful procedures, such as repeated chest drain insertion, are required. If it seems that distress and pain is continuing indefinitely and cannot be adequately controlled, it may be appropriate to stop such intensive treatment even though life is shortened as a result.

In practice there may be professional or personal pressures which make it difficult for health care staff to withdraw intensive care once it has been started. Some babies may receive weeks or months of treatment even if the outlook is hopeless. On occasions like these, intensive care can change from being a source of healing and restoration and can become a source of harm, even a strange form of child abuse. It is the responsibility of every health professional to ensure that the powerful and invasive technology at our disposal is only used for good and not for harm. Sometimes we need the courage to say 'enough is enough'.

Implications for practice

It is important to remember that there are times when intensive care become a source of harm or even abuse rather than a source of healing.

Coping with uncertainty

One of the most troubling aspects of these critical care decisions is that, when assessing the future outcome for a child, we are nearly always dealing with probabilities and very rarely with certainties. In some cases we may be fairly certain that the brain injury is so devastating that the future outcome will be extremely poor. But there may be a small chance that the outcome will be better than we think. The very nature of

neonatology means that we cannot predict the future with complete accuracy. My own experience over 25 years of trying to predict long-term outcome in newborn babies with brain injury has convinced me that confident predictions based on brain scans and other information are often inaccurate. Therefore we have to be honest with ourselves and also honest with parents about the degree of uncertainty in any particular case. On the other hand we have a duty to help parents to have a balanced and realistic understanding of what the future may hold for their child.

If there is a significant degree of uncertainty about the future outcome, then it is generally agreed that health professionals should decide in favour of life, and continue intensive treatment. As health professionals we have a moral and legal 'presumption in favour of life'. Similarly, if there is substantial disagreement between different members of the health care team, it is better to continue treatment for the time being. Although sometimes staff may feel under some pressure to make a decision rapidly to withdraw treatment, in my experience it is unwise to yield to this pressure. Clinical situations often become clearer with time and a consensus can usually be reached after further review and discussion.

Philosophical and religious perspectives

Fundamental values and attitudes towards newborn babies have varied dramatically in different cultures and historical periods. In the classical Greek and Roman cultures, newborn babies were often regarded as having little intrinsic value. Infanticide or exposure of unwanted or abnormal neonates was a frequent occurrence, and the practice was approved by several philosophers and commentators. The earliest textbook for midwifes written by a Roman physician in the first century AD, has a chapter entitled, 'How to recognise the baby that is worth rearing', listing the characteristics by which congenitally malformed or sick infants could be identified so that they could be allowed to die. The underlying philosophical view was that the value of a baby's life lay in the future potential to be a productive citizen. If the baby was abnormal the future potential was limited and hence the value of that life was minimal. It was only adult lives that carried real value. It is not surprising that medicine and nursing for sick babies and children did not develop in this culture.

By contrast, the Jewish and Christian cultures of the same historical period had a radically different perspective. Babies and children were seen as being made in 'God's image', just the same as adults. Hence, even the life of an abnormal or sick baby was regarded as uniquely precious and to be protected from abuse and neglect. The early Christian churches and monasteries established orphanages and 'foundling hospitals' in which unwanted and abandoned babies and children could be cared for[5]. The Islamic culture, which developed some centuries after the early Christian era, adopted the same attitude of respect and protection for babies and children.

The concept of the 'sanctity of human life', which is still a foundational principle of modern Western law, derives historically from the religious perspective shared by the Jewish, Christian and Islamic cultures, that all human beings, including newborn babies are made in God's image. Similarly, the internationally accepted principle of Universal Human Rights can be traced historically back to the religious perspective of the unique value and dignity of each human life.

However, recognising the unique value and dignity of every baby does not mean that we are obliged to provide intensive treatment in every conceivable condition. We do not have an absolute moral duty to attempt to prolong life even when there is no prospect of recovery. Despite spectacular advances in medical technology, there are some babies who cannot benefit from medical treatment and death is inevitable. In such cases it seems clear that withdrawing

or withholding intensive care is an ethical and appropriate option.

The concept of the sanctity of human life leads on to the view that the intentional killing of newborn babies is always morally wrong. In current UK law, and in professional guidelines provided by the General Medical Council and the Royal Colleges, a clear distinction is drawn between the withdrawal of life-sustaining treatment when it is futile or excessively burdensome, and intentional killing by administration of lethal medication or other intervention (neonatal euthanasia). In the first case the intention is to remove treatment when it becomes burdensome and damaging. In the second case the intention is to kill. The first is accepted as an important part of medical practice whereas the second is generally regarded as both illegal and immoral.

Is there a distinction between 'allowing to die' and 'intentional mercy killing'?

This distinction has come under increasing attack both from a number of philosophers and from some paediatricians, particularly in the Netherlands. Several philosophers have argued that the distinction between allowing to die and intentional killing is meaningless. Since death is the end result in both cases, they argue that the precise intention of the doctor is irrelevant. Instead we should accept that doctors have a duty to save life sometimes and to end lives in other situations.

In 2005, a group of Dutch paediatricians published the so-called 'Groningen Protocol', which outlined circumstances in which euthanasia or mercy killing could be carried out in severely ill newborns[6]. The criteria included the following:

- The diagnosis and prognosis must be certain
- Hopeless and unbearable suffering must be present
- There must be confirmation of the diagnosis and prognosis from an independent doctor
- Both parents must give informed consent

- The procedure must be performed 'with the accepted medical standard'
- The case must be referred to the coroner after death

It is reported that a small number of cases of neonatal euthanasia occur annually in the Netherlands; although this action is technically illegal doctors have been exempted from prosecution provided that the published protocol is adhered to.

The neonatal working party of the Nuffield Council on Bioethics specifically addressed the issue of whether neonatal euthanasia or intentional killing should be accepted in the UK. After intensive discussion the working party concluded that neonatal euthanasia should not be legalised[7]. They argued that intentional killing was a violation of the professional duty to protect the life of the patient and was a breach of the generally accepted ethos of health professionals. They also argued that permitting intentional killing would have a detrimental effect psychologically on health professionals and may lead to a loss of trust from parents and the general public. Finally, they argued that if euthanasia of newborn babies were to become an accepted part of medical practice it was logically inconsistent not to extend this to brain damaged children and adults.

Caring for the dying baby

See also Chapter 15.

When health professionals and parents recognise the point that intensive treatment should be withdrawn or withheld, it is important to realise that although medical treatment may stop, caring must never stop. We must provide the highest quality of terminal care for dying babies just as we should provide terminal or palliative care for every dying adult.

Basic care includes adequate pain and symptom relief, so that not only is pain adequately treated but also distressing symptoms such as breathlessness or convulsions are controlled. Second, except in extreme cases where there is no gastrointestinal function, milk and fluids should be given via a nasogastric tube. Allowing babies to die from starvation and dehydration is not compatible with treating them with respect. However, these infants will not require the amount of feed given to healthy infants (100–150 ml/kg/day) as they will not be as physically active and nutrition will not be needed for growth but only maintenance of cellular function and comfort. A reasonable amount to consider is 30–50 ml/kg/day. Finally, and equally important, each dying baby deserves tender loving care. Loving cuddles, where possible from the mother or another close relative, is a physical demonstration of the tender care and respect which we owe to each baby. Many parents look back with sadness but also with fond memories to a special time they spent cuddling their dying baby. Caring for dying babies and their families is costly and difficult but it is an important and rewarding part of modern neonatal care. Staff working in the field of neonatology need to understand that enabling a baby to die peacefully in their mother's arms, free of pain, can be as much a triumph of modern neonatal care as ensuring the survival of an extremely preterm baby. The recent report of the Nuffield Council on Bioethics recognised the importance of this aspect of care and recommended mandatory training in palliative care for all professionals working in neonatology.

The death of a newborn baby is one of the most devastating psychological traumas a parent can sustain, often with lifelong consequences. Siblings can also be profoundly affected by the death of a long expected brother or sister. Health professionals need to ensure that emotional and practical support is provided for parents and for siblings before, during and after the death. Many professionals, too, suffer from the emotional costs of providing this level of care and it is important that appropriate support mechanisms are in place for them.

Conclusion

The overriding ethical principle of all neonatal
care is the duty to act in the individual baby's
best interests. The parents have a central role in
participating in all treatment decisions and staff
need to develop an open, respectful and collaborative relationship from the outset. Health
professionals start with a primary orientation
towards the protection and preservation of life.
However, there are situations in which the consequences of disease or developmental abnormality are so severe, that it may be appropriate
to withhold or withdraw life-sustaining treatment with the knowledge that death is likely to
follow. In these critical decisions it is important
to balance the burdens and benefits of intensive
treatment, and to seek a consensus both between
the professional staff caring for the baby and
with the parents. Recourse to the courts is necessary if no consensus can be reached or if there is
clear evidence that the parents are not acting in
their baby's best interests. Although withdrawal
of life-sustaining treatment may be appropriate,
euthanasia or intentional killing is not an
accepted part of neonatal care in the UK.

References

1. UNICEF Convention on the Rights of the Child
    http://www.unicef.org/crc/
2. Department of Health, 'Reference Guide to con-
    sent for examination or treatment' and 'Consent –
    a guide for parents': http://www.dh.gov.
    uk/PolicyAndGuidance/HealthAndSocialCareTopi
    cs/Consent/ConsentGeneralInformation/fs/en
3. The Royal College of Paediatrics and Child
    Health (2004) *Withholding or Withdrawing Life
    Sustaining Treatment in Children: a Framework
    for Practice*. 2nd edn. RCPCH, London.
4. Nuffield Council on Bioethics (2006) *Critical Care
    Decisions in Foetal and Neonatal Medicine; Ethical
    Issues*. Nuffield Council on Bioethics, London.
5. Wyatt J (1998) *Matters of Life and Death*.
    InterVarsity Press, London.
6. Verhagen E, Sauer PJ (2005) The Groningen pro-
    tocol. *New England Journal Medicine*, **352** (10),
    959–962.
7. Nuffield Council on Bioethics (2006) *Critical Care
    Decisions in Foetal and Neonatal Medicine; Ethical
    Issues*. Nuffield Council on Bioethics, London.

Chapter 20

DISCHARGE PLANNING AND THE COMMUNITY OUTREACH SERVICE

Sylvia Gomes

Learning outcomes

After reading this chapter and studying the contents the reader will be able to:

- Identify when to begin discharge planning
- Identify other professionals who should be involved in the discharge process
- Identify the importance and role of the neonatal outreach team
- Discuss the discharge learning needs of parents and carers
- List the babies likely to need nursing support following discharge home
- Describe the learning needs of parents with infants with some specific conditions

---

Introduction

The discharge home of a previously sick infant can be a very anxious time for parents and Merenstein and Gardner suggest that the parents have five psychological stages to complete before they are ready to take the infant home[1]:

(1) Working through the traumatic events related to the infant's delivery
(2) Grieving for the infant they had anticipated during the pregnancy
(3) Acknowledging feelings of guilt and failure
(4) Adaptation to the intensive care environment
(5) Making a relationship with the new baby

Most parents will work through these stages with the help of supportive family members and the neonatal unit staff; once the relationship is developing between the infant and his/her family discharge may be anticipated and preparations begun. This chapter will look at the plans and preparation for discharge once these stages are well developed.

Preparation for discharge

It is important that preparation for discharge should begin well in advance of the possible discharge date. Most parents eagerly look forward to discharge as this is a sign that their baby has made good progress and is well enough to be cared for at home. Although taking their previously sick baby home is a happy and exciting time it is also an anxiety-provoking event.

Whilst their baby has been resident on the neonatal unit parents have had consistent support from medical and nursing staff and the withdrawal of this support promotes anxiety. There is a transfer of responsibility as to the action to be taken if their baby becomes unwell after discharge and this should be a gradual transfer rather than a sudden one.

Birth and subsequent hospitalisation of a very premature infant evokes considerable psychological distress in parents[2]. They will need to have come to terms with traumatic events associated with the early delivery and admission to the neonatal unit before they are ready to take their baby home. Most parents will work through these with the help of family members and support from the neonatal unit team and some will have taken advantage of professional help from a psychologist or counsellor.

It is well recognised that increasing parental involvement in the caregiving throughout hospitalisation and working with families to facilitate the discharge process allows parents to emerge from the NICU experience with increased competence and confidence in infant care giving[3]. The high-tech neonatal environment and sophisticated machinery used to provide care can be frightening to parents. They are initially often scared to handle their sick baby and worried that they may knock lines or interrupt monitoring. Staff should help parents adapt to the neonatal environment by explaining unit routines and giving them information on the equipment used to provide care to their baby.

Parental confidence can be improved by encouraging parents to help with both the physical and emotional care of their baby right from the very beginning. Some parents may be scared to do this initially. This fear needs to be recognised to ensure neonatal staff can help parents overcome their fears and improve their confidence in caring for their baby.

Discharge preparation should ideally start from admission. The mother's community midwife, family GP and baby's health visitor should be informed of the baby's admission to the neonatal unit as soon as possible. Parents should be encouraged to visit their baby on the unit and to talk to their baby and they should be taught basic tasks like changing nappies and providing mouth care. As they become more familiar with their baby and neonatal unit routines they can be encouraged to take on more tasks, like feeding their baby via a nasogastric tube. Parents should be consulted when planning the baby's routines, i.e. nappy change and feed times, to allow maximum participation in meeting their baby's needs.

Implications for practice

The preparation for discharge should begin with admission.
There should be a gradual handover of caring roles from the nursing staff to the parents as the infant becomes more stable and ready for discharge.

Communication with parents

Infants admitted to the neonatal unit should have a named/lead nurse who will act as a main coordinator for the baby and family. This will improve the approach to discharge planning and teaching of essential skills by making it more structured and specific to meeting the needs of the family. Parents need to build up a therapeutic relationship with the lead nurse caring for their baby, who will be a very important source of support.

To help meet the needs of parents of NICU infants, parents need to be informed of the infant's diagnosis/medical problems, treatment plan and procedures. Staff should answer parents' questions honestly, actively listen to parents' fears and expectations and assist parents in understanding their baby's responses to treatment and other effective nursing interventions[4]. This will encourage parental involvement in decisions about care and increase parental confidence in the staff caring for their infant.

It is good practice to keep parents informed of their infants' condition on at least a daily basis. Most units have a communications policy to ensure parents are regularly updated with their infant's condition, medical findings and treatment options by medical staff. It is essential that the nurse caring for the baby attends these sessions to support parents and help them understand new information. Although the neonatologist's role in parent education is important, parents have identified the nurses as the primary source of information[5]. A survey on 'How parents of premature infants gather information and obtain support' concluded that nurses are the main source of support and help for parents in understanding and adapting to their baby[6].

Implications for practice

Good communication with parents is vital at all stages of the infant's stay on the neonatal unit, daily updates should be provided.

Role of outreach service

A neonatal outreach service consists of experienced neonatal nurses who plan discharges with the families of infants admitted to neonatal units and the medical and nursing team looking after them. The main role of a neonatal outreach service is to ensure seamless transition of care from the hospital to the community. This can be achieved by the early identification and involvement of community health professionals that will provide support and care for the infant after discharge. The service also acts as a resource for general practitioners, health visitors and community services.

Outreach nurses help parents to identify their learning needs and help them gain the essential skills and knowledge needed to care for their baby at home. They work in partnership with parents, helping them to gain confidence in caring for their infant independently at home and they also provide some of the initial support in the community in collaboration with community midwives, health visitors and GPs.

Community neonatal services provide an invaluable service to families, particularly if the person delivering the care possesses advanced skills and knowledge in neonatal/ family care, and is able to integrate care from the neonatal unit into the community[7]. The results of a multicentre survey looking at the impact of community neonatal services suggested that community neonatal services may reduce the length of stay without any subsequent increase in readmission[8].

Communicating with outreach service

Most neonatal outreach services are based on the unit and the neonatal outreach nurse should be able to meet with the parents within a week of admission. Outreach nurses can work with the lead/named nurse in gathering relevant information about the family and identifying their needs.

Initial discussions should encapsulate information about the family and the ongoing commitments that parents have whilst their baby is resident on the neonatal unit and include:

- Family details
  - Health of parents
  - Relationship details
  - Number and health of other children
  - Employment, maternity and paternity leave
- Family support: availability of grandparents or friends
- Other caring commitments
  - Other children
  - Sick or dependent relatives
- Arrangements for travel to neonatal unit

These sessions should help the outreach nurse understand the family dynamics and the level of support the family will need whilst their infant is resident on the unit and after discharge. It may also help to appreciate the level of additional caregiving responsibility the family could cope with.

It is vital that this is recognised before planning for discharging a baby with ongoing medical needs home, for example oxygen dependent infants.

Later discussions may include:

- How parents would like to be involved in planning to meet the baby's physical and emotional needs
- Housing and financial needs

Parents can be offered help with housing and financial needs by referring the family to social services for benefits advice and guidance on applying for housing.

Implications for practice

Early introduction to the outreach team is vital.

Communication with community health professionals

Community midwives, health visitors and GPs should be informed of the baby's admission to the neonatal unit at the earliest opportunity. Midwives, health visitors and GPs can be a good source of support for parents whilst their infant is resident on the neonatal unit as well as after discharge. They can support the family outside the unit and help meet the family's own individual health needs. Community health professionals involved with the infant and family should be regularly updated about the infant's condition and response to treatment. They should ideally be involved with the discharge planning. Health visitors should be encouraged to visit the parents and baby on the unit and can give parents advice on how to introduce siblings to the new baby and manage any behavioural changes within these siblings.

Specialist health visitors, community paediatricians and community children's nurses will need to be involved with those infants who have complex medical needs that are likely to be long term. Involving community health professionals early can help ease the transition of care from hospital to home. Community health professionals should be informed of the proposed plan of care at home when the baby is discharged.

Implications for practice

Ensure that the GP and health visitor are informed of the infant's delivery and admission to the neonatal unit as soon as possible after delivery.
Involve these and other relevant professionals in the discharge process.

Discharge planning

The aims of discharge planning are:

- To promote parental confidence in caring for their infant
- To reduce the readmission rate to hospital
- To minimise infection risk by promoting handwashing and other hygienic measures
- To reduce the risk of cot death
- To promote optimal growth and development

Discharge planning should focus on helping parents gain the confidence and competence in providing infant care independently at home. Parental anxiety often centres on forgetting what has been taught, making a mistake in the treatment and coping in a crisis if their child becomes ill. This is why it is so important to begin discharge preparation at admission by actively involving the parents in the infant's physical and emotional care as this active participation will maximise their learning. There should also be clear guidance on who will be available for support following discharge.

Most units use a discharge checklist to help parents gain the basic skills needed to care for their newborn infant. Ideally, these checklists should prompt staff to take into account the previous experience of parents and to discuss what parents wish to learn. Parents can date and sign the checklist once they can perform a task independently.

The children's charter for health and social care recommends: '*Treatment at home for children and young people who have complex health needs, so that they can manage their illness and still have a fulfilling life*'.

There are major benefits in discharging medically stable infants home early with neonatal outreach support. These benefits include:

- Promotion of parent-infant bonding
- Enhancement of normal growth and development
- Reducing the risk of nosocomial infection
- The establishment of oral feeds and promoting breast-feeding

Infants that are medically stable, not needing continuous monitoring, maintaining their temperature in a cot and gaining weight should be cared for by their parents, preferably at home.

Most parents are willing to accept additional caregiving responsibilities and are eager to take their infant home with community support. The advantages and risks associated with early discharge should be discussed with the parents if the baby is medically stable and early discharge is being discussed. Parents should then be given the time and opportunity to discuss their views and feelings. It is an enormous commitment and the baby should not be discharged before the parents feel able to care for and deal with their infant independently.

To plan for early discharge the additional knowledge and skills parents will need to care for their infant at home safely should be identified. A plan is then made in partnership with parents to help them gain the knowledge and skills identified. Most parental teaching involves the discussion/explanation of the task, followed by a demonstration and supervised practice sessions. The teaching plan should allow time for repeat sessions, be systematic and run at the pace desired by parents. Written information should also be given to the parents for future reference. Well designed and executed discharge plans will help parents care for their infant with confidence.

Implication for practice

Early discharge of infants to parents who are supported and skilled in the care of their infant requires careful planning with both written and verbal information.

Neonatal outreach nurses should contact the health visitor and relevant community health professionals to inform them of the plan for discharge and to discuss the plan of care after discharge. Where possible, community health professionals should be involved and given the opportunity to offer support and visit the infant at home. Outreach nurses should facilitate a 'joint visit' at home with the health visitor and relevant community health professionals after discharge to discuss further management and plan of care.

Outreach nurses should contact the family by phone or visit the infant at home within 48 hours of discharge. Most infants are a little unsettled initially after discharge as they take time to adjust to their new home environment. This changes their normal feeding/sleeping pattern and can worry parents. A phone call can help reassure parents and if there are more serious concerns the outreach nurse will visit or advise on a medical review. Outreach nurses should liaise with community health professionals to plan for individual family needs and level of support required. This should prevent a barrage of health workers descending on a family at one time which can cause confusion and be looked upon as an unwelcome invasion of privacy.

Outreach nurses should ensure families of all infants discharged from the neonatal unit are offered support. Families of infants with no ongoing medical needs can be supported by health visitors. Before the infant is discharged outreach nurses should have a plan to handover the infant's care to community health professionals. This will prevent overloading of the service and ensure community health services are used effectively and efficiently (see Box 20.1).

> ### Box 20.1　Criteria for neonatal outreach visiting
>
> - Babies on tube feeds
> - Poor feeders
> - Babies under 2 kg at discharge
> - Oxygen dependent babies
> - Babies who need withdrawal treatment from maternal drug abuse
> - Babies who require palliative care
> - Poor parenting ability
> - Babies with tracheostomy
> - Babies needing stoma care

Sudden infant death syndrome (SIDS)

Parents must be updated on how to reduce the risk of cot death. Current information from the FSID includes:

- Location of cot: the safest place for your baby to sleep is in a cot in your room for the first six months. Do not share a bed with your baby if you or your partner:
  - Are smokers (no matter where or when you smoke)
  - Have been drinking alcohol
  - Take medication or drugs that make you drowsy
  - Feel very tired
  - If your baby was born premature or was small at birth

Never sleep with a baby on a sofa or armchair (Foundation for Study of Infant Cot Death, What is Cot Death? (FSID), 2006, www.sids .org.uk)

- Infant sleeping position
  - Place your baby on their back to sleep and front to play (see below)

  - Place your baby with their feet to the foot of the cot, to prevent wriggling down under the covers
- Do not let your baby get too hot: keep baby's head uncovered.
- Do not let anyone smoke in the same room as your baby.
- If your baby is unwell, seek medical advice promptly.

Sleeping position

The 'back to sleep' campaign is familiar to all neonatal professionals and to many parents. Infants nursed on neonatal units are often nursed prone in view of the evidence that it decreases respiratory effort. However, on the neonatal unit these infants are likely to have heart rate and saturation monitoring or be regularly monitored by nursing staff.

> ### Implications for practice
>
> Teaching parents the recommendations for sleeping position is an important part of any neonatal nurse's role.

Resuscitation training

Premature and low birthweight babies have an increased risk of cot death (FSID, 2006). Many infants admitted to the neonatal unit have episodes of bradycardias, desaturations or apnoeas. Parents find these episodes distressing and feel anxious about taking their baby home. Research has indicated that offering infant resuscitation training improves parental confidence and decreases anxiety[9]. All parents of infants admitted to the neonatal unit should be given the option of resuscitation training to equip them with the necessary skills to respond in an emergency[10].

The risk of apnoea or collapse increases if a baby becomes unwell. Therefore all infant resuscitation training sessions should equip parents with the information on recognising signs and symptoms of their infant's ill health with the recommendation that they seek medical advice promptly.

Resuscitation training aims to provide parents with the following clinical skills:

- Assessment for signs of life
- The ability to recognise when a baby is not breathing
- Providing gentle stimulation
- Opening the airway
- Giving five rescue breaths
- Reassessment for signs of life
- Delivery of effective ventilation breaths
- Delivery of effective cardiac compressions
- To continue CPR until help arrives

The training begins with a discussion of the initial assessment for signs of life and the ABC (Airway, Breathing and Circulation) of resuscitation. Parents are then advised on how and when to obtain help. Advice regarding the ratio of cardiac compressions to ventilation breaths is currently 3:1 (neonates) and 15:2 (infants and children) for resuscitation by health professionals, but 30:2 for lay people[11]. Many neonatologists and neonatal nurses are concerned at this development in view of the fact that it de-emphasises the importance of airway management and oxygenation.

An effective method for teaching resuscitation using four stages as used on the resuscitation council courses is outlined below:

(1) Silent demonstration using a manikin in real time by the neonatal nurse
(2) Slower demonstration with explanation/dialogue
(3) Trainer demonstrates on manikin under instruction from parent
(4) Parent practices/demonstrates on manikin; this stage allows the trainer to informally assess resuscitation knowledge and skills gained by parents

Once parents feel confident in their ability to perform resuscitation the trainer can proceed to care/management of an infant who is choking. Initially, signs and symptoms of choking are discussed. This is followed by a demonstration on the manikin using the four-stage technique.

Parents should be given the opportunity to ask questions and handouts are given to reinforce training and for future reference.

Implications for practice

Any parent who has had an infant admitted to a neonatal unit should be offered resuscitation training.

Home oxygen

With increased survival of extremely low birth-weight premature infants, it is most likely that the incidence of chronic lung disease will also increase[12]. This will increase the number of infants discharged home under oxygen therapy. Infants with other neonatal lung conditions, such as pulmonary hypoplasia, congenital heart disease with pulmonary hypertension, neuromuscular conditions requiring non-invasive ventilation and pulmonary hypertension secondary to pulmonary disease may also be discharged home on oxygen.

Infants dependent on oxygen can be safely cared for at home by their parents. Oxygen is usually supplied via a concentrator at home. An oxygen concentrator is a machine about 60 cm square and 75 cm high. It plugs into the ordinary household electricity supply. It filters oxygen from the air in the room, and this oxygen is then delivered by plastic tubing to a mask or nasal cannula. Long tubing can be fixed around the floor or skirting board, with two points where the user can 'plug in' to the oxygen supply.

Lightweight portable oxygen cylinders are supplied for use when the infant is ambulatory.

Sending infants home whilst they need oxygen therapy requires careful planning to ensure success, taking into account a number of patient, family, financial, home and community factors. This is best done in the context of an organised programme of discharge planning and parent education[13].

Before the infant is discharged home on oxygen:

(1) Oxygen requirements must be stable with mean SaO_2 of 93% or above, without frequent episodes of desaturation and CO_2 retention.
(2) No apnoeic episodes for at least two weeks.
(3) Infants should be able to cope with short periods in air without being at risk of rapid deterioration in case their nasal cannulas become dislodged. Generally this will apply to those requiring < 0.5 l/min, but this does not mean that some babies with a higher oxygen requirement cannot be on home oxygen.
(4) No other clinical conditions precluding discharge should be present and the infant should be medically stable with satisfactory growth.
(5) Parents should be willing to taking the baby home while still on oxygen.
(6) Home conditions must be satisfactory and preferably a telephone should be installed (or use of a mobile phone available).
(7) Home and car insurers will need to be informed[14].
(8) A discharge planning meeting involving the multidisciplinary team, including the social worker, community children's nurse, health visitor, GP and any other relevant community health workers should be organised. Plan for respite should be made at these meetings.

A structured parent teaching plan should be made after discussions with parents about their learning needs. Teaching sessions will involve awareness of the infant's normal breathing pattern, recognising change in breathing pattern and respiratory distress, recognition of hypoxia and action to be taken, use of equipment needed to deliver oxygen, including low flow meters and nasal cannulas, resuscitation training, safe use of oxygen at home, and travelling with oxygen safely. Written information to support the training package is essential.

The outreach service should involve appropriate community health professionals and communication with the general practitioner should take place to discuss the plan of care after discharge and to clarify roles for delivering clinical care. Parents must have a list of telephone numbers for advice and emergency help, including equipment breakdown. Arrangements should be in place for open access to the local paediatric unit[14].

Care at home
Outreach nurses should endeavour to visit the infant at home within 24 hours of discharge. An infant who needs the oxygen flow rate to be adjusted frequently due to desaturations while an in-patient should not be discharged. The issue of giving parents saturation monitors at home continues to be widely debated and research continues into alarm settings that should be used to provide the most predictive clinical data in these situations[15]. There is no evidence that provision of saturation monitors improves the outcome of babies on home oxygen, and in practice it may lead to excessive adjustments of the flow rate by the carers[16]. The infant's respiratory status and saturations should be checked by the outreach nurse at each visit. Additional spot checks of oxygen saturations are of limited value but can be used to reassure parents. They are insufficient to guide oxygen therapy, and prolonged monitoring of oxygen saturation by pulse oximetry while the child is awake, feeding and asleep is likely to provide a more accurate picture of the child's respiratory status. Modern software will rapidly analyse the data stored in pulse oximeters and, according to preset parameters, identify episodes of hypoxaemia as well as the average oxygen saturation[17]. Prolonged monitoring of saturations (for approximately 12 hours) should be done within the first week of discharge and repeated every four weeks. It will need to be done more frequently when weaning the infant off oxygen therapy. Feeding and growth are important indicators in monitoring the infants' health.

It is essential that outreach nurses support parents and promote well-being. Caring for an infant at home on oxygen can be an isolating experience for mothers. Observing for signs of post-natal depression and facilitating access to counselling services is recommended. Looking after a child with chronic lung disease on home oxygen requires appreciation of the emotional impact on the families and ensuring they are provided with social support[18].

Outreach nurses should also facilitate joint visits with the GP and health visitor at home to involve them in providing care and support. The GP may wish to examine the infant when well and record information which will be useful if he/she has to provide clinical care when the infant is unwell.

Implications for practice

Caring for infants at home on oxygen requires time to provide skills and confidence; introduce the possibility early in the infant's care to facilitate this.

Discharging a baby home on nasogastric tube feeds

Babies who are slow to feed or unable to suck can be discharged weeks earlier if parents are taught how to give nasogastric feeds. These babies include very premature babies as well as those with cerebral impairment or congenital abnormalities. The involvement of parents in offering nasogastric tube feeds from the outset will allow discharge preparation to be quicker and parents will gain the confidence and competence in feeding their baby via a nasogastric tube.

A discharge plan should be made in partnership with parents, acknowledging their fears and taking into account their learning needs. A structured plan will assist parents in gaining skills needed to care for their infant at home.

The teaching plan should involve:

(1) Measuring and passing nasogastric tube
(2) Checking position of the tube
(3) Feeding baby safely via a nasogastric tube
(4) Action to be taken if the baby vomits during feed
(5) Action to be taken if there is difficulty obtaining aspirate to test on pH paper

Care at home

A plan to encourage sucking and establishing breast or bottle feeds should have been made before discharge. Outreach nurses should liaise with the health visitor and dietician to monitor weight and to calculate subsequent increases in feed. Outreach nurses will also need to ensure parents have adequate supplies of equipment needed for feeding. This can be arranged via local primary care trusts or children's community services.

There is evidence that infants on a discharge programme with home gavage feeding had a mean hospital stay that was 9.3 days shorter than infants in the control group. Infants in the early discharge programme also had a lower risk of clinical infection during the home gavage period compared with the corresponding time in hospital for the control group[19]

Implications for practice

A small, well infant who is not able to complete all feeds for optimal growth would benefit from early discharge with tube feeds and outreach support; discuss this with the parents/carers.

Discharging a baby home with a colostomy or ileostomy

Babies with congenital malformations of the gastrointestinal tract, necrotising enterocolitis, or Hirschsprung's are likely to be discharged home needing stoma care. Early involvement of the parents in providing stoma care is essential for discharge to succeed. Parents should first be familiarised with the stoma and given time to prepare mentally and physically. Their fear and anxiety should be discussed so that nurses can help them overcome these. A structured training plan should be made after discussion with the parents.

Preparation is important to ensure that a suitable, comfortable, leak-proof appliance is fitted to contain effluent. A template should be made of the size and shape of the stoma and the bag cut using this as a guide[20]. Parents can practice preparing stoma bags under guidance.

Teaching focuses on how to:

(1) Drain stoma bag and secure with clip
(2) Change stoma bag
(3) Protect skin around stoma
(4) Action to be taken if stoma output is very watery (indicating diarrhoea) or formed (constipation)
(5) Action to be taken if stoma prolapses

When applying the bag the opening of the bag should be directed towards the side of the abdomen for ease of draining and so as not to lie uncomfortably in the baby's nappy.

Drainable bags can stay in situ for two to three days. Skin care should involve cleansing skin using warm water and soft cloth/gauze and drying thoroughly after. Barrier cream/paste can be applied to the skin to protect it from effluent. Parents should be able to recognise early signs of irritation/inflammation of skin. Bags should be drained before they are removed. Lifting them from the top will minimise trauma to the skin.

Outreach nurses should arrange stoma care equipment via the GP or primary care trust before the baby is discharged.

Implication for practice

Ensure that parents have adequate supplies of equipment and are able to access new supplies easily.

Discharge of a baby home on palliative care

Babies with conditions incompatible with life or with life-limiting illnesses can be safely discharged home with support. Community health professionals (GP, health visitor, midwife) should be informed of the plan of care. Decisions should be collaborative and clearly communicated. A copy of the care plan should be kept with parents to ensure information can be shared with emergency services when needed. The family should be provided with 24-hour access of support and professional advice. The discharge plan should also be flexible to allow parents access to the hospital or local hospice at short notice where palliative care can be continued.

Providing palliative care at home gives parents and the infant family time and privacy.

It is vital that outreach nurses liaise with the multidisciplinary team to ensure the family is supported, without overloading them with too many home visits or phone calls. A plan to support the bereaved family should be made in conjunction with a counsellor/psychologist to ensure family support is continued after the infant has died. Parents should be provided with contact telephone numbers of relevant services and written information on what needs to be done on death.

Implications for practice

Choices should be given to the parents at this difficult time, which may include taking their infant home after the death.

Discharge home of a baby with a tracheostomy

In neonates tracheostomies are most often indicated in order to provide a stable airway for infants with congenital or acquired airway obstructions, or to provide long-term mechanical ventilation. Learning to care for an infant with a tracheostomy can be challenging for both professionals and families.

A comprehensive discharge plan to support the family, to familiarise them with tracheostomy care and to link them with resources available after the baby is discharged will ensure successful transition of management of a tracheostomy from hospital to home[21].

One of the primary goals of discharge preparation is to promote positive adaptation to the tracheostomy. The family must be trained to develop the knowledge and skills needed to competently and independently provide tracheostomy care prior to discharge as listed below:

- Understand the reason for tracheostomy tube placement
- Describe the tracheostomy tube, how it functions and the resulting changes in the infant's airway, e.g. inability to cough
- Be able to competently perform the skills of stoma care, suctioning, and tracheostomy tube change
  - Stoma care: how to clean and protect skin around stoma
  - Suctioning: correct suctioning technique, use and care of suctioning equipment, recognising signs and symptoms that indicate need for suctioning and complications associated with suctioning
  - Tube change: how to prepare tube, change tube and secure it
- Recognise signs of breathing difficulty and respond appropriately
- Demonstrate how to respond in an emergency, resuscitation training, emergency tube changes

Initial training can be done using a doll to allow parents to become familiar with equipment. This will promote confidence and decrease anxiety. Parents can then observe the nurse performing tracheostomy care. When parents have had time to prepare themselves mentally and physically they can begin to provide tracheostomy care with assistance.

Families should be provided with an opportunity to practice these skills in a non-threatening environment. Nurses should foster ongoing discussions to address any issues or concerns and help the family identify specific learning and skill acquisition needs[22].

After the basic technical skills are mastered, the focus should shift to appropriate decision making and helping parents to identify their infant's cues[23]; this is the foundation for competent caregiving[24]. Written instructions should be provided to reinforce bedside teaching. Utilising structured discharge teaching and refining the discharge process can decrease the length of stay, benefiting the infant, the family and the institution.

Discharge should be planned using the multi disciplinary team to ensure comprehensive care is provided to the infant and family. Arrangements to support the family and respite care should be made before discharge. Outreach nurses must ensure a regular supply of disposable equipment needed for tracheostomy care via local health services.

Implications for practice

Ensure parents have sufficient opportunity for practice at suctioning and changing the tube on their infant prior to discharge to develop skills and confidence in its management.
Resuscitation training is vital in these infants.

Summary

Discharge from the neonatal unit and transfer of the responsibility for a neonate's care from the neonatal staff to the parents, can be a worrying time for parents. They need to be carefully prepared for this transition, with appropriate advice and support so that they can be confident in their ability to care for their infant. Involving parents in providing care for their infant from the outset will increase parental confidence and competence and increase the likelihood of a successful transition from the neonatal unit to home.

In the hospital the parents often do not feel like a family, a feeling that should change when they return home with their baby. This is one of the reasons why it is so important that the infant is discharged as early as possible from the hospital[25]. Early discharge is also known to promote bonding and breast-feeding, to reduce the risk of nosocomial infections and enhance growth and development.

Although standardised discharge procedures are very useful, Individualised discharge plans for infants that take into account parents learning needs make the discharge process efficient and effective. Neonatal outreach services provide an invaluable service to families of infants discharged from neonatal units in the transition from hospital to home.

Conclusion

As with many other areas of neonataology, a systematic approach together with an individualised plan of care is essential in planning discharge and community services. This should be done in partnership with the parents and should begin almost at the point of admission so that there is gradual handover of medical and nursing care to the parents throughout their neonatal stay. This should enable them to be discharged with the confidence and competence to care for their infant even when that infant has specific needs, such as effective management of a tracheostomy or ileostomy.

References

1. Merenstein GB, Gardner SL (1993) *Handbook of Neonatal Intensive Care*, 3rd edn. Mosby, St Louis.
2. Davis L, Edwards H, Mohay H, *et al.* (2003) The impact of very premature birth on the psychological health of mothers. *Early Hum Dev*, **73** (1–2), 61–70.
3. Griffin T, Abraham M (2006) Transition to home from the newborn intensive care unit: applying the principles of family-centered care to the discharge process. *J Perinat Neonatal Nurs*, **20** (3), 243–249; quiz 250–251.
4. Ward K (2001) Perceived needs of parents of critically ill infants in a neonatal intensive care unit (NICU). *Pediatr Nurs*, **27** (3), 281–286.
5. Kowalski WJ, Leef KH, Mackley A, Spear ML, Paul DA (2006) Communicating with parents of premature infants: who is the informant? *J Perinatol*, **26** (1), 44–48.
6. Brazy JE, Anderson BMH, Becker PT, Becker M (2001) How parents of premature infants gather information and obtain support. *Neonatal Netw*, **20** (2), 41–48.
7. Bissell G (2002) Follow-up care and support offered to families post discharge from the neonatal unit: who should give this care? *Journal of Neonatal Nursing*, **8** (3), 76–82.
8. Langley D, Hollis S, Friede T, *et al.* (2002) Impact of community neonatal services: a multicentre survey. *Arch Dis Child Fetal Neonatal Ed*, **87** (3), F204–F208.
9. Clarke K (1998) Infant CPR-The effect on parental anxiety regarding SIDS. *British Journal of Midwifery*, **6** (11), 27–30.
10. Davies PJ, Jenkins L (2004) Teaching parents infant resuscitation within a special care baby unit: report of twelve month trial. *Journal of Neonatal Nursing*, **10** (6), 206–209.
11. The International Liaison Committee on Resuscitation (ILCOR) (2006) The International Liaison Committee on Resuscitation (ILCOR) consensus on science with treatment recommendations for pediatric and neonatal patients: pediatric basic and advanced life support. *Pediatrics*, **117** (5), e955–e977.
12. Hack M, Fanaroff AA (2000) Outcomes of children of extremely low birthweight and gestational age in the 1990s. *Semin Neonatol*, **5** (2), 89–106.
13. Brown KA, Sauve REST (1994) Evaluation of a caregiver education program: home oxygen therapy for infants. *J Obstet Gynecol Neonatal Nurs*, **23** (5), 429–435.
14. Balfour-Lynn IM, Primhak RA, Shaw BN (2005) Home oxygen for children: who, how and when? *Thorax*, **60** (1), 76–81.
15. Gelinas JF, Davis GM, Arlegui C, Cote A (2008) Prolonged, documented home-monitoring of oxygenation in infants and children. *Pediatr Pulmonol*, **43** (3), 288–296.
16. Primhak RA (2003) Discharge and aftercare in chronic lung disease of the newborn. *Semin Neonatol*, **8** (2), 117–126.
17. Kotecha S, Allen J (2002) Oxygen therapy for infants with chronic lung disease. *Arch Dis Child Fetal Neonatal Ed*, **87** (1), F11–F14.
18. McAleese KA, Knapp MA, Rhodes TT (1993) Financial and emotional cost of bronchopulmonary dysplasia. *Clin Pediatr (Phila)*, **32** (7), 393–400.
19. Collins CT, Makrides M, McPhee AJ (2003) Early discharge with home support of gavage feeding

for stable preterm infants who have not established full oral feeds. *Cochrane Database Syst Rev* (4), CD003743.

20. Parry A (1998) Stoma care in neonates: improving practice. *Journal of Neonatal Nursing*, **4**, 8–11.

21. Parry A (1998) Stoma care in neonates: improving practice. *Journal of Neonatal Nursing*, **4**, 8–11.

22. Fiske E (2004) Effective strategies to prepare infants and families for home tracheostomy care. *Adv Neonatal Care*, **4** (1), 42–53.

23. Barnes LP (1992) Tracheostomy care: preparing parents for discharge. MCN *Am J Matern Child Nurs*, **17** (6), 293.

24. Bryant KD, Lagrone C (1997) Streamlining discharge planning for the child with a new tracheostomy. *Journal of Pediatric Nursing*, **12**, 191–192.

25. Jonsson LF, B (2003) Parents' conceptions of participating in a home care programme from NICU: a qualitative analysis. *Vard I Norden Nursing Science and Research in the Nordic Countries*, **23**, 35–39.

INDEX